PATHOLOGIES OF THE WEST

Pathologies of the West

An Anthropology of Mental Illness in Europe and America

ROLAND LITTLEWOOD

Cornell University Press
Ithaca, New York

Copyright Roland Littlewood 2002

First published in the United States in 2002 by

Cornell University Press
Sage House
512 East State Street
Ithaca, New York

Cloth 0-8014-3934-5
Paper 0-8014-8743-9

Library of Congress Cataloging-in-Publication Data
Littlewood, Roland.
Pathologies of the West: an anthropology of mental illness in Europe and America/Roland Littlewood.
    p. cm.
Includes bibliographical references and index.
ISBN 0-8014-3934-5 (cloth) – ISBN 0-8014-8743-9 (pbk.)
    1. Cultural psychiatry—Europe, Western. 2. Cultural psychiatry—North America. 3. Cultural psychiatry—Australia. I. Title.
RC455.4E8 L583 2002
616.89–dc21

2001047036

Contents

Acknowledgements

I am grateful for research fellowships from the Leverhulme and Nuffield Trusts, and to Wolfson College and the Oxford Institute of Social and Cultural Anthropology for their hospitality during 1993 during which I started working on the themes which comprise this book. And to my departments at UCL for sabbatical leave.

Among the numerous colleagues, friends and others whose criticisms here I have valued are Nick Allan, Shirley Ardener, Neelam Bakshi, Mukulika Bannerjee, Jonathan Benthall, Audrey Cantlie, Morris Carstairs, Ajita Chakraborty, Jacques Charles-Nicolas, Veena Das, John Davis, George Devereux, Robin Dunbar, Armando Favazza, Raymond Firth, Ronnie Frankenberg, Bill Fulford, Clifford Geertz, Maurice Greenberg, Byron Good, Alma Gottlieb, Ezra Griffith, Cecil Helman, Tim Ingold, Wendy James, Bruce Kapferer, Jafar Kareem, Susie Kilshaw, David Kirby, Laurence Kirmayer, Arthur Kleinman, Britt Krause, Jean La Fontaine, Helen Lambert, Murray Last, Sing Lee, Gilbert Lewis, Jenny Littlewood, Leti Littlewood, Margaret Lock, Louis Mars, Carole MacCormack, Mark Marchetto, Nalaka Mendis, H. B. M. Murphy, Charles Nuckolls, Yemi Oloyede, David Parkin, Mary Petevi, Raymond Prince, Paul Richards, Roy Porter, William Sargant, Edward Schieffelin, Ulrike Schmidt, Elaine Showalter, Ron Simons, Vieda Skultans, Leslie Swartz, James Thompson, Mitchell Weiss, Simon Wessely, Lewis Wolpert, Michael A. C. Wood, Allan Young; a number of editors and anonymous referees, my clinical colleagues at St Bartholomew's Hospital, Guy's Hospital and University College Hospital; and participants at meetings of the universities of the West Indies, Colombo, Stockholm, Oslo, Beijing, McGill and Melbourne, The Oxford Centre for Cross-Cultural Research on Women, the Transcultural Committee of the World Psychiatric Association, the British Medical Anthropology Society, the Association of Social Anthropologists, the Royal Anthropological Institute, the Royal Society of Medicine, the Royal College of Psychiatrists, the American Psychiatric Association, the Nafsiyat Inter-Cultural Therapy Centre, the Society for Psychosomatic Research, and at various other medical and anthropological seminars. For continual and provocative debate, I am indebted to my graduate students at UCL, particularly to Simon Dein and Sushrut Jadhav, now my colleagues, and to my UCL colleague Murray Last. My intellectual debts here to the figures of Gregory Bateson and Victor Turner will be evident.

Especial thanks are due to Ioan Lewis, Godfrey Lienhardt and Maurice Lipsedge for demanding conversations continued over two decades. This volume is a development of some ideas which have emerged in various papers since 1985: two of these were written with Dr Lipsedge and in what may be argued to be the central argument here (Chapter 3), it is difficult to distinguish the contributions we each made to an animated discussion back in 1985. He has had a central role in calling my attention to innumerable sources, medical and historical, popular and academic. Among my own papers on which I have drawn are: (1985) La migration des syndromes liés à la culture, *Psychopathologie Africaine*, *20*, 5–16; (1987) The butterfly and the serpent (with Maurice Lipsedge), *Culture, Medicine and Psychiatry*, *11*, 289–335; (1990) From categories to contexts, *British Journal of Psychiatry*, *156*, 308–27; (1991) Gender, role and sickness, in Pat Holden and Jenny Littlewood's book *Nursing and Anthropology*, London, Routledge; (1991) Against pathology, in *British Journal of Psychiatry*, *159*, 696–702; (1993) Symptoms, struggles and functions, in Maryon McDonald (ed.), *Women and Addiction*, London, Routledge; (1997) Psychopathology and its public sources (with Maurice Lipsedge), *Anthropology and Medicine*, *4:1*, 25–43; (1996) Reason and necessity in the specification of the multiple self, RAI Occasional Paper 43; (1996) Psychiatry's culture, *International Journal of Social Psychiatry*, *42:4*, 245–68; (1997) Military rape, *Anthropology Today*, *13:2*, 7–16; (1991) Post-adoption incest and phenotypic matching (with Maurice Greenberg), *British Journal of Medical Psychology*, *68*, 29–44. To avoid excessive cross-referencing, these papers are generally not cited here. I thank my publishers and colleagues for permission to use argument, and in some instances text, again.

I owe much to my patients, many of whom have been subjected to reading sections from these chapters. For their tolerance, criticism and support, thanks. If I have offered here interpretations of their experiences with which they might not always agree, I have tried to do the same for the doctors with whom they have been involved, myself included. Clinical cases cited here are heavily disguised and, of course, with pseudonyms.

A terminological note

I use the term *Euro-American* to refer to societies whose dominant culture is of White European origin – Britain and the rest of Western Europe, as well as Canada, Australia, the United States – not just to what is currently termed *Anglo-American*.

Preface

During the riots of 1986 in the English city of Birmingham, I was working as a university psychiatrist in Handsworth – the area particularly involved. Two days after the violence ended in a wary peace, I was telephoned by a local family doctor who asked me to visit a patient at her home: a 15-year-old girl, born in Bangladesh, who had now been in Britain for two years. She lived with her family, spoke English well and attended the nearby mixed secondary school. She had, he said briefly, become 'hysterical'. The local violence had initially been described by the press as a race riot, directed by Blacks against the predominantly White police force, and against shops and businesses owned by South Asians. An Asian postal worker was burned to death when his post office was gutted. One well-known Birmingham psychiatrist argued in evidence to the official inquiry into the looting that it was the action of cannabis-intoxicated, young Afro-Caribbean men. This inquiry, re-examination of television news and police video film, together with publication of the ethnic origins of those who were eventually prosecuted, suggested, however, that the rioters comprised White and Caribbean youths in a proportion fairly representative of the local population. And some women. And indeed a few young men of South Asian origin. The eventual public and media opinion was that this was less a race riot than the frustration of the unemployed in a neglected ghetto area who in despair of any economic change, had called attention to their situation by attempting to destroy their own neighbourhood.

The streets near my hospital were still full of debris being cleared up, littered with charred timbers, bricks and shards of broken glass. Down the neighbouring main road many of the shops had been burned down, and those that remained still had their shutters fastened up or boards nailed across the windows in case of further looting. The police had withdrawn to a discreet distance, and people were now gathering on the broken pavements to assess the damage and exchange their stories. The smell of burning still hung as an acrid smoke in the air but daily life was cautiously re-establishing something like its previous pattern. I stopped to talk with a cafe owner I knew who had just opened up again for business: he was complaining of a story on the local radio which said that the Asians had burned down their own shops to collect the insurance. Turning the corner I eventually found the terraced house. Little damage at least in this side street. The family warily opened their door and I introduced myself.

I met Hasmat (as I shall call her here) in the downstairs room lying on the floor, eyes firmly closed, occasionally thrashing about with her arms and legs, and shouting out something nobody could quite understand. Her parents stood about rather helplessly, placing cushions under her head, holding her hands and trying to calm her down. Every now and then this seemed to work: she got up and quietly denied any knowledge of what had been happening, assuring her family that she was now feeling quite well, appearing puzzled by their concern but taking some tonic drink they offered. She refused food, saying she was not hungry. Then, without warning, she would slide back onto the floor.

The father told me Hasmat had been like this, on and off, for two days; she was seriously ill with these fits and he was glad that I had finally come to take her to the hospital. He was certainly distraught but also, I thought, rather angry. Her elder brother then called me aside and in the stairway whispered that Hasmat 'was just putting it all on' because she had been arguing with her father for months about going out in the evening with a schoolfriend who said she wanted to be a fashion model and whom the parents distrusted. Recently the two girls had quarrelled after the other one had apparently told a friend that Hasmat was too fat. He told me later their mother had become upset when Hasmat then bought a glamorous slimming magazine saying she proposed to go on a diet. Another brother stood at the side, watching his concerned family with what to me seemed ironic amusement. Having greeted Hasmat – she responded quietly and appropriately – I asked her father what they had been able to do to help her. He reluctantly agreed with my query about whether he had taken his daughter to the local mosque when she had started talking strangely. (Their GP, who was a Muslim of Indian origin, had sardonically told me about this, and said that he had told the father off for such nonsense.) Someone at the mosque – the father didn't know them – had said some Qu'aranic verses over his daughter to force any intruding evil power to leave, and had given her something special to drink – he wasn't sure what – but it had not worked, of course, because she was really physically quite unwell as the GP had carefully explained to him that morning. Or perhaps some evil force had now gone but left her physically ill? Had the family lost anything in the riots? I asked. No, he was only a foundry worker: no property. No, no one they knew had been hurt. The riots were nothing to do with them. I persisted: all the same, could the riots (still very much on my own mind) be the cause of Hasmat's distress? He disagreed: how could riots, however dreadful, cause people to become physically sick in this way?

I asked the family to leave the room, saying I wanted to talk with Hasmat alone. Conventional medical practice fifteen years ago. I told her I thought she was upset by something. She gazed quietly at me, past me. I felt uncomfortable, almost embarrassed. Speaking normally she abruptly asked me to promise to keep something confidential. I agreed reluctantly. If I was really a doctor, Hasmat then said, shouldn't I now examine her? I hastily declined: what was this secret? What had happened? She told me how, on the morning after the rioting ended, she and her elder brother's new wife, aged nineteen, had secretly unpadlocked the door (her father had secured it firmly from the inside when the looting approached down the neighbouring roads), and had gone out to have a look 'for fun'. Terrified – deliciously terrified I suddenly thought – at the devastation, the two young women had returned home immediately without anyone else in the family knowing. She had seen in the street a boy from her school and thought he might attack her. Why? Just thought he might. Had he? No. Was he a relative? Was he White, Black? No response. Back in the house she had then felt dizzy and was still unwell. That was all. Could I now tell her father she had been sick but that it was not serious and she did not need to go into the hospital? And certainly not tell him about her going out? I called the family back and told them that Hasmat had become ill – I chose the word 'ill' – because of the awful things which had been happening, but that I thought she would soon be well without needing to take any medicine.

What did the doctor think the sickness was then? Well, I said, she was 'weak'. They looked nonplussed. I suggested she should have something to eat and said I would call again the next day together with a Bengali community worker, a neighbour of theirs, who was working with me as a part-time counsellor. That afternoon I got a telephone call from the family doctor who had been round to see how I had got on. Hasmat seemed much better. He congratulated me ironically on my successful intervention, saying that he had tried to reinforce my advice but that the family had felt let down because I had not seemed properly concerned: no real treatment, no physical examination, no hospital, nothing. So he himself had given her some sleeping tablets to keep everybody happy, a placebo for the whole family as he put it. Did I agree? Well, why not? The next morning the father left a message for me at the hospital: his daughter was now much better, thanks, and they didn't need a psychiatrist or anyone else coming again. I telephoned back and said all right but could they make an appointment with my secretary for the next week? He said unenthusiastically he would try. They didn't. The GP dropped by my office and told me everything was now back to normal, and I forgot about the whole business. About two months later I was contacted by the local casualty department with a request for the clinical records of my 'depressed patient who has just taken an overdose of tranquillizers'.

The argument

Perhaps not such an unusual medical encounter. As yet, a thin description: the bare bones of some choreography seen from the outside, for the details of the family dynamics, its social context, and its eventual resolution (on the whole I think happy) are beyond the scope of a preface. I merely want to note here the ambiguities of power for doctor and patient (and parent), and the choices and personal identifications which are available in different understandings of illness, each with their own characteristic experiences and medical perceptions, including, of course, my own as a European and male physician, embedded in and in some part controlling the process – and also, in these pages, as its not so disinterested narrator. The events seem to condense down in a single story what one might well define as quite distinct understandings – the religious, the medical, the psychological, the gendered and the political. And yet there is a unity. The biography of an individual? The medical gaze, as Michel Foucault termed it? My own prosaic attempt here to make sense of the encounter as a narrative? To justify myself to you?

Hysteria, and other medicalized dissociations of our customary consciousness, self-starvation, overdoses of medical drugs, chronic fatigue and phobias, multiple personality disorder, depression: such 'minor psychiatric disorders' – as they are called by psychiatrists to distinguish them from psychoses like schizophrenia and manic-depression – are common in Western societies and have been estimated to be part of the life experiences of over 20 per cent of contemporary Americans and Britons. Beyond the pragmatics of its actual resolution, the encounter I've recorded opens up a number of questions with which this book is concerned:

(i) How do patterns now recognized as psychiatric illnesses occur at particular cultural and historical moments? Are they perhaps symptomatic of wider social changes, say of increasing individualism or of changing relations between women and men, between children and parents? Do they represent an increasing 'civilising process' as Elias called it, or a less robust assertion that certain traumata are no longer to be borne without question but are frankly abnormal? Are illnesses like eating disorders or agoraphobia standardized to the extent that we may consider them as representative of a particular society's concerns or social structure, perhaps institutionalized as something like established rituals which shape personal distress while at the same time declaring our public values? Do these patterns have any coherence across time, and across societies, or should we argue that there is something particularly 'modern' and 'Western' about them? (And for the moment let us take these two characterizations as relatively unproblematic.)

(ii) And if they are Western in some sense, how do they fit with any psychological and biological differences in the individuals in whom they manifest? Are they reflections of some more universal psychological or biological cause which can be simply shaped by any culture? Beyond that, how does 'culture' interact with or reinforce an individual's biological predisposition?

(iii) Can one distinguish the physician's observation of illness from the medicalized context through which these patterns emerge and are treated? Do doctors and patients understand matters in similar ways such that medical understanding can do any sort of justice to the personal experiences of those it treats as patients?

(iv) How should we take the popular recognition that, at some level, such patients are responsible, in that we can hold them in part accountable for their illness? For these people are not regarded as insane in any conventional medical sense.

I attempt in this book some ways of clarifying these questions. My approach may be characterized as anthropological in that I seek to understand personal experience as meaningful within a particular social and political context. I am not concerned here with adding further to the already extensive repertoire of statistical clinical information assembled by psychologists and psychiatrists about these illnesses, but rather with elaborating ideas by which we might interpret them. A purely psychological or psychopathological approach misses out the shared values through which these experiences emerge, in particular with an ambiguity in human life which I argue seems true for all societies. For we understand our bodily experiences, our thinking selves and our actions sometimes as the free exercise of our will, yet on other occasions as constrained or even caused, and thus as external to our intentions and perhaps to our responsibility. We seem to be both the active agents and the passive recipients of our lives. In different situations one or other seems particularly true, but we are often ambivalent about deciding which. Is our self-righteous anger, our feeling of bodily tension, the lump in our throat, the tension in our stomach, really just some reflection of stress? Or are we perhaps letting ourselves go, slipping too easily into the not-so-uncomfortable role of victim, maybe indeed somehow fabricating the whole business to gain sympathy and some perverse type of power? How could we know the difference? Something like this dilemma seems true not only in our own experience, but in our understanding of another person, and in the collective response of our culture. Do we consider the person who takes a dangerous overdose of medically prescribed drugs to be somehow intending this action because of their anticipation of how others will respond, and thus they are to be held morally responsible? Or is their action simply the symptom of some underlying problem for which they cannot, in any everyday sense, be held accountable? Are they helpless victims or moral agents? Patients or malingerers?

There is no answer to this through an empirical study which seeks the elusive biomedical essence of an illness. For we are always both, the active maker of our life and the victim of contingency. To use now conventional terms, we can understand ourselves *personalistically*, the usual perspective of historical, literary or other humanistic studies; and also *naturalistically*, mechanistically, as favoured by the natural sciences. And in everyday life we do both. Neither is false, nor fully true. To deny personal decisions and experience is to reduce medicine to a veterinary science, the body to an arbitrary happenstance beyond our intentions; yet to deny the natural is to take human life as a disembodied flow of cultural inscriptions. In certain situations we move from one understanding to the other: when as women or Black people or psychiatric patients we realize that what we have taken as our own intentions is merely the working-out of some other structuring – of another's political power or of biological disease, moments when we might then turn to reaffirm ourselves again as active agents, striving to resist and transcend these structurings.

In Chapter 1, I offer an overview of how many social patterns of experience and action have been recognized by contemporary Western medicine as sicknesses. While psychiatry has avoided attributing any cultural significance to illness in European societies, not only preferring here mechanistic models but generally ignoring any personal meaning to the experience, it has produced an extraordinary, and generally exotic, literature on other societies. Indeed, it has argued that some cultures (but not the European) have illnesses which may be described as simply 'cultural' – as representations of a society's way of life or of its transitions. I look at these 'culture-bound syndromes', as doctors call them, through the recent critiques of comparative psychiatry which have been made by social anthropologists. This is developed through looking at our notion of 'pathology' and its apparent resolution in 'therapy' to argue that while these ideas have powerful practical resonances for members inside a society, they obscure any attempt to give us some more distanced view (Chapter 2). Western illness can only be understood in the context of a wider look at 'psychological distress' in other societies. In the next chapter I argue that we can derive a general schema for Western patterns of 'distress' derived from anthropological approaches to situations of spirit possession in small-scale and non-industrialized communities. Rather than follow psychiatrists in labelling spirit possession as hysteria, we can approach hysteria through the idiom of spirit possession. I use comparative evidence from different societies to reflect on common phenomena which have a certain family resemblance to each other without claiming that they are identical, such that possession *is* mental illness, or indeed the converse.

This way of looking derives in part from a number of earlier anthropologists who have offered structural and systemic ways of understanding, and I argue that for industrialized and Western societies it appears equally useful when we incorporate the biomedical context within which Western patterns develop and within which they are studied. Chapters 4 to 9 examine the value of this approach for interpreting certain patterns which have been identified in the West, including drug overdoses, agoraphobia, eating disorders and other less common reactions including some which are identified especially in nurses and in men, and the more common, but hardly distinctively Western, war-time sexual violence. The last two chapters assess my theoretical assumptions in placing them together in this way, and the extent to which they may have some general validity beyond my instances through looking at one of our latest diseases – multiple personality disorder.

I make associations between eating disorders and both our conceptualizations of the body and the current fragility of the modern family, between agoraphobia and ideas of space as a representation of gender, between overdoses and the social response to any sickness, between posttraumatic stress disorders and our experience of time and causality, between multiple personality and our currently fragmentary sense of self; but each identified pattern is not intended to be reduced to some isolated one-to-one index of a salient set of embodied social or cultural constraints. A woman's place may certainly be in the home but agoraphobia is not just a gendered prison: men, too, may become agoraphobic. I do not assume that each change in pattern automatically presumes a corresponding change in society as a whole, but rather that all the patterns are associated together as cultural schemata which allow individuals who are temporarily or permanently dislocated as powerless or distressed to achieve some redress of their immediate position through the dominant social structurings. For we all seek to adjust our situation through the available strategies: to insist on distinguishing these patterns as either 'unconscious desire' or 'intentional deceit' – as hysteria or malingering, to use the doctors' dichotomy – is to miss that it is through this very distinction that people can adjust their situation without overtly challenging the superordinate structures, and this in turn allows all societies to mark symbolically our double identity. You indeed do 'have' agoraphobia as much as you 'are' agoraphobic.

Most of these patterns are more commonly identified by doctors in women, and through many of them run powerful images of sexuality and motherhood. While I have drawn here on recent feminist critiques of psychiatry, I am not simply offering what has come to be known as a social constructivist model, whereby women – essentialized and gendered by historical status – are the hapless cyphers of male medical concerns, but rather some account of embodied action through and against such ideologies. That these patterns are perceived as diseases is essential to their very occurrence, yet 'minor psychiatric illness' shades into our everyday response to the world in which we find ourselves – thinking, feeling, suffering, anticipating, acting, resisting, deceiving, escaping. Unlike recent sociological critiques of psychiatry, this volume does not seek to demonstrate that the concerns of psychiatry can be rewritten as sexual politics alone. Nor are biological differences between individuals irrelevant. Yet, while biological differences make much sense in explaining our recognition of psychotic patterns such as schizophrenia, this is not to claim that they are the appropriate way of making primary sense of all of psychiatry's concerns.

Indeed I suggest here that it is the ambiguity between the biologically constrained and the humanistic which provides the legitimacy for many of these patterns in the West and elsewhere. It is not just that physicians' discomfort with an overtly moral perspective gives them a limited understanding of such patterns, but that such discomfort is integral to their very possibility. As the social anthropologist Ioan Lewis suggested many years ago, we can recognize resonances between the idiom of 'spirit possession' and that of 'disease'. My central schema is fairly simple. I argue that a subdominant individual may experience possession (or disease) which enables everyday dislocations of normal experience to be understood as an external intrusion of some other power, as a relative loss of our own agency which thus provides personal exculpation from immediate responsibility, while the recognition of this by others constrains them to restitution through restoring us to moral agency. Both possession and disease replay and confirm the moral values within which such action is possible. And in both, biological differences are best understood as supplying a repertoire not a causality – but also as the social presumption which provides personal exculpation.

Another incident, perhaps a necessary warning. Some months after Hasmat and I first met, a group of hospital physicians asked me to give a lecture on the value of anthropology for clinical medicine. I read a short draft of the original paper from which the ideas of this book derive. The response was alarming but in retrospect fairly predictable. I was warmly congratulated for being the first psychiatrist they had met to finally come clean. For of course other doctors had always known that neurotic patients were simply putting on an act and playing games with doctors, even if it was professionally unwise to say so. At last someone on the inside had produced the choreography of their performances. Now there *is* something in this – but at the time I was naive enough to be surprised by the implication of my arguments. It is part of the psychiatric tradition in which I was educated that until Freud's elaboration of psychodynamic therapy the patients we now term neurotic were dismissed variously as malingerers or diseased. The humanistic claims of modern psychiatry are that it now recognizes how individuals may frequently act against their 'real' interests, and that they should not necessarily be held accountable for doing so. Against the ambiguities of what I term here the personalistic and naturalistic understandings of ourselves, as experiencing ourselves as intentional agents yet constrained by events beyond our control or awareness, the psychoanalytical notion of the unconscious has attempted to dissolve the contradiction. If, in the following chapters, like that early critic of psychoanalysis, Karl Kraus, I wonder if the treatment might not be part of the very problem which it claims to resolve, this is not to agree with the psychoanalysts that the naturalistic must always be replaced by the personalistic, that one must at all costs seek to be held responsible for one's actions. Indeed my argument on genetic sexual attraction is largely naturalistic.

Dissolve the question then or resolve it? Our intellectual history since the eighteenth-century Enlightenment seems a gradual Western disenchantment with our given structurings as essential or inevitable – whether they are regarded as divine or natural – yet some recourse to an understanding that misfortune is beyond our willed intentions seems inevitable. This volume is an attempt at understanding, not a discourse on ethics. If, as I argue here, those people medicine terms neurotic are playing a game, then (to paraphrase Engels) it is a game whose rules are set by others, and a game in which participation is hardly to be considered a free choice but rather the best available under the circumstances.

The idea of sickness as some sort of wilful act is hardly new. Is our child's headache 'real' or just a way of avoiding school? Is the perpetrator of sexual violence who claims his own childhood abuse as the cause providing an explanation or an exculpation? Hasmat's brother and the hospital doctors to whom I gave my paper, like libertarian lawyers and right-wing psychotherapists such as Szasz and Berne, have all argued for an intentional approach in which we freely choose (or should choose) our actions out of the variety of available choices. Rather, I prefer here the idea of something akin to the anthropological sense of a ritual – a standardized way of proceeding which represents core idioms and which constrains and transforms the way we experience ourselves but which does allow us to have access to some other power without demanding that we be held fully accountable. And through which ambiguity, our responses reaffirm the meaning of everyday life for our fellows. And its power.

It is very likely that a hypothetical Sri Lankan who had observed a hysterical female in Victorian Europe would probably state that hers was a case of 'spirit possession', for this is the only category term in the culture that could embrace the overt behavioural signs of 'hysteria'. This, of course, would be ridiculous ...

Gananath Obeyesekere, *The Work of Culture: Symbolic Transformations in Psychoanalysis and Anthropology*

Data from a New Guinea tribe and the superficially very different data of psychiatry can be approached in terms of a single epistemology – a single body of questions.

Gregory Bateson, *Naven*

1. Psychiatry's Culture

Everyday distress at the beginning of the twenty-first century often appears to have some unknown cause hidden away beyond personal awareness – but a cause which can be found and identified by the scientist or physician. In the industrialized societies of the West our distress is an aspect of our life which, to a considerable extent, is already medicalized: it is seen through a lens which encourages us to experience, and indeed shape, individual concerns in medical ways – such that our misfortune often seems something like an illness which suddenly comes upon us from outside our immediate intention, that it has a particular cause (often governmental malfeasance) and a characteristic pattern which can be recognized by experts, and that there is perhaps some treatment available to cure it. Is our experience of bereavement perhaps a cause of sickness? Or even itself a sickness? The impact of unemployment, or environmental degradation, or civil disaster or incestuous abuse? The impulse to steal or hurt others? Or even the pace and confusions of contemporary life?

In its modern attempt to become recognized as a purely naturalistic science, independent of the particular historical context and moral traditions in which it has developed, Western medicine since the nineteenth century has played down the social relationship between patient and doctor, and between the experience of suffering and the local understandings through which suffering occurs. Medicine appeals to the laws and regularities of a physical world immune to changes in historical frames of reference or in human cognitions. It objectifies human experience as if our experience was constructed out of natural entities and, ascribing to them the conditions of our clinical observation, it reifies our personal contingencies as biological necessity; as the French anthropologist Pierre Bourdieu has put it, 'The observer transfers into the object the principles of his relation to the object.'[1] As indeed we do when, as patients or doctors, we talk of 'psychiatry' as some entity rather than as the actions of particular individuals in their ethical and political world.

If we want to understand patterns of psychological distress not simply as biological changes which appear from beyond our awareness until they are diagnosed but also as part of meaningful experience and action – as what we might term cultural patterns – we need to pay some attention to psychiatry's own culture: to the historical origins and politics of its nosologies, to its clinical engagement with its subjects, and indeed to its very understanding of 'culture', whether in the case of Hasmat (page viii) or anybody else.

When psychiatry developed as a clinical speciality in late eighteenth-century Europe, physicians recognized that certain of the concerns which (by analogy with physical disease) they examined as sicknesses could appear more commonly in one physical environment rather than in another. Psychiatry took up existing speculations on a nation's 'manners and spirit': in his *Poétique* of 1561, the Italian humanist Julius Scaliger had identified the character of his compatriots as 'cunctatores, irrisores, factiosi'.[2] England was described by its physicians as a country particularly liable to the *morbus anglicus* (despair and suicide) as a consequence of its climate (cold and wet), its diet (beef) and the pace of its commercial life (fast), all contributing to the vulnerabilities of the national character (melancholic).[3] Illnesses like melancholia, spleen or neurasthenia were, however, recognized not only as the consequence of climate but as the cost of accepting new public responsibilities by men of the emerging middle classes in the period of early industrialization and extending political representation. Other sicknesses – hysteria and moral retardation – were rather a distressing inability to accept such responsibility, an outward manifestation of the weaker bodily or moral constitution of European workers, criminals and women, or of African slaves and other colonized peoples, when they were threatened with the possibility of similar obligations.[4] Mental abnormalities were taken as characteristic of life in one or other nation or social strata, more immediately to be understood as the manifestation of physical environment, occupation, age, gender, temperament, habit and bodily constitution, as individuals variously conformed to or neglected their necessary obligations.[5] Or more generally through some idiom which tried to put together the physical environment with those obligations and sentiments, social organization and history, modes of sustenance and technical knowledge, individual character and family life, rituals and symbolizations which seemed to characterize a particular society: what has become known as its 'culture'.

Together with the Romantic idea of the nation as an entity which demonstrated shared patterns of thought and emotion, language and customs, 'culture' – once the idiom for individual self-development – became accepted as a term to place together all those moral and aesthetic characteristics attributable to living in a particular society, through acquiring which, children, like botanical specimens in a nursery, were cultivated into maturity.[6] Johann Herder proposed that each national culture resembled a plant, distinct and destined to grow in its own way. Whether each human group could be said to have a separate physical creation remained debated until Darwin, but 'culture' was generally placed in opposition to the existing term 'nature'; once the physical world created by divine action, 'nature' now denoted those features of human life which were found in other living beings – physical form and function, growth and reproduction; or which more specifically were shared only with animals – including the passions, sexuality, aggression and even such propensities as benevolence and sociality, all animal attributes which could be found in human societies in differing degrees.[7]

The term 'nature' seems to carry a number of related meanings for contemporary Europeans: the archaic and the chronologically presocial; our internal bodily processes; the universal and inevitable order of the organic and inorganic; and (identified or imagined) technologically primitive peoples.[8] By contrast, 'culture' argued for the moral and aesthetic moulding of natural growth, for a precarious binding of that which was more elemental and basic but which still sought expression in human life. Non-Europeans and European proletarians, women and children, inaccessible to culture or still to be cultivated, remained 'in a state of nature'.[9] Donna Haraway has argued recently that in the early industrial period Europeans took as nature 'only the material of nature appropriated, preserved, enslaved, exalted or otherwise made flexible for disposal by culture in the logic of capitalist colonialism'.[10] Culture was not only a historical process in human time but, like nature, some correlate thing which could be accumulated for use, and thus commodified. And taught. The more culture, the less significant was nature in a human society – and the converse. As in the earlier Christian schema, nature in herself was independent of willed human intention but she could be mastered by man's agency; the development of European civilization demonstrated that Man had gradually acquired dominion over nature, both as an industrial resource 'out there', as raw material or slaves, but also in his own body; as Francis Bacon put it, in a 'truly masculine birth of time [in which Man] would conquer and subdue Nature'.[11] And if Man had eventually learnt that he could not control the natural depredations of bodily diseases by an act of magical speech or sorcery, nor even by divine supplication,[12] he could often effect bodily healing through culture's technical power over nature: in Prince Albert's words, to 'conquer Nature to his use'.[13]

The actual relationship between nature and culture – what we might now prefer to consider as modes of thought taken for concrete entities – was and remains problematic. Different professional disciplines developed to specialize in each: what from Germany became known as the natural and the moral (or human) sciences. The pervasive notion of a hierarchy within nature – initially ordered as the Creator's Great Chain of Being, later as an unfolding evolutionary struggle – placed together what we still distinguish as the biological and the moral into a unitary schema: certain races had particularly high rates of one sort of psychological illness or another through their position in the evolutionary chain and their ability (or failure) to dominate their given nature. If melancholy was the fruit of European civilization's gradual accumulation of culture and self-consciousness, then primitive mental illness – a lack of control over instinct and impulsivity – was demonstrated by tribal peoples.[14] Yet one's 'psychic energy', the measure of mental health, reflected the number of the (newly discovered) brain cells. If biological and cultural were variously elided in different ways, the common conclusion was that 'culture' was primarily an attribute of Europeans, a function of their 'development'. Illnesses like Down's mongolism or mass hysteria warned Europeans of their possible degeneration to an earlier and more protean nature.[15]

Core and periphery, form and content

Clinical psychiatry developed as an academic discipline in the nineteenth-century hospitals and clinics of Europe where a new industrial order had confined those recognized as insane, and the majority of hospitalized patients still remain diagnosed as psychotic – as demonstrating diseases which, if pathological changes in the brain cannot readily be demonstrated, are at least presumed to be present.[16] And which reduce responsibility and thus legal accountability. The scientific ambitions of hospital medicine, and its identification of an illness which corresponded to what was popularly recognized as chronic insanity (and which by the early twentieth century came to be known as schizophrenia), tended to make the predominant understanding of mental illness the medical.[17] When the new 'nervous specialists' and 'alienists' were called to deal with patterns of distress or unusual behaviour among people who could not be obviously recognized as physically diseased or insane, they were faced with a practical issue of deciding if the patient was responsible for their symptoms; and whether they were accountable when making a will or giving evidence in a court of law, or if they could be expected to take responsibility for criminal acts or for rearing their children. If members of the upper or middling classes, some disease-like category such as hysteria or nervous prostration (neurasthenia) might be advanced which minimized the patient's responsibility for the condition itself but not for their other actions.[18] Doctors in private practice had realized that to challenge a patient's own ascription of illness too radically was to lose a resentful client, as sardonically illustrated by Molière and Proust. When deciding accountability for criminal acts where the individual claimed to be ill, doctors might, or might not, hold the prisoner accountable; decisions had to be made as to whether the illness was 'real' – caused by physical changes which were independent of the prisoner's awareness and whose actions were unintended – or feigned as they might be among those awaiting trial or sentence. The simulation of insanity under such circumstances might itself be reasonably considered an illness, it was concluded, yet not one which should provide exculpation for past crimes.[19]

Not every person who was diagnosed as having a particular mental illness reported exactly the same experiences. To deal with variations in the symptoms between individuals, while maintaining the idea of a uniform disease, clinical psychiatry still makes a distinction between the essential *pathogenic* determinants of a mental disorder – those biological processes which are held to be necessary and sufficient to cause it – and the *pathoplastic* personal and cultural variations in the pattern.[20] These two are still distinguished in everyday clinical practice by the particularly nineteenth-century German distinction between form and content.[21] To distinguish form from content was once a virtually ubiquitous practice in comparative studies in art history, ethnology, literary criticism or archaeology, indeed in the humanities in general; but in those areas it has been superseded by looser thematic, mimetic or emergent approaches, in part because of the inevitable uncertainty over deciding what was properly form and what content, together with the problem of justifying whether one or the other was somehow more fundamental, whether (ontologically) in a pattern's historical appearance or in its immediate causation, or (epistemologically) in its observed configuration and scholarly typology. It has been argued that the form/content dichotomy is facilitated by Indo-European subject-predicate syntax, or more specifically that it is characteristic of the scientific method whose advances have been fuelled by the analysis of apparent wholes through the underlying natural properties of their presumed parts, together with an empiricist theory of linguistic realism in which names simply label distinct entities such as diseases which are already present in the external world.[22] To which we might add the modern imperative to objectivize experience; so our experience of hotness, translated into temperature, became something recalling a natural entity which, like the idea of manic-depression, could easily be rated as a linear scale.[23]

However this may be, the form/content dichotomy continues in psychiatry as a medical proxy for distinguishing the biological (which we claim we can explain) from the cultural (which we can only seek to understand).[24] It has seemed most applicable when abnormal experiences and actions were associated with a recognized and presumably ubiquitous disease such as brain or thyroid tumour, anaemia, or with traumatic and vascular damage to the brain. The hallucinations which were experienced during the delirium of the brain-damaged alcoholic were taken as directly reflecting the biological form which was expressed through an insignificant content which simply reflected their particular character and the standard preoccupations of their society. Thus, looking at persecutory ideas in the West Indies, one study in the 1960s argued that for the local Blacks, paranoid suspicions (the form) were directed against their relatives and neighbours (the content), following local ideas of sorcery in an egalitarian village community; while for the White Creoles, preoccupied with retaining control as a precarious elite, the phantom poisoners were identified among the surrounding Black population.[25]

If nature was form and culture content, treatment was to be directed to the underlying biological cause, relatively easy – at least in theory – if it was identified by neuropsychiatrists as an object like a tumour or a bacterium. But to distinguish form from content was problematic in psychological illness where there were seldom any evident biological changes, and thus where the distinction had to be made on the basis of the patient's symptoms as presented to the physician. Hallucinations and delusions contrary to shared everyday reality were nearly always regarded as primary and thus biological; their particular themes had even less bearing on the cause (and thus treatment) of the disease than the way patients might understand pain had any significance for ascertaining the origins of the pain. To take an example from the German psychiatrist Emil Kraepelin: that a patient said he was the Kaiser rather than Napoleon (in other words, a variation in the content of his illness) was of little clinical value compared with the fact of a delusion of grandiose identification (the form). Now this left the shared social world fairly redundant in psychiatric illness as it was observed in the hospital; except in as much as a society might facilitate one or other physical cause – as patterns of drinking might encourage alcohol-induced dementia, or local perceptions of risk increased the likelihood of traumatic accidents to the head, or in a less direct way through a society's transformation of the physical environment and thus of human biology through genetic selection (as with malaria susceptibility and sickle cell anaemia). If cultural values could thus sometimes cause disease through transforming natural causes, they could not cause serious mental illness directly in the way that Christianity, Islam and popular understandings might still identify moral turpitude as the immediate cause of insanity.[26]

The form/content schema worked fairly smoothly in European mental hospitals where the scope of what counted as clinical observation was limited by the institutional context; but by the beginning of the twentieth century psychiatry began to extend its practice to the peoples of the colonial empires. Many local patterns which suggested novel types of mental illness had been previously recorded by travellers, missionaries and colonial administrators, sometimes indeed as illnesses but often as examples of the criminal perversity of native life or just as picturesque if rather troublesome oddities. Most notable among these was *amok*,[27] a Malay word which has passed into the English language for indiscriminate and unmotivated violence by one person against others. In one of the first discussions of the problems of comparing psychiatric illness across societies, Kraepelin, after a trip to Java during which he collected accounts of amoks and also observed hospitalized patients, suggested that the characteristic symptoms of a particular mental illness – those which one could find everywhere in the world – were the essential pathogenic ones which directly reflected its physical cause.[28] Yet, as he noted, 'reliable comparison is of course only possible if we are able to draw clear distinctions between identifiable illnesses'. This proved difficult given the variety of local patterns, together with the intention, which Kraepelin enthusiastically shared, to fit them into the restricted number of categories already identified in European hospitals.

Eugen Bleuler, the Swiss psychiatrist who had coined the term 'schizophrenia', argued that those symptoms by which we can distinguish this illness from other patterns directly reflect the underlying biological process.[29] This coalesced with Kraepelin's idea that the characteristic features are the universal ones, to produce the still current model of psychiatric illness which may be described as something like a Russian doll: the essential biological determinants which specify an illness are surrounded by a confusing series of cultural and idiosyncratic envelopes which have to be picked away in diagnosis to reveal the real disease.[30] As Kraepelin's pupil Karl Birnbaum put it, these pathoplastic envelopes just give 'content, colouring and contour to individual illnesses whose basic form and character have already been biologically established'.[31] Wittgenstein critically likened the same sort of approach in the psychological sciences to our picking away the leaves of an artichoke in a hopeless attempt to uncover some real artichoke, on the assumption that (to use the anthropologist Clifford Geertz's sarcastic aphorism) 'culture is icing, biology cake ... difference is shallow, likeness deep'.[32] The medical observer was to focus on those symptoms which seem distinguishing and characteristic, and thus biologically determining: symptoms notably elusive in psychiatry where anxiety, irritation, insomnia, anorexia, depression, self-doubt and suicidal preoccupations are common to virtually all identified illnesses, and which themselves shade into everyday experience. Such common features tend to be ignored in diagnostic practice, more by an act of faith in the Kraepelin–Birnbaum model than through an empirical consideration of all the available evidence. And even the statistical attempt to develop a nomenclature favoured by epidemiologists in the 1970s and 1980s resulted in circular and quite varied arguments about categorization and universality.[33] Psychiatric illnesses have not been shown to fit neatly bounded monothetic categories (which supposedly 'carve nature at the joint' as Young rather nicely puts it[34]), and multivariate analysis of a multitude of possible symptoms produces rather different schemata for

classification, depending on the statistical procedure adopted, on whether
one includes or omits shared symptoms, and indeed on what is to count as
a symptom.[35]

The local understandings of illness which a society shared were ignored
by colonial doctors who, as in Europe, restricted themselves to examination of those admitted to prison or later to the psychiatric hospital.[36] When
faced with patients from a society or minority group with which they are
unfamiliar, British and American psychiatrists still complain of the
culturally confusing factors which obscure the elusive disease process.
With European patients in a predominantly European society they have
fewer problems in finding universal categories because 'culture' is always
there, tacit, to be implicitly omitted in what counted as the clinical
assessment, for, being fairly uniform, it does not seem to contribute to
variability between patients. Indeed, any differences within the shared
social context of Western patterns, say between women and men, have
been ignored until recently in favour of biological or bio-psychological
aetiologies to explain variation (and thence 'causation'). Thus there has not
seemed anything immediately 'cultural' in those patterns identified
particularly in the West – eating disorders, panic reactions, phobias, self-
harm or shoplifting. And thus these could be easily presumed to be world-
wide patterns. Socially appropriate ways of experiencing and demonstrating distress, like everyday notions of personhood and responsibility, have
not been taken as causal, for what appeared as a constant could not
determine a variable like illness. Ignoring the full range of symptoms across
societies and their relationship to the patients' own beliefs and expectations
(and to the therapeutic context) did not seem inappropriate for practice
within apparently homogeneous societies, because there doctor–patient
interactions and the process of diagnosis were already significant and
taken-for-granted aspects of daily life. Diagnostic decisions were followed
by generally accepted patterns of social response – by medication, hospital
admission and, on occasion, suspension of civil rights.

Imperial psychiatry

It was when they took their diagnostic systems with them to their colonies
at the beginning of the twentieth century that psychiatrists first recognized
some of these difficulties. And this brings us to their current understanding
of 'culture'. Dysphoric moods and unusual actions were locally recognized
in Africa or Asia, not necessarily as something recalling a physical illness
but often as part of totally different patterns of experience and order – as
spirit possession or rituals of mourning, or as events in the course of
initiation, sorcery and warfare. Those patterns that recalled the psychoses

of the West seemed generally recognized as unwelcome but not always as akin to sickness.[37] Yet, when colonial doctors turned to writing reports and academic communications, local understandings of self and illness which might now seem to us as analogous to psychiatric theories were described, not as self-contained, meaningful and functional conceptions in themselves, but rather as inadequate approximations to Western scientific knowledge. At times, however, the local understandings of small-scale rural societies, like the more recognizably medical traditions of India and China, cut dramatically across European experience. The anthropologist Charles Seligman, who had trained as a doctor, reported that there seemed to have been nothing in New Guinea before European contact which could be said to resemble schizophrenia.[38] As cases analogous to schizophrenia have been later identified by psychiatrists, he has been criticized for what is known as 'the Seligman error' – missing a universal illness because local understandings and social response did not allow it to appear objectivized through social extrusion as in a Western hospital but which rather incorporated it into some shared institution where it lay unremarked by the medical observer. And similarly, Amerindian and circumpolar patterns of healing, religious inspiration and leadership, in which election to the shamanic role might be signalled by a sudden illness, accident or other troubling experience, were thought to mask underlying schizophrenia.[39]

Patterns like amok or *piblokto* ('arctic hysteria') were initially taken as rather odd – generally simpler – variants of the psychiatric disorders described in Europe. Mental illness in Java, said Kraepelin, showed 'broadly the same clinical picture as we see in our country ... The overall similarity far outweighed the deviant features'.[40] Individuals locally regarded as amoks were thus really demonstrating epilepsy or perhaps catatonic schizophrenia.[41] But what were to be taken as these 'deviant features', and what was being compared with what? – presumably the form of the illness, the basis for categorization of the pattern as some clinical entity. If one looked, for instance, at a Malay patient who had an unjustified belief that she was persecuted by her neighbours, then her delusion was the form, and the neighbours provided the content, but the persecution seemed variously one or the other. That she was deluded is important for arguing that she is mentally ill; the neighbours are of no diagnostic significance, but that her delusions were persecutory could be or not, depending on the selected illness. The assumptions made by Kraepelin in his studies in Java remain the dominant paradigms in comparative psychiatry: how similar do patterns have to be before we can say that we are talking about the same pattern? How do we distinguish between those features which appear to be generally the same and those which vary? And what are our units of categorization going to be when deciding sameness and difference, normality and pathology? Does something similar to 'depression' occur everywhere? Or perhaps just a less specific experience such as 'distress'?

Psychiatric textbooks have generally argued that locally recognized patterns like amok are 'not new diagnostic entities: they are in fact similar to those already known in the West'.[42] This equivalence has often been extraordinarily optimistic. To take one pattern which attracted considerable interest because of its exotic salience, *windigo*, the 'cannibal-compulsion' syndrome of the North American Ojibwa and Inuit, was locally described as an individual becoming possessed by a cannibalistic vampire and then attacking other people in an attempt to devour them. Windigo was identified by psychiatrists confidently but quite variously with known patterns as disparate as depression, schizophrenia, hysteria and anxiety. Similarly, amok was explained not only as the local manifestation of either epilepsy or schizophrenia, but as malaria, syphilis, cannabis psychosis, sunstroke, mania, hysteria, depression, disinhibited aggression and anxiety.[42] *Latahs*, women of the Malay Peninsula who uttered obscene remarks when startled and who parodied the speech and actions of others apparently without intent,[43] were identified as demonstrating a 'psychosis [or] hysteria, arctic hysteria, reactive psychosis, startle reaction, fright neurosis, hysterical psychosis [or] hypnoid state'.[44] Identifying symptoms rather than the local context meant that amok and latah have generally been regarded not as autonomous cultural institutions, but simply as erroneous Malay explanations which shaped one single universal disease, although the psychiatric observers disagreed radically as to which disease this might be. The extent to which such patterns could be fitted into a universal schema depended on how far the medical observer was prepared to stretch a known psychiatric category, and thus on the preferred theoretical model. By the 1970s, Weston La Barre and Georges Devereux, psychoanalysts who were much less attached to purely biomedical arguments, had gone further in including as instances of schizophrenia a wide variety of local institutions – possession states, shamanism, prophecy, millennial religions and indeed, for La Barre, social change in general. They argued not just that schizophrenia might typically appear in these social institutions but that the institutions exemplified the schizophrenic experiences from which they originated;[45] everyday culture in non-Western societies could be understood, as it were, as insanity spread out thin.

If psychiatrists of the colonial period remained puzzled about the cultural encrustations they saw adhering to the essential symptoms, they could be struck by the opposite: the 'barrenness of the clinical picture ... In more primitive culture schizophrenia is "a poor imitation of European forms"'.[46] Culturally obscured, or simply a primitive form, in neither case did culture determine anything but rather acted as a sort of indeterminate soup which passively filled in or distorted the biological matrix. And yet 'culture' itself could be a proxy for biological 'race'. Categorizations of illness, professional or popular, are adjacent to other social classifications – to those of character, ethnicity, gender, the natural world and historical experience – on which they draw and which they plagiarize. The distinction, and indeed opposition, between form and content had depended on a fairly clear distinction between universal biology and the variant culture which constrained it, yet by the end of the nineteenth century descriptive psychiatry was increasingly influenced by Social Darwinist ideas of racial biology in which, while humans now were agreed to have once had a common origin, neurological, psychological, social and moral variations were all considered as reflections of each other at a particular level on the linear scale of 'development'. Allan Young has recently proposed the term 'the normalisation of pathology' for the Victorian topology (associated particularly with the neurologist Hughlings Jackson and thence found in Herbert Spencer, W. H. R. Rivers and Freud) in which the central nervous system, like the colonial order, was organized in a series of levels of control in which the 'higher' could generally override the 'lower'.[47] (Jackson's analogy was a rider and a horse.) Hysteria was recognized as dysfunctional at the 'lower' level, and Kraepelin explained the unusual symptomatology of mental illness among the Javanese as reflecting their 'lower stage of intellectual development'.[48] Variations in (what doctors called) the 'presentation' of illness in different societies have been attributed until recently not just to particular historical and political experiences, as we might have expected from the pathoplastic model, but to the existence of a fairly uniform primitive mentality (more nature than culture) which was shared with European children and with the 'degenerate', 'deviant', 'regressed' or 'retarded' adult European, governed by impulse, deficient in foresight, and which manifest symptoms characteristic of a loss of higher control: 'hyperidic states', 'catastrophic reactions', 'malignant anxiety', 'simple responses available to psychologically disorganised individuals' and 'primitive reactions corresponding to outbursts of psychopathic persons in developed countries'.[49] Not altogether unrelated physiological explanations attributed *piblokto* and *kayak angst* to the undeveloped mind reflecting on 'the stillness and the sense of impending doom that are so characteristic of the Arctic climate'.[50]

Depression

This topological psychology of linear development, put together with the assumption that symptoms observed in Europe were somehow more real and less obfuscated by cultural values, led to the common argument that depression did not yet occur in non-Europeans for its essential Western characteristic of self-blame (a consequence of mature selfhood) was not observed.[51] The absence of depression was sometimes directly attributed to a less evolved brain where the 'primitive layers' predominated, an idea which might have had (but practically didn't) implications for the Colonial Office when it considered the possibility of independence for colonial Africa, as recommended in a report by the colonial doctor J. C. Carothers.[52] Guilty self-accusations of the type found in clinical depression in the West had in fact been identified in colonial Africa in the 1930s, not by the doctors in the colonial hospitals but by an anthropologist looking at witchcraft and the distribution of shrines.[53] Reactions which recall Western depression are now frequently described in small-scale non-industrialized communities but the issue depends, not only on the frequency with which people with less socially disturbing problems come to the hospital to be treated and thus studied, on medical failure to empathize with another's experience, nor on a rather cursory epidemiology based on colonial hospital statistics, but on what one means by 'depression'. Is it something like the misery which we might identify in various situations of loss or bereavement, or the pattern of rather physical experiences such as loss of interest, waking up early, and poor appetite, which are recognized as clinical depression (and which appear likely to be universal), or else some more specific expressed sentiment of Judaeo-Christian guilt and a wish to die? Greater psychiatric familiarity with the experience of personal distress in the former colonies has suggested that 'depression' may be simply a variant of widespread patterns of what we might term dysphoric mood which in depression is represented through a particularly Western moral psychology which assumes an autonomous self as the invariant locus of experience, memory and agency. When looking across societies, a more common experience of everyday distress than 'depression' (which figures a phenomenological sinking downwards of the once active self into an inertia for which we remain responsible[54]), may be one of depletion and the loss of something essential which has been taken out of the self – a pattern well glossed in various Latin American idioms of 'soul loss'.[55]

The culture-bound syndromes

In the 1950s, following revulsion at German academic psychiatry's 'eugenics' under the Nazis and its development into ethnic extermination,[56] the social and medical sciences gradually discarded the ideas of biological evolution and psychological development as explanations for differences of experience and action between contemporary societies. All societies were now recognized as having 'a culture' in similar ways, and biological differences between groups as a whole – that between men and women still excepted – could not explain their different types of mental illness. The recognition that many non-Western illnesses could no longer be subsumed as primitive forms of universal categories led comparative psychiatry (or as it now came to be called, cultural psychiatry) to propose a new sort of illness altogether whose study did not entail the biological form/cultural content dichotomy. Patterns like amok and latah, which had recalled the idea of psychological illness in Europe yet remained unclassifiable, came to be known as 'culture-bound syndromes'.[57] They were usually episodic and dramatic reactions, limited to a particular society where they were locally identified as distinct patterns of action very different from those of everyday life. And which, we might now note, had been of colonial concern because they were bizarre, outrageous or frankly troublesome. Less dramatic patterns of distress – personal withdrawal from shared activities, troubling thoughts, chronic pain, bereavement, despondency – which did not come to the attention of the colonial administration or the local police were ignored until the development of medical anthropology in the 1980s.

A large number of such 'culture-bound' illnesses have now been catalogued[58] as distinctive and consistent patterns, transmitted to each generation in a continuing cultural tradition, and which are taken as closely related to a society's distinctive understanding of self and its prescribed norms.[59] Thus, however high the incidence of reactions like grief or terror might be in war-torn communities, they were not regarded as culture-specific unless they continued in some consistently recognizable form in successive generations as part of an enduring identity. What exactly was it that was 'bound' in culture-bound syndromes? Had 'culture' now achieved the master status of 'biology' in the international nosology? There is a continuing debate as to what the category 'culture' refers: usually restricted to a pattern found only in the society in question and which symbolizes and represents fundamental local concerns, on occasion it has been applied to apparently universal and biologically understood illnesses which are shaped, distinguished and treated in a local content.[60] Thus one might include *kifafa*, *malkadi* and *moth madness*, locally recognized patterns in Tanzania, Trinidad and among the Navaho which closely recall the medical description of epilepsy.[61] A locally recognized reaction in New Guinea, *kuru*, was however once regarded as a culture-bound syndrome akin to hysteria, but no longer, given the likely role of a slow virus in its aetiology. (And which has made it even more exotic through recognition that it could be transmitted through cannibalism.) Patterns like kuru or the restricted abilities of senescence, or such apparently motivated patterns as homicide and rape, the deliria of malnutrition or alcohol intoxication, or the use of other psychoactive substances have certainly been regarded as characteristic of a particular society but are seldom described as 'culture-

bound' because they appear potentially available in any society or else do
not immediately recall European 'mental illness'. Yet, if these patterns
persisted – like the alcohol abuse, *anomic depression* and suicide consequent
on the relocation of Native Americans onto reservations – they were taken
as manifestations of 'American Indian culture', ignoring the political
relationship between colonizer and native, and thus the context of the
psychiatric observation. 'New illnesses' identified by more sophisticated
epidemiological techniques in urban populations or through the expansion
of psychiatric observation to a wider population have been termed 'culture-
change' or 'acculturation illnesses' exemplified by the *brainfag syndrome*
identified in some West African students.[62]

Conflict and resistance

If these local patterns were distinguished as 'culture-bound' by the
European psychiatrist only in that they occurred in (other) cultures, how
then did a culture lead to illness? Did 'culture' mean simply shared
conceptualizations so that the psychiatrist could identify local concerns and
sentiments either in the type of person who was vulnerable, or else in the
actual symptoms which represented the culture in a way that recalled
seventeenth- and eighteenth-century ideas of a national character? Or
could 'culture' be located in social and biological stressors which occurred
in a particular society but were not necessarily recognized there as
problems? And anyway how could such illness be clearly distinguished
from the other cultural patterns in which it was embedded? A later
question, reserved for the 1980s, was whether to extend the category to
illnesses such as eating disorders which were apparently only to be found in
European societies.[63]

In part, the continuing problem of 'culture' for psychiatrists lay in its
double-edged connotations. 'Culture' was still a valued commodity, that
constraint on nature which distinguished human from animal, educated
European from the primitive (and which thus often referred to 'high
culture' alone).[64] Yet, for Western psychiatrists establishing their discipline
as a medical speciality, 'culture' remained secondary to scientific biological
reality. As frank biological racism became disreputable after the Second
World War, and the unifying idiom of 'development' separated out into the
distinct fields of child psychology, economics and technology, the
psychological differences between European and non-European could
again be perceived only in rather uncertain 'cultural' terms: as a medical
proxy for the other's 'difference' (or even for the lingering idea of biological
'race') and which still immersed the individual in some undifferentiated
other, now less their biological level than their way of life. As medicine had

little idea of how to deal with 'culture', it drew on other disciplines, particularly psychoanalysis and social anthropology, which claimed to be able to relate the interests of medicine to the inter-subjective social world in a more empirical and humanistic way than had evolutionary medicine. The new cultural psychiatrists generally held appointments in Western university departments, away from the poorly funded and intellectually marginal concerns of colonial psychiatry which still remained close to popular Western ideas of race.[65] Psychoanalysts and anthropologists interested in providing a 'cultural psychiatry' of local patterns in British Africa based on intensive fieldwork in local communities were seldom interested in examining hospital statistics, unlike the epidemiologists associated with the World Health Organization who until recently have preferred to stick with the presumed biomedical universals, and thus with the form/content idioms of hospital psychiatry.

Particularly in the United States where a strong inclination towards psychoanalysis was apparent in medicine and the social sciences from the 1930s, psychiatrists emphasized the similarity of local illnesses to the 'modal personality' which an individual developed in their culture. The affected person was now suffering less from something recalling a medical disease with a bit of culture tacked on, so much as demonstrating in an exaggerated form those psychological conflicts established in the course of childhood socialization. So *windigo* (the Ojibwa cannibal-compulsion psychosis) was interpreted as a local preoccupation with food in a hostile environment, fuelled by residues of infantile resentment at the mother for the early weaning necessitated by the scarcity of food. After an indulgent childhood, the young boy was precipitated into early adulthood by brutal tests of self-reliance and encouraged to fast in order to attain ultrahuman powers. Dependence on his parents was replaced by a precarious dependence on spirits which encouraged solitary self-reliance in hunting. The mother, feared and hated for her violent rejection of her son, returned to possess him in the form of the windigo.[66]

Psychoanalytically orientated anthropologists proposed in this sort of way that any culture was a dynamic compromise between conflicting interests – ecological, physiological, between self and others, between parents and children, men and women. Symptoms, dreams, religious symbols and social institutions could all be taken as aspects of the same conflicts refracted through an individual's psychological functioning.[67] Was the European observer now to take the locally identified illness as the expression of such conflicts in unconscious motivations as a society's symptoms? Or, given the incorporation of personal conflicts into local institutions, was the 'illness' to be considered as a type of collective psychological adjustment, indeed as a sort of healing? Psychoanalysis agreed with psychiatry that one could distinguish problem, causation and treatment,[68] but differed as to how to go about it. Devereux, perhaps the most sophisticated of the psychoanalytical anthropologists, eventually proposed that institutions like shamanism (which had often been taken as employing altered states of consciousness to facilitate something akin to Western psychotherapy[69]) were themselves the expression of psychological disturbances in what he called the 'ethnic unconscious': disturbances which could then be enhanced by a society to produce 'ethnic psychoses' as he called these pathological institutions.[70] Criticizing the historian Edwin Ackernecht who had argued for a clear distinction between cultural meaning and medical terminology,[71] Devereux argued that the local healing of unconscious social conflicts simply exacerbated them: 'There exist societies so enmeshed in a vicious circle that everything they do to save themselves only causes them to sink deeper into the quicksand.'[72] The British biological psychiatrist William Sargant, a former Methodist who had taken to arguing that religious experience and spirit possession were a type of brainwashing, emphasized the cathartic function of culture-specific patterns which allowed the individual, when in a state of dissociated consciousness, to express otherwise socially forbidden inclinations in a non-threatening and relatively sanctioned manner – as if they were half-way between an 'illness' and its 'treatment'.[73] Like Devereux, he still regarded it as all distinctly unhealthy. Alternatively, Weston La Barre, Ari Kiev and Thomas Scheff took the cathartic expression of hidden desires as a resolution rather than an exacerbation of cultural conflicts – as something closer to healing.

This all got rather circular and, like hospital psychiatry, ignored local conceptions of healing in favour of Western assumptions of normality and illness. Paralleling the earlier assumption that non-Western pathologies were masked or incomplete forms, non-Western healing was now taken as an elementary version of psychoanalytical therapy but one which employed 'suggestion' rather than 'insight'.[74] What remained constant in all of this was the conviction, however muted, that Western categories were still the appropriate way to frame the question; and that these provided universal criteria by which one could agree that certain local patterns were justifiably termed dysfunctional or maladaptive.[75] On rare occasions analysts carried out formal psychoanalysis with their African and Amerindian informants,[76] even if they still presumed Freudian ideals of psychological maturity to be universally valid.[77] Few of the classic culture-bound syndromes were not at some time explained as the projection of unconscious fantasies and thwarted incestuous wishes, as the consequences of traumatic weaning, or simply as the overwhelming existential anxiety of tribal societies which followed from their unsophisticated psychology.[78]

Eliding the conventional distinction between pathology as an individual phenomenon and treatment as a social response, the cost to the psychoanalysts was, as Ackernecht had warned, 'the wholesale pathologisation of cultures'. Equivalence between modal personality, characteristic personal illness and social structure led to an interpretation of small-scale communities as paranoid, obsessive or whatever – even if the implication of these terms was evidently less 'strong' than the clinical usage from which they derived.[79] During and after the Second World War, American psychoanalysts were funded to study the 'cultural pathologies' of enemy nations.[80] Psychoanalysis still subscribed to those positivist ideals of the late nineteenth century which had sought a moral understanding of human society in science rather than in religion; like the French neurologists under whom he had studied, Freud had explained the medieval persecution of Europe's witches on the grounds that they had really been suffering from mental illness, and psychoanalysts like Devereux took with them the assumption that spirit possession was a variant of hysteria when they turned to look at non-European cultures. The presumed universality of the Oedipus complex even in matrilineal (mother-descended) societies which did not recognize a male role in procreation was a matter of particular interest;[81] not unlike the hospital psychiatrist Kraepelin, the psychoanalysts took a European pattern for which theories had been elaborated as the basic form which other societies then manifested as evident, masked or incomplete.[82] And they tended to the evolutionary idioms of late nineteenth-century psychiatry, if in a less biologized way, still arguing developmental parallels between archaic ancestor, contemporary primitive, child and neurotic, all as early, arrested or regressed levels characterized by an infantile psychology in which 'psychic omnipotence' and 'magical thinking' trailed behind the advancing line of mature rationality. Nor, with rare exceptions,[83] was colonial power of much psychoanalytical interest, whether as the rather unusual site for their observations or – occasional comments on the perils of imitating primitives for the Whites apart[84] – as itself pathogenic.[85]

More recently, local illnesses have been regarded by psychiatrists influenced by anthropology less as diseases or unconscious conflicts than as particularly salient everyday sensibilities and values or exaggerated idioms of distress:[86] as with the Hindu *suchi-bar* ('purity mania') and the related *ascetic syndrome*, or the Taiwanese *shen k'uei* and Japanese *taijin kyofusho* ('interpersonal phobia'). If these had been termed pathological or maladaptive by Western psychiatry, it was because normative institutions – Brahmanical obligations to avoid certain foods and preserve bodily purity, or Japanese expectations of self-restraint and the avoidance of inappropriate familiarity – were taken too enthusiastically by certain individuals, resulting in anxieties or interpersonal problems which could be recognized as disproportionate both in the local context and by psychiatric observers. Or alternatively, recalling the psychoanalytical view, the patterns represent in the individual a conflict or contradiction between the local institutions themselves: thus it has been argued that the continuing antagonism between the values of sexuality and asceticism in India generates the 'purity syndromes'.[87] Or else, as Sargant had argued, personal conflicts are expressed in limited contravention of role-specific norms in fairly standardized situations,[88] and that it is these contraventions which had been identified, correctly or otherwise, as pathologies. It has been suggested that all cultures have such loopholes which are themselves 'socially reinforced and have the same structural characteristics as other behavioural norms in the system'; and that at least in the case of latah and amok, we should employ a less medical term than 'syndrome': perhaps something like 'stylised expressive traditional behaviours' for those deviant patterns which are fairly standardized and limited in time, but which, whilst they certainly contravene everyday behaviour, are somehow culturally condoned to allow the expression of apparently repressed but not uncommon sentiments.[89] This does push the psychiatrist's normative question back even further, but if deviance (or pathology) is sometimes locally condoned or even encouraged, what is the frame by which one should term it deviant? – the lingering Western presumption of pathology, or some local 'don't do this but if you must, do it this way'? As with the earlier colonial psychiatry, the idea of 'a culture' has however remained one which is fairly homogenous, with values and social order accepted in the same way by all members: a model which followed the idea of a tightly bounded society once sought by colonial officers and anthropologists, and which ignored any unequal distribution of knowledge and power, of local contestation or global change.[90]

The limits of cultural psychiatry

The evolutionary schema did offer one mode of comparison by placing societies (or illnesses) as states of transformation along a historical spectrum driven by certain processes and thus 'normalising' pathologies as stages.[91] Few social anthropologists, some sociobiologists, Freudians and Marxists perhaps excepted, would now subscribe to the idea of a unilinear human development through which local institutions and mentalities are to be understood as determined by underlying processes, whether those of evolutionary selection or of the relations of production. Whilst it is still argued that the insights offered by psychoanalysts may provide a useful perspective when trying to understand psychological experience in non-European societies,[92] others have argued that Freud's followers have little to contribute to the critical or social sciences for they offer a moralized version of commonsense Western assumptions about the inevitability of European rationality with entrepreneurial autonomy as 'health' or 'adaptation'. On the whole, with the exception of a few psychoanalytically orientated anthropologists such as Melford Spiro and Gananath Obeyesekere, the ethnographic monographs written by anthropologists now place little emphasis on the early childhood experiences which the psychoanalysts had argued was significant in generating culture. They take particular patterns of childrearing as the manifestation rather than the cause of social knowledge.[93] The assumption that non-Europeans' thought is less rational has been superseded by recognition that all societies employ both deductive and inductive logic, both concrete and abstract reasoning, but that they do so within limits which are determined by their own social interests. Societies differ psychologically not in their capabilities but in their modes of thought – through cognitions and categorizations of space and time, the sexes and the natural world, their understandings of causality and invidia, and which are encoded in their systems of representation particularly language. What was once regarded as primitive (magical) thinking on the origins of sickness or misfortune appears now as a focus on the moral 'why' rather than the technical 'how', for societies differ in the focus of their immediate interests and practised knowledge. Indeed, in terms of the everyday understanding of sickness, Western medicine is less efficacious in relieving distress through its emphasis on the proximate mechanisms of misfortune, leaving the individual with chronic or serious illness little help in answering 'why me?'.[94] In the case of severe mental illness we might note that psychiatry remains unable to offer its patients any understanding, technical or moral, in terms of our everyday knowledge (or, indeed, of biology).

To recognize some other's pattern as especially 'cultural' is to assume a privileged perspective concerning it, whether colonial hubris or academic analysis. (As Pascal had put it, we have truth but they have customs.) By the mid-1980s culture-specific illnesses had become recognized by critics as psychiatry's 'twilight zone', 'what other people have, not us'.[95] Medical interest in isolated and disembodied exotic patterns was seen to have directed attention from more immediate questions of economic development, poverty, exploitation and nutritional diseases, besides providing yet another justification of the otherness of non-Europeans, and one which ignored the role of Western medicine once in facilitating imperial expansion and now in the global marketing of untested pharmaceutical drugs.

How directly relevant had psychiatry been to imperialism? Both evidently developed in the same period. They shared certain modes of reasoning: we might note, for instance, affinities between the scientific objectification of illness experience as disease and the objectification of people as chattel slaves or a colonial manpower, or the topological parallels between the nervous system and the colonial order. Both argued for an absence of 'higher' functions or sense of personal responsibility among patients and non-Europeans. The extent, however, to which any elaborated set of ideas which might be termed 'imperial psychiatry' provided a rationale for colonialism in British Africa or India is debatable: in a recent review I have argued that the evidence is meagre.[96] With remarkably few exceptions,[97] the small number of colonial psychiatrists barely participated in the debates I have outlined above. Segregated facilities, of course;[98] prejudice and neglect, undoubtedly; but hardly practicable ideologies for perpetuating racial or cultural inferiority.[99] (Indeed, we might more plausibly argue the case of contemporary psychiatric practice in Britain.) One possible exception was the common medical assumption in the 1940s that too rapid social change (that is access to schools and waged labour) were causing an increase in African psychiatric illness,[100] but this increase was often explained by others as a better access to hospital services. Whether this argument was taken seriously in London I am doubtful; it could of course be turned on its head by arguing that it was colonization, not 'change', that was pathogenic.[101] While the few colonial psychiatrists were quite tangential to the making of Colonial Office policy (and were themselves rather 'marginal' individuals within both British and colonial society[102]), in the francophone colonies and in Haiti, local Black psychiatrists developed radical critiques of European domination to argue for a distinct 'African identity' as against the White settlers, and one which was couched in terms of 'ethnopsychiatry'.[103] Ethnographers like W. H. R. Rivers and Bronislaw Malinowski, aspects of whose work developed into what was to become medical anthropology, while they relied on missionary evidence and colonial office support,[104] did not significantly influence British policy in Africa or elsewhere.[105] If diseases in the colonies were of any political interest to the metropolis, the concern was not madness but the acute infections which threatened to deprive the imperial administration of its labour force, or else the psychological health of the colonists themselves.[106]

Contemporary anthropologists have proposed that all illnesses may be said to be 'culture-bound' in that our adaptation to illness experience is always socially prescribed, while human behaviour can never be taken in independence from human action. The classic 'cultural syndromes' still remain as titillating relief in the margins of British psychiatric textbooks in the 1990s. Often the hearsay repetition of previous descriptions, travellers' tales and missionary anxieties, frequently in their most bizarre form, they distort local significance and context in providing a voyeuristic image of the other. The windigo cannibal-compulsion which still appears in these books has now been recognized as psychiatric folklore, a 'near mythical syndrome' with perhaps three reported instances and one which has never been observed by Europeans.[107] Similar doubts have been cast on the evidence for *voodoo death* ('pointing the bone') in which awareness that one had been ensorcered apparently precipitated sudden death through 'a fatal spirit of despondency'.[108] Psychiatrists concerned with establishing basic mental health services in post-colonial Africa and Asia have deplored the endless collecting of novel syndromes 'by a host of short-term visitors [producing] a wealth of data about some strange ritual of an obscure tribe, analysed with style and erudition, but without comment on general trends particularly as they relate to the more mundane aspects of clinical psychiatry'.[109] For those concerned with establishing basic medical services and providing humane treatment in situations of poverty and exploitation, debates on the cultural specificity of suffering may appear otiose.

And yet 'culture-bound syndromes' represent salient instances of a particular community's dilemmas, as extreme if sometimes contentious representations of human distress in its distinctive milieu. To essentialize such social dramas as medical diseases in independence of everyday meanings or other experiences of distress, or in independence of the political context of our observation, is to render them exotic curiosities. To ignore them altogether is to render human adversity bland and familiar, to affirm that the European's experience alone is true, and thus to naturalize the patterns of Western psychiatric illnesses, to affirm them as transcending our intentions, as necessary and immutable.[110]

2. A Chapter against Pathology

Hospital psychiatrists and those inclined to psychoanalysis both argued for unitary theories of the phenomena once observed by missionaries, army doctors and colonial administrators, even if, as we have seen, they disagreed as to what any such unity comprised: universally recognizable disease entity, exaggeration of norm, cultural conflict, social change, sanctioned rejection of the norm or even therapeutic response. Social anthropologists have objected that their error was to use a medical grid which inevitably objectified social action as disease entity. Rather, one should start by simply describing a society in its own terms, for societies are not traditional residues of some forgotten past which is passing away but always constitute themselves anew in their chosen memories and actions.

If the term 'culture-bound syndrome' is to retain value only as a concept of local sickness, whether or not psychiatry recognizes it as akin to Western disease, what, however, is to count as our very 'concept of sickness'? Social scientists are hardly immune from comparing one society with another to obtain regularities and general patterns, and in order to do that, they too define apparently analogous domains in each – whether those of social structure, kinship, religion or sickness. And these domains inevitably derive from Western terminology. Another society then simply comes to be read as an aggregate of such areas of comparison which have a structured and causal relationship to each other. The comparative problem is hardly unique to medicine. As the British anthropologist Edward Evans-Pritchard is said to have observed, 'If social anthropology is anything, it is a comparative discipline – and that is impossible.' It is not that psychiatry's inevitable grid, pathology, is necessarily inappropriate for comparing what looks to the European like 'suffering' or 'madness' in different societies, but pathology is just one possible grid and one which carries with it particular assumptions about normality and abnormality which explicitly ignore consideration of power and of the context of observation. And of what is observed, and how our 'observation' itself might shape it.

In the previous chapter, to some extent, I excused psychiatrists for seeking to understand social patterns in terms of sickness, for any approach to a complex system has to reduce complexity by imposing or seeking some grid of observation which presents us with patterns as intelligible, and for scientists ideally measurable. Our problems are then whether this misses too much of interest, or whether it actually transforms the system itself (and these two problems are hardly distinct). And of course what type of social power it is which is supported by medicalization. If we strip away the context and the differences within any new system we can always find 'universals'. Whether these are significant or not is up to us. We should perhaps not be too hard on the form/content solution (pp. 5–7), for similar problems arise in any comparative human science including social and biological anthropology. Do, for instance, the modes of thought in a particular society present us with a unitary schema, or do we need to distinguish shared representation (image or subject matter) from individual psychological mechanism? Is the avoidance of sexual relations with near kin by other primates the same sort of thing as the human prohibition of incest (Chapter 8)? Are we talking of homology or analogy?

It will be evident that I consider the application of a medical schema to social experience has only limited claims to provide us with some sort of analytical commentary; that it gets us into rather circular debates about normality and universality; and that it has failed to deal with the context of our observation as contributing to what we observe. Are these just problems inherent in any comparative study – say when examining the universality of such a practice as 'incest prohibition' or 'marriage' or 'taboo'? Or is there something particular about the pathological idiom that gets us into more inextricable difficulties? Can we even talk about something like 'the medical system' of a non-Western society as any sort of coherent subject? Is it truly homologous with Western medicine or just an analogy, or just a convenient way of initially marking out our area of interest?

The newer approaches in cultural psychiatry which have developed since the 1980s under the influence of social anthropology have been concerned with the relevance of psychiatric theory and observation to all contexts including Western societies. While a variety of perspectives has been adopted, from the Marxist to the postmodern, one particular idea which is hardly congenial to doctors is the suggestion that their very notion of 'pathology' might perhaps be usefully abandoned. For many psychiatrists, this seems a return to the 'anti-psychiatry' of the 1960s when R. D. Laing and David Cooper criticized medical explanations of mental illness as a dehumanizing reductionism.[1] Certainly there are some analogies – indeed some shared anti-medical sensibility – but in many respects our anthropological argument is rather different. It is less a return to the humanistic conviction that psychiatric diagnosis can only inappropriately match our lived experience (unless it becomes self-fulfilling through institutional power) than a concern with how this type of humanist critique itself or indeed any other position is itself associated both with its analytical procedures and with the political context in which our patterns of interest develop. As what we may term a meta-psychiatry – an investigation into how any psychiatry is itself constructed – it does not usually make any arguments about correct therapeutic procedures in themselves;[2] and the medical practice influenced by it – sometimes called clinically applied anthropology – has taken a variety of approaches from radical political activism to the psychodynamic. The essential difference is that psychiatry's own theories and social power are already part of what it claims to study.

The anthropological criticism is not just that cultural psychiatry's ambitious extension of medical categories outside their original Western context may be inappropriate, ethnocentric, or worse, but that its very inapplicability brings into focus some problems with the status of these categories themselves: in particular their collection together under some such unifying rubric of 'psychopathology' or 'mental illness'. For the Counterculture anti-psychiatrists like Laing and Cooper, the psycho-pathologies identified by doctors were an overextended application of the biomedical project outside its proper frame of reference, biological disease.[3] The objection to treating schizophrenia as a disease was, they argued, not that doctors should not be concerned with diseases of the brain which resulted in unusual experiences, but that schizophrenia had no biological origin at all, not even any consistent biological changes associated with it. Similar positions are those of the psychoanalyst Thomas Szasz and the sociologist Erving Goffman, who have both argued that we should restrict psychiatric illness to brain disease alone: psychiatry should be neurology.[4] The essayist Susan Sontag similarly argues for the reality of physical disease in a world to be truly understood only through biology as against its cultural extension as a popular rhetorical trope in which political opponents are characterized as mad, or immigration is vituperated as a cancer.[5] Social critics have examined how the ascription of pathology has been used to control social dissent or to define ethnicity and gender.[6] As psychiatry is a social practice, the debates on what properly constitutes its subject matter have been bound up with the question of its own social power and its legitimacy as an institution. Not surprisingly, solutions to the question 'what then is illness?', perhaps more of a defining question for psychiatry than for other branches of medicine, have for thirty years simply been subsumed under an anti-psychiatric or pro-psychiatric position.[7]

What I would propose here is something more – and in some ways less – radical. Does our idea of pathology and disease, in any system of understanding, whether it be the psychological, the sociological or even the biological, necessarily enable us to understand the phenomena in question any better? Not just the often criticized view of pathology as biological lesion but any more general, if pragmatic, focus on 'problem' or 'malfunction':[8] whether we see this as developmental, anatomical, physiological, social or whatever. Why should we need this sort of frame?

In its claims to be a scientific discipline, psychiatry is vulnerable because its area of interest encompasses not only the experiential and behavioural correlates of (statistically) unusual brain processes, but also patterns of individual response which may also be understood more simply in terms of gender or political antagonisms, or simply as common points of development along the socialized individual's life history or family cycle, or indeed even as standardized social drama.[9] We seldom find central or 'general' theories in psychiatry for it is more obviously social practice than are the natural sciences. Attempts to produce any unifying schema for psychiatry, any core procedure, have either had to jettison much of the traditional focus of interest and develop others (as has psychoanalysis, now taken by most analysts less as a treatment for illness than as an edifying conversation), or else have been so unwieldy as to constitute a procedure for clinical assessment rather than anything one can call a theory.[10]

Psychiatry in the twentieth century has drawn variously on virtually every likely discipline from ethology to biophysics, from existential philosophy to narratology, but its most consistent frame of reference remains that of clinical medicine. And it is organized as a medical discipline. The biomedical paradigm presumes that we can, independently of our eventual explanations, start from the conventional distinctions between aetiology (cause), pathology (whether we take this as some distinct entity or simply as a point on a quantitative gradient), symptoms and treatment. Indeed it seems difficult to envisage any system as 'therapeutic' which does not employ some schema of cause, problem and resolution.

It was the older sort of comparative psychiatry which suggested there could be some problems here. As we have seen, certain local categories of illness which were fitted into the psychiatric nosology turned out to be mythical tales, statements of local collective ideologies, rather than everyday experiences. Others seemed on closer examination to be moral values, or even new relationships between the colonial authorities and their subject peoples. In the case of what psychiatry has pathologized as 'possession states' in non-industrialized societies, it became difficult to distinguish preceding social events from individual experience and from the collective response. In many instances of 'possession', it is a collectively or individually initiated reaction to a locally perceived illness; what is illness and what is treatment for the observer may hinge on a local distinction between this type of 'therapeutic' spirit possession (as in Haitian *vodu*) versus unsolicited possession (an illness caused by malevolent forces), which may be difficult to distinguish phenomenologically.[11] Is the individual who becomes possessed by a spirit thereby exhibiting personal illness, or are they enacting some sort of drama on behalf of their community? Is possession a symptom or a treatment? Or both? An experience or an event?

It has been argued that amok (p. 6), the most notorious of the culture-bound syndromes, has only become what we might term 'a syndrome' under the influence of colonial psychiatry. Early descriptions by European travellers, prior to the establishment of permanent European settlements, used the term to refer to a way of seeking 'an honourable death'[12] in response to an unacceptable insult. The word *amok* originally meant aggressive fury of person, animal or natural forces, and was used to refer to acts committed in a state of confusion. Henry Murphy has suggested that amoks provided suicidal shock troops for local rulers while at the same time limiting their exercise of arbitrary authority – 'a recognised instrument of social control restricting the abuse of power'. The colonial administration established in the East Indies by the Dutch and British replaced amok as a form of retributive justice, but 'the heroic legend remained and offered a model frequently acted upon', a recourse for now increasingly eccentric and marginal individuals, including those who would be regarded by psychiatrists as psychotic. And in the post-colonial period an increasing number of those amoks who have been apprehended alive are now given a diagnosis of schizophrenia.[13]

What were once described by anthropologists as calendrical rituals – socially standardized and collective practices among colonized peoples – have gradually disappeared under the impact of imperialism or industrialization. Some psychological anthropologists have argued that periodic rites which express existing 'tensions' in a constrained manifestation – and thus resolve them – may in the breakdown of pre-industrial social formations become attenuated into individual patterns which psychiatrists might term 'neurotic'. Joe Loudon's example is the well-known *nomkubulwana* among the Zulu, a 'ritual of rebellion' in which, at the time of the new crops, women not only guaranteed the fertility of the land but could give expression to their resentments against men in adopting characteristic male dress, behaviour and obscene expressions: a pattern which 'acted out cathartically' local antagonisms between the sexes and resolved them ceremonially for a time.[14] By the earlier part of the twentieth century, the ceremony could no longer be performed, the men (the necessary active 'audience') having to leave their homes for up to two years at a time to seek work in the urban areas of Durban and Pietermaritzburg. However, the women, who now perforce became the household heads, started to develop a pattern of 'anxiety', *ufufunyana*, characterized by preoccupations with childbirth. Given the scanty information available to the White anthropologist, it would be unwise to claim a simple 'translation' of shared ritual into unresolved individual psychopathology, but Loudon's example does suggest that each may at some level be a social equivalent of the other, while it does (unintentionally) show how colonization not only induces what we might term 'external stress' in an existing system but pathologizes the whole field so that the very idiom in which the relations between the sexes (and the races) is expressed now becomes one of disease.

Are such collective ceremonies then to be understood as a sort of social support in a traumatic society for women and whose absence thus precipitated illness? If so, what is the 'aetiology' of the illness? Or is there a more intimate relationship between the two? Was colonization pathogenic (an empirical question)? Or did it reframe the whole social field so that, as in South Africa or the Malay Peninsula, conflict could become read as individual psychopathology (an interpretive question)? Maurice Lipsedge and I have argued that the European's encounter with African peoples through the development of slavery in the Americas was justified when necessary in the metropolitan capitals as a civilizing mission, but the whole practice was later challenged by liberal opinion and, as emancipation became a serious possibility, new theories of biological racism argued the natural impossibility of practical equality; with political freedom and an assumption of equality, this biological inferiority became transformed into a pathological idiom by which non-Europeans may be said to have (with medical encouragement) 'internalised' their political relations as a personal illness.[15] Rather than being a problem they had a problem – one which required treatment, intervention by psychiatrists, social diagnosticians and other agencies.

Can one explore such questions by using a framework similar to those of natural science? What sort of analysis could examine how such social forms are manifest in the individual, how 'struggle' may become 'pathology'? Psychiatry reads the political as the pathological; the moral as the biological; the collective as the individual. It has to, otherwise it becomes too evidently social work or policing. The contrary move occurs with the recent reinvention of 'ritual healing' within the women's movement in America where what doctors have identified as psychopathologies of women (premenstrual tension, eating disorders, agoraphobia, the consequences of rape, drug overdoses) are not simply alleviated but are reframed from individual pathologies into active attempts at political or spiritual resistance; and similarly with the reappropriation of traditional healing by once colonized peoples in new situations of oppression and identity conflict.[16] After the Chinese Revolution, opium addiction was reframed by the Communist Party from an individual pathology to a consequence of the colonial oppression which had its origins in the Anglo-Chinese opium wars: the addiction was less a personal failing than a collective oppression.[17] And the Cultural Revolution of the 1970s reframed family disputes and personal dysphorias into ideological errors, moral choices; after the death of Mao these have been replaced again by individualized health problems.[18] With the Islamic revolution in Iran and during the war against Iraq, mourning – previously a psychological coming-to-terms with a painful personal loss – was transformed into a public celebration of martyrdom.[19] Can we hold, as medicine would argue, some 'problem' or 'distress' as a constant, independent of changing experience and conceptions? And would such identity be demonstrated by a continuity of expressed themes or in our identification of a similar social context? What is happening when existing illnesses and locally undesirable behavioural patterns which are characteristic of relations between individuals within a community, say between men and women, become emblematic of the totality of relations between whole communities.[20] Do we maintain the pattern is constant and only its direction has changed? And if so, 'where' is 'it' located?

A wide range of minority ethnic groups in contemporary societies dominated by Euro-Americans have been found to have high rates of psychiatric illness.[21] Can we still employ the individual focus and simply argue that racism or disadvantage has caused 'more stress' or removed 'support', given that dominant European groups have pathologized (and thus individualized) the very context within which what might otherwise be seen as 'resistance' is expressed?[22] Responding to a European neuropsychiatrist's argument in the 1950s that Africans were 'lobotomised Europeans', the Martiniquan psychiatrist Frantz Fanon retorted by describing the Algerian uprising against the French as 'the logical consequence of an abortive attempt to decerebralise a people' and argued that its violence could be considered necessary, indeed therapeutic. Are pathology and ethnicity (or gender) really independent constructs, or does the very notion of pathology become internalized as part of personal selfhood, so that psychopathology and collective response are themselves part of the same general process?[23] If so, how could the sort of purely statistical approach favoured by medical epidemiologists disentangle them?

This is not just a question of medical practice or, if you prefer, malpractice. Social scientists themselves have frequently used the term 'social pathology' to collect together undesirable patterns of activity amongst marginal or oppressed groups.[24] Indeed, one of Britain's most influential sociologists has argued that the 'truly pathological [is] defined to include all those actions on the prevention of which public money is spent'.[25] Less ingenuously, the sociologists' idea of pathology usually invokes a model of society as a homeostatic organism by analogy with the physiological body with inputs and outputs, the whole regulated so as to preserve cohesion and a constant structure through time: a perspective which, of course, places a primacy on the notion of society at any moment as really being a fairly harmonious functioning whole, ignoring any questions of social change, innovation, oppression, unequal power or conflict. Like the physical body, the body politic is subject to imbalances, malfunctions and invasions; in the extreme case, it becomes prey to cancer, invasion and decay.[26] And thus the treatment, the surgery, has to come from outside the everyday political realm.

My argument up to this point is fairly unexceptional and indeed is similar to that of many academic psychiatrists.[27] Perhaps we only need to restrict ourselves to a more limited definition of 'pathology' (and 'healing'), away from the problematic social arena to situations where we find relatively invariate biological abnormalities, perhaps to what our transla-tion of the German psychiatrists terms 'coarse brain disease', or at least to the medical ideal of 'constituent characteristics [that] can be defined without recourse to social phenomena'.[28] Our problem is perhaps merely one of powerful metaphors extended too far, always a temptation for doctors involved in questions of public policy. (As Rudolf Virchow, the nineteenth-century German pioneer of cellular pathology, cheerfully put it: 'Politics is simply preventative medicine'.[29]) That the experience of physical suffering is so ubiquitous, so overwhelming and painful, so demanding of resolution, makes the arbitrary nature of sickness an apt vehicle for a variety of ills experienced as dangerous. The biological assumptions which psychiatry recalls through the idiom of pathology have a powerful natural (and hence objective) status and can serve to legitimate or initiate a variety of social control procedures, reinforced by the coercive power which treatment demands, for once we recognize a disease our everyday understanding of sickness presumes the imperative for treatment. Putting it another way, doctors should perhaps stick to biology. Yet, following Virchow, the Nazis recommended their eugenics programme as 'applied biology', and based it on genetics: do we then simply argue that this was rather poor genetics? And that now we have more accurate knowledge? The extended (weak) notion of disease in sociology is no more – or less – unreasonable than the restricted (strong) use of biologically orientated medicine. Both are 'figurative', both are 'real'. They are grounded alike in our assumptions as embodied social beings. And each may become transferred into the other.

Since the seventeenth century, Western academics have employed a disciplinary distinction between the human world of agency and the natural world of causal necessity. 'Pathology' in the strong (biological) sense is to be located as a pattern existing in the natural world as 'disease', independent of our knowledge of it. It is 'real', an entity not a social procedure. It is 'there'. It is experientially manifest to us through 'illness', depending on our bodily states, our values and expectations and the possibility of action, but it appears directly observable through the procedures of natural science. Psychiatry remains marginal within medicine precisely because it fails to achieve this in the same way as the other medical specialisms. This is less historical bad luck than that psychiatry is perhaps constituted as a subject by this inability; it is a residual area of clinical practice in which knowledge of biological structural change leads to the rapid transfer of one of its particular disease entities into the corpus of knowledge of another medical speciality, as has happened with general paralysis of the insane or thyrotoxicosis, now located in neurology and endocrinology. Psychiatry is a residual discipline, dealing it is true with the behavioural and experiential correlates of our presumed disease, but it is also marked by an absence – the absence of any accessible one-to-one correspondence between the subjective experience of illness and disease as identified by doctors, and thus an absence of correspondence between patients' and doctors' understandings. The attempt to establish such a one-to-one model within psychiatry was the conventional form/content distinction with illnesses closely associated (for the psychiatrist causally, if not necessarily so for the patient) with a biological process; but it becomes increasingly unhelpful in the marginal edges of a psychosis like schizophrenia or in other illnesses where a multiplicity of cultural meanings and experiences confounds any neat one-to-one causal linear relationship (Chapter 1). 'Pathology' is always a measure of difference: both between the normal and the abnormal, and between pathologies themselves. While this difference, or singularity, is the defining feature, it by no means follows that defining features should have a determining role in the sequence of preceding events, as Kraepelin assumed and as psychiatrists still do when they weigh the significance of Schneider's 'first-rank symptoms' against depression in a case of schizophrenia.[30]

If 'pathology' in the strong sense is to be understood as some sort of undesirable state of affairs in the natural world, independent of any necessary human apperception (although its personal consequences are potentially unpleasant), how is this undesirability generally conceived? Psychiatry has considered an extraordinary variety of choices: pathologies as entities, processes or events, as a disturbance of functional balance (whether psychological, social or physiological), as anatomical changes, as evolutionary and developmental processes, as failures to achieve ideal or statistical norms of health or autonomy, or simply as the perceived cause of our experience of suffering.[31] Such attempts at value-free conceptualizations themselves are not, however, given by the subject matter 'out there' but are justifications within a particular clinical and historical context. A particular pathology may be understood as all of them.[32] But they are not arbitrary tropes; for they return us to the personal experience of illness, to everyday pain and suffering. Yet such experiences are themselves socially constructed in that 'pain', for instance, is not always perceived as an illness or indeed as an unalloyed evil.[33] When challenged, psychiatrists respond that the ultimate aim of medical diagnosis is to alleviate immediate suffering, and psychiatric research then defends itself as 'practical'.[34]

Anthropological critiques would hardly quarrel with the notion that as embodied social beings we bring to our afflictions an urgency and certain powerful assumptions which are shared with our fellows. And that we are compelled to act in order to be 'practical'. And that psychiatry is a practice.

This book takes a more traditional view: that we are not just embedded in our immediate problems but that we can make an attempt to attain some more distanced knowledge of social and biological phenomena. The question is not the ultimate reality of biological data, but the choice of frame through which to generate and interpret them, and how independent this frame is of social institutions with their own need for categorical action. What is questionable is whether the current methodological individualism of psychiatry invariably leads to the most satisfactory procedures for comparing illness experience in different contexts and at different times, and for understanding the mutual construction of what we distinguish as causation, experience, diagnosis and therapy. Is contemporary medicine's practical distinction between these always analytically helpful? The objection is less the old one that psychiatry is simply only empirical and physical in its thinking but rather something like the reverse. It is too socially embedded in the sense that it cannot examine its own institutional assumptions, and mistakes the particular for the universal, and mistakes what it can conveniently examine for alternative constructions of the phenomenon. It is not that such embedded (and embodied) human sciences are invalid, but merely that they cannot have the particular level of generality we claim without our reflexively examining their social origins and our observations.

If the questions for psychiatry are really practical, then what does the notion of 'pathology' (in either the strong or the weak sense) usefully achieve? Some practical constraints on the limits of the phenomenon which doctors could study and alter, defining 'it' as a phenomenon? Certainly. Some notion that the phenomenon is ultimately undesirable? This hardly seems necessary unless we feel unable to act without assuming our therapeutic or penal procedures must have the power of reinforcing some almost inevitable, natural order of things. Through identification and extension we recognize pathologies in animals akin to ourselves (hence we can talk of veterinary medicine for domesticated mammals and pets), but the limits of our sympathy fade when applied to unicellular organisms. Are phages the 'disease' of sick bacteria? In what environment can we help the tapeworm develop most humanely and fruitfully? The idea is absurd because the idea of disease is so radically rooted in our personal, mammalian concerns.[35]

Does this anthropocentrism matter? Would we lose if medical theory became a type of comparative ecology, independent of our compelling human interests? The implications are moral. They are about the way we recognize suffering in ourselves and empathize with it in our fellows. And what we then propose to do about it. One psychiatric justification for preferring a more precise 'biomedical' term is when an existing popular recognition seems associated with stigmatization of the individual: thus we replace 'idiocy' or 'retardation' with 'learning disability' (or, as was briefly fashionable in the 1970s, 'alternatively abled'), 'mongolism' with 'Down's Syndrome', 'senility' with 'Alzheimer's Disease'. There are, however, uncertainties here as to whether the original term is really responsible for the stigmatization or whether each new term becomes stigmatizing in turn. 'Idiocy' and 'imbecility' became replaced by 'retardation' and thence perhaps 'handicapped', 'disability' and 'learning difficulty'. The newly preferred terms are more likely to refer to the disease rather than to the person (as an incomplete moral agent): he is an idiot, you have a learning disability. To specify the disease is to assume that 'underneath' it lies the same sort of moral agent as any other person. There is a continuing struggle between such destigmatizing campaigns as 'normalisation' in the case of mental handicap and the popular perception of them as only euphemistic if a 'normal' moral agent cannot be easily identified 'underneath', particularly when mental illness (or abnormal EEGs or XYY chromosomes) serves as legal exculpation for criminal acts – such as when the British press ridiculed psychiatric evidence for a criminal court that a mass murderer, the Yorkshire Ripper, was psychotic.

A more neutral perspective can enable us to ask certain new questions about any theme within that area of interest which we conventionally call 'psychopathology'. One is our distinction between aetiology and pathology, which becomes more problematic because of the loss of the immediate frame, as in the vexed question of distinguishing *stress* from *stressor*, or of neurotic illness in its social context from the therapies elaborated within the same context.[36] As we shall consider in Chapter 9, do we say Charcot's nineteenth-century hysterics were suffering from an illness, a treatment or a lifestyle? Were they even 'suffering', or 'enacting', or simply 'representing'? What are the criteria by which we distinguish? Krauss' acerbic declaration that psychoanalysis is really a symptom of the sickness it claims to cure has a wider generality: if our contemporary focus on illness has shifted to examining undesirable limitations on an increasingly Cartesian indexical and autonomous self which is given in advance of any external relations,[37] then the therapies derived are manifestations of the same historical shift.

This is not, as some psychiatrists have suggested, a reassertion of the anti-psychiatric argument 'that schizophrenia is not a break-down but a break-through'.[38] Schizophrenia is neither. To argue the one or the other is equally arbitrary, depending not on the biological or social data in themselves but on a particular morally embedded point of view.

Schizophrenia, like left-handedness or dyschromic spirochaetosis,[39] can be perceived in a variety of ways depending on our own frame of reference, our personal identification and sympathies, our compelling social urgencies. 'Break-through' and 'break-down' are equally moral positions constrained by their particular powers of social representation. This is not to deny that from the clinical perspective schizophrenia appears as a biosocial phenomenon which is relatively invariate across cultures, and whose local meaning is generally of something undesirable. But potential meanings do not necessarily reflect the biomedical paradigm, for meaning is not a phenomenon of the natural world but, biologically speaking, arbitrary. If the experiences of schizophrenia are taken on occasion as meaningful then they are meaningful in that context. If they are not, then they are not. The anti-psychiatrists of the 1960s Counterculture failed to institutionalize any social patterns in which schizophrenia could be a valid experience.[40] Particularly in periods of rapid social change it does seem that valid meaning may be ascribed to experiences which recall those which at other times would be perceived as simply insane.[41] Occasionally, we find situations in which everyday insanity is consistently recognized as especially meaningful, although these seem to be rare, while the 'fey' or the 'touched' can certainly be taken by groups as authentic emblems of their own identity.[42]

Deafness and sign language provides a powerful contemporary instance. There is a biological difference here certainly, but the 1980s saw a dramatic shift in the United States from the perception of deafness as a deficit state – as simply a failure or an absence – to a recognition that American Sign Language had validity as a self-sufficient communication in itself.[43] *Signing* is not some compensatory pantomime of spoken languages, nor does it follow their syntactical structures. It too is powerfully expressive, with its own subtleties and metaphors, spatial representations of agency and of pronouns, and not least its own dreams.

Biology is not some substance external to normal human life which only needs to be dragged in to explain patterns we decide are undesirable anomalies. Take the instance of recent debates on the relevance of her mental illness to the writings of Virginia Woolf. Empathically described as frequently depressed through intelligible past experiences (incest by a stepbrother; an overbearing father; similar husband), her periods of overactivity (writing) by contrast have either passed without comment, or been attributed to a biological process.[44] Yet both her underactivity (depression) and overactivity (mania) are biosocial processes. Normality is as biologically and morally problematic as abnormality.

The allocation of meaning to what is otherwise dismissed as madness has a long history, not restricted to the anti-psychiatrists. Indeed, in the form of psychobiography and psychohistory, it has frequently featured in the evening interests of psychiatrists themselves, as a rather Romantic interpretation of 'creativity' as something external to self and society, descending on the individual like a divine muse. Sometimes mocked as the 'Napoleon's glands' view of history' (St Paul was epileptic, Joan of Arc hysterical, and so on), in literary criticism this sort of reductionism is criticized as a form of the 'biographical fallacy' (the meaning of a text is to be found in the life experiences of its author). What I am suggesting here is something rather different, not 'biological causality' but, to use Steven J. Gould's phrase, 'biological potentialism'. The meanings that are placed on natural phenomena as they appear to us, whether these meanings are disease or creativity, are by no means determined by the phenomenon itself. None of this argument is especially novel in those cross-disciplinary studies which take the human potential for sociality and culture itself as both a biologically and a historically given attribute.[45] By contrast, for psychiatrists the only alternative to reductionism seems to be to regard humans as biology plus society, as genes topped up with culture. This mistakes our understanding of biology as much as that of culture. Biology is a discipline, a social procedure, a way of examining what is going on in the field in which organic forms are located, not a kind of stuff.

If our modern scientific project attempts a perspective which is independent of a particular observer's point of view at a particular place and time, then our abandonment of 'pathology' is surely exemplary. The attempt to exclude social meaning and context from psychiatric theory itself does not automatically render that discipline value free and universal. Rather the converse.

3. The Butterfly and the Serpent

Let me start this chapter from the situation of women. The more frequent diagnosis of mental illness among women, particularly married women, in many societies has been subject to numerous feminist critiques over the last twenty years.[1] Is her illness to be properly located in the woman as a patient or else in the politics of her society? We can note two very general, and different, explanations:

A The preconditions for psychological distress in women are essentially the same as they are for men, but either because women are somehow more vulnerable or because they are exposed by men to more 'stressors' they experience more illness.[2] But can women's experiences and political context be so easily approximated to those of men?

B The validity of the psychiatric diagnoses of women is questionable because the very notion of something like mental illness in Western societies closely relates to dominant male – and hence medical – conceptions of female identity and behaviour as characteristically 'other' to psychological normality.[3] And what is taken as their illness is then just an exaggeration of this professional ascription. But if so, how can women authentically act and suffer?

Very similar responses have been proposed in relation to the greater frequency of mental illness among Europe's minority ethnic groups.[4] Both for women and Black people, older ideas of innate biological vulnerability to psychological illness (Chapter 1) are now generally played down; yet for both, the idea that 'the illness' may be regarded as an intended response on the part of the patient to her situation is seldom considered (except as 'malingering' by unsympathetic doctors). Recognition of, and resistance to, male dominance is postulated rather in the new radical therapeutic responses – generally to be yet devised – rather than in 'the illness' itself.[5] And how can the idea that misogyny runs through both explanations be applied to the illness of men? Do they have to be simply ignored?[6]

There would certainly seem to be a problem here. Understanding any illness as a biosocial pattern requires both an interpretation of how individuals choose – or see themselves as constrained – to engage in the pattern for certain ends, explicit or otherwise, together with an explanation of its preconditions and influences. Psychiatry, like social theory in general, remains undecided as to the relationship of the instrumental to the causal.

How much do people strategically 'employ' available patterns? Alternatively, how much can one say these patterns invariably 'reflect' particular social or biological causes? And are these two modes of thought inherently contradictory either in theory or in experience? Are moral agency and causality to be taken as additive categories, as mutually dependent, or as incommensurate? Is our accepted idea of human agency itself cultural, perhaps particularly masculine as some recent feminist jurists and philosophers have argued?[7] In the case of those patterns conventionally termed *psychopathology*, which is more useful in examining incidence and variation: interpreting the inter-subjective meanings and values which are situationally deployed by individuals out of their local cultural repertoire at a particular historical moment, whether instrumentally or otherwise; or employing such objectivized explanations as prescriptive class and gender norms, social 'stress', relative power, economic and technical development, ecological constraints and biological imperatives? This distinction between instrumental ('pull') and causal ('push') factors is arguably one of scale as well as epistemology; it is elided, perhaps not altogether successfully, in psychoanalysis and ethology. In clinical practice, the issue is one which appears not only in medico-legal debates on criminal responsibility but in everyday encounters when patients may see themselves as 'ill', and thus not accountable for their symptoms, while to the medical observer their actions and reported experiences may well appear motivated. Or the converse.

An adequate interpretation of women's illness requires an understanding of personal subjectivity and action as well as the social field – and of male illness as well as female. Gender is certainly an element in psychological illness but it cannot in itself be essential. In this chapter I examine particularly parasuicide with medically prescribed drugs: a pattern common among Euro-American women. I suggest that we can gain an understanding of such 'overdoses' through a comparison with patterns found in less pluralistic small-scale societies; and that we look not just at the person involved but at the local meaning of the act in the political context in which it happens.

Overdoses: woman's violence against herself

The starting point here is that women in Western societies are already identified with mood-modifying pharmaceutical tranquillizers.[8] A study of such prescriptions in a North American city showed that 69 per cent of them were given to women; and a similar pattern is found in Britain.[9] Certainly, more Western women than men consult doctors and receive prescriptions, but there is an even greater disproportion in the number of women receiving such psychotropic drugs.[10] During a single year preceding a national sampling of North American adults, 13 per cent of the men and 29 per cent of the women had taken medically prescribed drugs, especially minor tranquillizers and daytime sedatives, 10 per cent of the women in the previous two weeks.[11] These American rates are consistent with other Western industrialized nations: physicians apparently expect their female patients to require a higher proportion of mood-altering drugs than do more phlegmatic male patients.[12] These are perhaps the 'attractive healthy women who thoroughly enjoy being ill' as the *Daily Express* sardonically put it in 1984.

That this is not reflecting simply a 'real' (biological) gender disparity in psychological distress prior to the doctor's interpretation and intervention is suggested by the symbolism of medical advertising. Women outnumber men by 15:1 in advertisements for tranquillizers and anti-depressants.[13] One advertisement depicted a woman with a bowed head holding a dishcloth and standing beside a pile of dirty dishes represented larger than life size; the medical consumer is told that the drug 'restores perspective' for her by 'correcting the disturbed brain chemistry'. Employed women are rare in drug advertisements, and women are usually shown as dependent housewives and child-rearers: the world acts on them, they do not act on the world. Psychotropic drug advertisements emphasize women as passive patients; they are represented as failing in their role in life, dissatisfied with marriage, washing dishes or attending parent–teacher association meetings.[14] The treating physician is never depicted in the advertisement as a woman, and all the female patients appeared helpless and anxious. Doctors' advertisements for psychotropic drugs tend to portray women as patients, while those for non-psychiatric medicine often show men; within the psychotropic drug category alone, women are shown with diffuse emotional symptoms, while men were pictured with discrete episodes of anxiety because of specific pressures from work or from accompanying organic illness.[15]

Deliberate 'overdoses' of medical drugs have been said by social critics to be a communication of powerlessness for they are up to five times more common among the unemployed and among women, especially in the 15-to-19 age group. Among young women of this age in Edinburgh during the 1970s, more than one in every hundred took an overdose each year. (Since then, the incidence has declined somewhat.) At the same time, of those patients who attended hospital following a non-fatal act of deliberate self-harm, 95 per cent had taken a drug overdose. Half of these episodes involved interpersonal conflicts as the major precipitating factor. Only a minority of women had made definite plans to prepare for death, to avoid discovery or subsequently regretted not having killed themselves. Suicidal intent and risk to life thus appear to be relatively low, especially as overdoses are usually taken with somebody close by: 59 per cent occur in the presence of, or near, other people.[16] And yet family concern is, of course, motivated by the fact that sometimes people who take overdoses do die, and these have generally made previous attempts to harm themselves.

While the reasons given by the individual for 'taking overdoses' are often expressive (explaining the overdose as a result of personal predicament and associated feelings such as self-hatred at the time of the act), they may often be instrumental – that is, they are explained by the woman in terms of the desired consequences of the act, usually increased support or understanding. That they are socially learned patterns is supported by the finding that they are concentrated in linked clusters of individuals. A study of young women who took overdoses suggested they viewed their act as a means of gaining relief from a stressful situation or as a way of showing other people how desperate they felt; hospital staff who assessed their motives regarded them as symptomatic of psychological distress but also noted that adolescents took overdoses in order to punish other people or change their behaviour. Typically a teenage girl took tablets after a disappointment, frustration or difference of opinion with an older person (usually a parent); many patients afterwards reported that the induction of guilt in those whom they blamed for their distress was a predominant motive for the act.[17] While overdoses can be seen in this way as strategies designed to avoid or adjust certain specific situations, the experience of the principal is primarily one of distress, social dislocation and extrusion; the overdose exaggerates this extrusion, offering a threat of refusing member-ship in the human community altogether: attempted suicide is, amongst other things, a dangerous adventure.

The conventional resolution of this inversion of shared life-enhancing assumptions involves its complement: medical intervention and family response endeavour to return the patient into everyday relationships. Not surprisingly, the overdose meets with little professional sympathy, particularly when it is recognized as an instrumental mechanism rather than as the representation of underlying hopelessness or psychiatric illness. 'Expressive' explanations (resulting from despair or depression and aiming at withdrawal, escape or death) are more acceptable and evoke more sympathy or readiness to help in both doctors and nurses than apparently pragmatic motives.[18] Doctors tend to distinguish acts as either suicidal or 'manipulative', and are more accepting of a wish to die. Nurses, themselves predominantly female, are somewhat more sympathetic than are doctors to instrumental motives; they are more likely to perceive overdoses as legitimate attempts to manage distress.[19] Patients taking overdoses are regarded by hospital doctors as a nuisance, extraneous to the real concerns of medicine and less deserving of medical care than patients with physical illnesses, especially if the self-poisoning episode appears 'histrionic'.[20] As the *British Medical Journal* once put it: doctors 'feel a sense of irritation which they find difficult to conceal'; for, to use the language of attribution theory, doctors trained in biomedicine prefer the more individualized 'dispositional' to 'environmental' attributions of human suffering.[21]

Comparative perspectives

As we noted in the first chapter, psychiatric research is carried out principally in urban industrialized societies where mental illness tends to be regarded by the medical profession as if it were culture free. Certain contemporary biomedical conceptualizations and their associated patterns of social action are, however, closely tied to the cultural politics of age and gender, particularly where these invoke notions of personal identity and attribution. Conceptualization, therapy and the illness itself are all articulated by a shared set of values in action. While the notion that biomedicine is essentially different from other theories of disease is being abandoned, there remains an assumption that Western science cannot be submitted to the type of symbolic analysis which has proved so fruitful in the study of small-scale non-industrialized societies; for industrialized societies are supposedly too complex, pluralistic and pragmatic to allow us to do so. In an attempt to minimize the reduction of our subject, which includes biomedical concepts, to such concepts themselves, and to achieve a greater degree of 'universality', I shall, however, employ a model derived from non-Western analogues of what psychiatrists term 'psychological illness'. Where I differ from other sociological critics is in proposing the older sort of structural–functional model which allows us to articulate simultaneously context, ascription, action, institution and political change.

While biomedical and 'traditional' illnesses and therapies have been compared before, the points of similarity have assumed the primacy of the physiological or psychodynamic mechanisms of Western understandings. The converse – the direct mapping of Western categories onto traditional systems – has seldom been attempted because of the cultural contextuality of the latter as they appear to Western professionals (which has not prevented the latter from conducting the reverse procedure, that is, mapping traditional categories onto Western systems, still the character-istic practice of cultural psychiatry (pp. 9–10). To attempt to identify something resembling traditional non-Western patterns in a Western population demands more than claims, based on superficial phenomen-ological similarities, that spirit possession or amok may occur in the West; it requires the application to the West of the comparative models we have developed for small-scale communities. To the extent that such models are derived from within a Western academic perspective they still remain culture bound but perhaps at a higher degree of universality than clinical

explanations which themselves form part of the everyday Western
construction of the reactions.

'Overdoses' appear to be a relatively discrete reaction which appears,
historically and geographically, culturally specific to industrialized societies, especially to the United States and Europe, that is to those with easy
access to pharmaceutical drugs. While culture-specific patterns may, of
course, have a distinct biological component (as with kuru or with
amphetamine psychosis), the psychiatric idea of a *culture-bound syndrome*
classically described among small-scale communities has usually been
taken to refer to: patterns of time-limited behaviour specific to a particular
culture which, while regarded as undesirable, are recognized as discrete by
local informants and medical observers alike; few instances of which have a
biological cause; in which the individual is not held to be aware or
responsible in the everyday sense; and where the behaviour usually has a
'dramatic' quality (p. 12). And these characteristics will be my starting
point.

Such patterns frequently articulate personal predicament but they also
represent public concerns, usually what we may take as core structural
oppositions between age groups or the sexes. They have a shared meaning
as public and dramatic representations in an individual whose personal
situation demonstrates these oppositions, and they thus generally occur in
certain well-defined situations. At the same time they have a personal
expressive meaning for the particular individual for whom they may be
regarded as individually functional ('instrumental'): 'in situations of
deprivation or frustration where recourse to personal jural power is not
available, the principal is able to adjust his or her situation by recourse to
"mystical pressure"' as the anthropologist Ioan Lewis puts it:[22] that is,
through appeals to values and beliefs which cannot be questioned because
they are tied up with the most fundamental and taken-for-granted political
understandings and structures of the community. How 'conscious' the
principal is of pragmatically employing the mechanism as a personal
strategy is debatable but it may be noted that medical observers have
frequently described these reactions as 'dissociative'. Victor Turner aptly
calls this sideways recourse to tacit pressure 'the power of the weak';[23] the
disparaging medical term for an illness which cannot be seen as a disease is,
of course, 'manipulation'.

To consider in more detail my analogous instances: *wild man* behaviour
(*negi-negi, nenek*) is a term given to certain episodes of aggressive behaviour
in the New Guinea Highlands.[24] The affected man rushes about erratically,
threatening other people with weapons, destroying their property,
blundering through the village gardens and tearing up crops. Episodes
last for a few hours, or at most days, during which the wild man fails to
recognize people and, on recovering, claims amnesia for the episode.

Behaviour is locally attributed to possession by spirits, and treatment may include pouring on of water as a sort of exorcism, although Western observers have felt these measures were applied half-heartedly if not theatrically.[25] The incipient wild man's initial announcement that he no longer wishes to eat and his rejection of his share of the prepared food, advertise his coming performance.[26] This is always public: 'It would be possible for a man to run wild in seclusion but no-one does.'[27] The audience participate by feigning terror, attempting to mollify the principal or ostentatiously hiding weapons. To Western observers the wild man retains a high degree of control. Like the shaman in his trance, 'though he flings himself in all directions with his eyes shut [he] nevertheless finds all the objects he wants'.[28] In negi-negi and similar reactions there is 'a disproportion between the injury threatened and actually inflicted. It is generally more alarming to the white onlooker than the native', the anthropologist and physician C. G. Seligman wrote in 1928. (Similar episodes of spear throwing by Western Desert Aborigines remain constrained and relatively safe; only participants with organic brain syndromes are 'out of control'.[29]) The pattern typically occurs among young men, politically powerless, in situations such as despairingly working to pay back a bride-price debt raised through a network of their elders. Negi-negi exaggerates this social dislocation to the point where the young man dramatically declines membership of his social community altogether. Resolution may include latitude in repayment. The net result is to restore and legitimate the status quo, not to question it.

What we might term audience participation is essential to negi-negi and to certain more evidently 'suicidal' behaviours. In the Western Pacific island of Tikopia, aggrieved or offended young women and men once swam out to sea.[30] As an islander commented to the anthropologist: 'A woman who is reproved or scolded desires to die, yet desires to live. Her thought is that she will go to swim, but be taken up in a canoe by men who will seek her out to find her. A woman desiring death swims to seawards; she acts to go and die. But a woman who desires life swims inside the reef.'[31] While completed suicide is locally regarded as a revenge on the community, the pay-off for the survivor of a suicide swim includes enhanced status together with a renegotiation of the original problem. Thus an adolescent girl who is rebuffed or censured by parents reacts by exaggerating this extrusion, detaching herself further from the community, and the resolution restores the immediate equilibrium. For the community, the tension between parental authority and filial independence is presented as dramatically as the account of a lovers' suicide pact in the British popular press.

Sympathy for the Tikopian suicide swimmer wanes with repetition; like *saka* among the Kenyan Wataita, the reaction can occur 'once too often'.

Approximately half of married Taita women were once subject to saka (which we might gloss as 'possession') after a wish was refused by their husband, typically for an object that is a prerogative of men.[32] It was locally recognized that saka was clearly something to do with relations between men and women. While women provided food for the family they were also expected to supply domestic objects which could only be purchased through access to the profits of the sale of land or livestock, yet such access was denied to women.

> Women are said to have no head for land or cattle transactions. They do not have the right sort of minds for important community affairs because they have little control over emotions and desires. Indeed femininity is made synonymous with an uncontrolled desire to acquire and consume ... In saka attacks, women are caricatured as uncontrollable consumers ... They are shown as contrasting in every way with men and the contrast is symbolised as a personal malady.[33]

Their anthropologist suggested in the 1950s that 'women can acquire male prerogatives or the signs thereof through illness', and compared the reaction to a European woman's 'sick headache' or 'pregnancy cravings'. While observers feel the reaction can be considered either 'real' or 'simulated', some local men say the whole reaction is a pretence. Saka is variously regarded by the Wataita as an illness, as a possession by spirits, and as the direct consequence of a woman's personal wishes and her social role. Possession ceases when the woman's wish is granted by her husband or when he sponsors a large public ceremony in which she wears male items of dress or new clothes.

Pastoral Somali women similarly became possessed by the *sar* spirits who demanded gifts and attention;[34] 'Therapy really consists in spoiling the patient while ostensibly meeting the demands of the spirit as revealed to the expert therapist.' In a patriarchal Islamic society (before the recent civil war) in which women were excluded from the public realm, the outrageous behaviour of possession coerced husbands into gestures of reconciliation and consideration while at the same time the formal public ideology of male dominance remained unchallenged. The cost of sar ceremonies has been such as to preclude the purchase by the husband of additional wives. The typical situation was a

> hard-pressed wife, struggling to survive and feed her children in the harsh nomadic environment, and liable to some degree of neglect, real or imagined, on the part of her husband. Subject to frequent, sudden and often prolonged absences by her husband as he follows his manly pastoral pursuits, to the jealousies and tensions of polygamy which are

not ventilated in accusations of sorcery and witchcraft, and always menaced by the precariousness of marriage in a society where divorce is frequent and easily obtained by men, the Somali women's lot offers little stability or security ... Not surprisingly the sar spirits are said to hate men.[35]

Function and opposition

To summarize, these patterns appear to occur where major points of political and cultural oppositions are represented in a particular sub-dominant individual's rather drastic situation and thus, not surprisingly, where the everyday resolution or affirmation of power relationships are inadequate as perceived solutions to the problem. Such oppositions may occur between elders and younger people (*negi-negi*, Tikopian swims) or between men and women (swims, *sar*, *saka*). Employing our own psychological way of thinking, these contentious points may represent what we might call 'social tensions'. Victor Turner insists such tensions do not imply that society is about to break up; instead they 'constitute strong unities ... whose nature as a unit is constituted and bounded by the very forces that contend within it.[36] [The tension becomes] a play of forces instead of a bitter battle. The effect of such a "play" soon wears off, but the sting is removed from certain troubled relationships.' As Harris comments about the saka attack, it 'allows a round-about acknowledgement of conflict, but in the saka dance there is again peace, dignity and festivity';[37] indeed key symbolic elements of this resolution are included in other public rituals of the community. 'The use of symbols in ritual secures some kind of emotional compromise which satisfies the majority of the individuals who comprise a society and which supports its major institutions.'[38]

The patterns I have described may be shown as demonstrating three stages. First, the individual is first extruded by others out of normal social relationships in an extension of what is already a devalued or subdominant social status. This is followed by a prescribed role, deviant yet in some sense legitimate, which represents further exaggeration of this dislocation (and in this becomes a direct contravention or 'inversion' of the social values supposedly held in common by the whole community) to unbalance the social equilibrium to such an extent that it is succeeded by restitution back into conventional and now unambiguous social relationships; for a society cannot let its subdominant individuals out of the human schema altogether. 'The saka dance [the resolution] turns the saka attack on its head.'[39] The Tikopia suicide voyager's 'attempt at detachment has failed, but he has succeeded in resolving his problem. He is once again absorbed and an effective catharsis has been obtained'.[40] Let me place the 'women's reactions' – saka, sar, swim parasuicide – in the common (but hardly universal[41]) symbolic field in which women are regarded as more 'natural' and less 'social' than men. We can summarize the process analytically as a function:

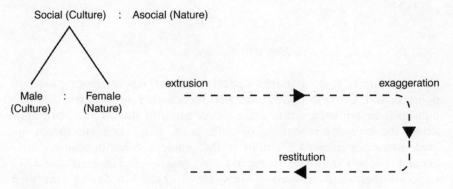

Figure 1

The curved dotted line represents a 'degenerative causal loop' (to use cybernetic terminology) which returns the relationship to a more complementary form. Matters may alternatively be represented structurally as a signed digraph (Figure 2) in which positive lines represent complementary relationships and dotted lines represent antithetical relationships. (The line *de* is dotted because of the hierarchical nature of the 'Nature/Culture' distinction at different levels where *d* expresses male interests; thus the graph is 'unbalanced'.[42]) Arrows represent the accepted assertion of dominance at the three stages between the principal actors.

A similar three-stage model of separation, transition and reintegration has been postulated for those psycho-social transitions usually glossed as 'rites of passage', including certain types of shamanic trance possession and women's cult groups in Africa.[43] While Western medical convention distinguishes 'symptoms' from 'treatment' within such patterns, I propose here to consider them a single complex: '[Possession] attack and [therapeutic] dance are two manifestations of a single situation ... [they] can be translated into one another,' Harris notes of saka.[44] Edmund Leach has suggested that what we generally recognize as ritual may be 'normal social life ... played in reverse', and he offers the terms formality, role reversal and masquerade to represent near-equivalents of my three stages (*b*, *c*, *d* in Figure 2).[45] The prescribed deviant role *d* amplifies the rejection by the community, frequently taking the form of behaviour which contravenes the core values of the society, female modesty or decorum. During this period the principal is regarded as the victim of external mystical power (which must be placated) and is not held accountable;

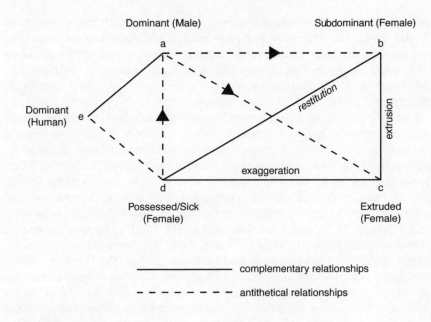

Figure 2

when negi-negi, 'a man does not have a name':[46] like a pig gone wild, he is a once-domesticated being now escaped from everyday social control.[47] While I am emphasizing here the instrumental, rather than the expressive aspect of this behaviour, we may gloss the personal experience for the principal (and audience) by the Western psychological term 'catharsis', similar to the collective experience of social inversions found in public humour, carnivals, licensed rituals of rebellion and contravention of norms in certain specific and tightly controlled situations.

Such functionalist explanations of symbolic inversion by anthropologists stress both group catharsis and the social marking of a norm by its licensed and restricted contravention. The audience is placed between distress and safety, the position of 'optimal distancing' and balanced attention suggested for group catharsis.[48] Because the behaviour is in one understanding a 'performance' is not to say that the 'actors' may not fully identify with their new parts – suffering, engaged in self-discovery, perhaps exploring new identities. For the community as a whole, potential social oppositions are dramatically demonstrated yet shown to be susceptible of a solution, albeit a temporary and restricted one (for they are not 'ultimately' resolved). The spectacle of reversal of values in, say, negi-negi, articulates the structural opposition between affines and kin, wife-givers and wife-receivers, and between older and younger men. The performance embodies social oppositions cognitively and experientially for all members of the audience but also permits individual identification with the protagonist; that sex-specific performances appear appreciated equally by both sexes suggests that close individual identification is perhaps less important than psychodynamic writers have suggested: ritual derives its efficacy and power from its performance.

I am not proposing a simple and invariably homeostatic function which neatly cements a society's fracture lines. Diagnosis of sar possession is certainly in the hands of women and its treatment groups provide an organization for women in clear opposition to the public practice of Islam dominated by men. The participation of women in such healing groups (which may encourage further possession but now in a solicited and controlled female ritual setting) may be said to 'allow the voice of women to be heard in a male-dominated society, and occasionally enable participants to enjoy benefits to which their status would not normally entitle them'.[49] Ogrizek and Boddy suggest that the healing rituals associated with possession trance may sometimes enable women to explore and develop an 'oppositional' female identity howbeit not in evidently political terms such as 'resistance'.[50] Such groups may indeed maintain the woman's stigmatized ('sick' or 'vulnerable') identity in opposition to complete reversion to normative values, but elsewhere new spirit possession therapy groups, especially those for men, may develop to take on dominant roles including taxation, redistribution and welfare;[51] their organization may then provide, in contrast to a hypothesized 'homeostatic' function, whether individual or communal, a dynamic mechanism for social mobility and even institutional change;[52] and we can here offer parallels with 'consciousness raising' and political activism in Western women's therapy groups.

In large-scale literate societies (with, we might argue, something more like a linear rather than a cyclical expectation of social time[53]), individualized reactions of 'hysterical conversion' may come to succeed the periodic and carnivalesque rites of role reversal of smaller and more homogeneous groups; Loudon (p. 26) described such a 'pathologising' shift for isolated Zulu women in the 1950s. Lee shows how the analogous symbolic inversions found in amok, latah and possession states continue in a now industrialized Malay society, although the attribution of responsibility has now been transferred from supernatural agencies onto an acquired Western notion of individual psychopathology.[54]

Spirits and diseases: the 'mystical pressure' of Western medicine

My model of these patterns involves non-dominant individuals who display in their immediate personal situations certain basic contradictions (for example in saka and zar that women are socialized humans, yet they cannot be regarded as truly accountable), which is expressed through the available intellectual tools, with recourse to 'mystical pressure' permitting personal adjustment of their situation by a limited contravention of society's core values. Each pattern involves dislocation, exaggeration to the point of inversion of the shared norms and then restitution. An attempt to look for analogous reactions in Britain or the United States would appear quite straightforward apart from the notion of 'mystical pressure'. What unquestionable 'other-worldly authority' equivalent to the spirit world, standing outside everyday personal relations might serve to explain and legitimate them, and thence reduce human accountability both in the starting situation of subdominance and in its later exaggeration? And then compel social restitution?

For small-scale and non-literate communities, social organization and normative principles, along with the categorization of the natural world and human relations to it, are referred to a fairly tight system of cosmology which we generally refer to as 'religion'. Religion is an ideology: it both describes and prescribes, allocating the individual to the natural order. Through its other-worldly authority it legitimates personal experience and the social order. By contrast, in the secularized West, Christianity has lost its power of social regulation and competes both with other religions and, more significantly, with a variety of alternative ideologies, both moral and political. Where then can we find an equivalent 'mystical' sanction which integrates personal distress into a shared conceptualization of the world?

I would suggest that the legitimation of our present world view lies ultimately in contemporary science. In its everyday context as it relates to our personal experience, science is most salient in the form of medicine which offers us core notions of individual agency, responsibility and action. In all societies illness is experienced through an expressive system encoding indigenous notions of social order. As Allan Young argues, while illness 'is an event that challenges meaning in this world, ... medical beliefs and practices organise the event into an episode which gives form and meaning'.[55] The power of an illness reality is derived from its ability to evoke deeply felt social responses as well as intense personal effects.[56] This obligation to order abnormality is no less when it is manifest primarily through unusual behaviour. The person whose behaviour is seen as being unpredictable not only becomes an object of fear; she becomes endowed with the potential for a perverse form of power. Her power lies not only in the threat of contagion but in the unstated assumption that it is a medicalized society who will be ultimately responsible for what she does.

Young women who take overdoses still gain access to hospital, despite the physician's antipathy, since the popular understanding of suicidal behaviour is of 'something that happens to one', rather than something one intentionally brings about.[57] The patient's family accept that her problems are outside her direct personal control, and responsibility is thereby attributed to some agency beyond the patient's volition.[58] Thus we have the continuing popular use of (quasi-accidental) 'overdose' as opposed to (active) 'self-poisoning' or 'attempted suicide'.

Professional intervention in a sickness involves incorporating the patient into an overarching system of explanation, a common structural pattern which manifests itself in the bodily economy of every human being. Accountability is transferred onto an agency beyond the patient's control: diseases now rather than the spirits. Both are 'other', outside our usual social world (Figure 1). Both compel the intervention of others. Becoming sick is part of a social process leading to public recognition of an abnormal state and a consequent readjustment of patterns of behaviour and expectations, and then to changed roles and altered responsibility. Expectations of the sick person include exemption from discharging some social obligations, exemption from responsibility for the condition itself, together with a shared recognition that it is undesirable and involves an obligation to seek help and cooperate with treatment.[59] Withdrawal from everyday social responsibilities is rendered acceptable through some means of exculpation, usually through mechanisms of bio-physical determinism: 'When faced with a diagnosis for which he has equally convincing reasons to believe that either his client is sick or he is not sick, the physician finds that the professional and legal risks are less if he accepts the hypothesis of sickness.'[60] To question the biomedical scheme itself involves questioning some of our most fundamental assumptions about nature and human agency. Because of its linking of personal experience with the social order, its standardized expectations of removing personal responsibility and initiating an institutionalized response, and its rooting in ultimate social values through science, biomedicine offers a powerful and unquestionable legitimate inversion of everyday behaviour – as disease. It will thus not be surprising to find many non-Western equivalents already included by medicine in psychiatric nosologies. Others, like chronic pain, chronic fatigue, 'factitious' illness and eating disorders we may suspect lie hidden more effectively in the fringes of physical medicine rather than in psychiatry.

Why women?

This model emphasizes a discrepancy in power and opportunity between the dominant and the subdominant groups within a community. In most societies women are 'excluded from participation in or contact with some realm in which the highest powers of the society are felt to reside'.[61] They are excluded by a dominant ideology which reflects men's experiences and immediate interests. As the anthropologist Jean La Fontaine notes, 'The facts of female physiology are transformed in almost all societies into a cultural rationale which assigns women to nature and the domestic sphere, and thus ensures their general inferiority to men.'[62] The core aspects of the female role in Western society are reflected in the ideals still held out to women: marriage, home and children as the primary focus of concern, with reliance on a male provider for sustenance and status. Beveridge, one of the founders of the British Welfare State, put it like this: 'Her home is her factory, her husband and children a worthwhile job.' There is an expectation that women will emphasize nurturance and that they live through and for others rather than for themselves. Even at the beginning of the twenty-first century women are still often expected to give up their occupation and place of residence when they marry and are banned from the direct assertion and expression of aggression. Women of reproductive age are biomedically 'normal', against which their menopause is seen by doctors as a sickness,[63] yet through childbearing every woman in the West becomes a potential patient. Their lack of power is attributed to their greater emotionality and their inability to cope with wider social responsibilities, for dependency and passivity are expected of a woman; her image in standardized psychology tests is of a person with a childish incapacity to govern herself and a need for male protection and direction.[64] Contemporary Western women are permitted greater freedom than men to 'express their feelings' and to recognize emotional difficulties, enabling the woman to define her difficulties within a medical framework and bring them to the attention of her doctor.[65]

Jordanova has suggested that medical science is characterized by the action of men on women; women are regarded as more 'natural', passive, awaiting male ('cultural') organization.[66] As a standard British gynaecology textbook put it not that long ago, 'Femininity tends to be passive and receptive, masculinity to be more active, restless, anxious for repeated demonstrations of potency.'[67] In the emblems of Britain's Royal College of Psychiatrists, as sported on the ties and cuff-links of its members, women continue this tradition as the wayward Butterflies of disordered Psyche, awaiting the Serpents of the healer Aesculapius.[68] Serpent and Butterfly are each an opposed complement to the other. Ingelby and others have argued that there is a close historical relationship between the psychiatric notions of 'woman' and 'patient', and many critics of psychiatry have noted the similarity between neurotic symptom patterns and normative expectations of female behaviour.[69] Thus we may summarize the Serpent/Butterfly relationship as complementary pairs:

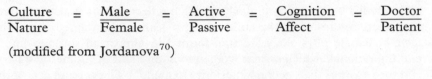

$$\frac{\text{Culture}}{\text{Nature}} = \frac{\text{Male}}{\text{Female}} = \frac{\text{Active}}{\text{Passive}} = \frac{\text{Cognition}}{\text{Affect}} = \frac{\text{Doctor}}{\text{Patient}}$$

(modified from Jordanova[70])

To this Bryan Turner adds:[71]

$$= \frac{\text{Public}}{\text{Private}} = \frac{\text{Production}}{\text{Consumption}} = \frac{\text{Desire}}{\text{Need}}$$

A polythetic classification of this type means that it is the *relationship* between each pair of elements which remains constant, not that there is equality between individual superordinate or subordinate elements considered horizontally.[72] Clearly not all doctors are men (indeed, medicine has a greater proportion of women than other professions) but the woman doctor's role in relation to her patient replicates the male/ female relationship: a male patient may flirt with his nurse but hardly with his doctor. To decide when 'complementarity' becomes 'dominance', 'opposition', 'tension' or 'conflict' depends on our understanding of individual action lived through such a schema.[73] If my schema emphasizes gender difference, we can replace Male/Female by Older/Younger or even by Employed/Jobless: an unemployed man is in many ways feminized.

To take an earlier Western instance which I shall consider in more detail in Chapter 9: the dominant male versus passive female idiom which similarly embodied the nineteenth-century hysterical reaction was mirrored in the therapy – the rational male physician actively treating his passive patient in the grip of her nature. In the nineteenth century, hysteria was a well-recognized pattern, mainly found in women. The middle-class woman was taught that aggression, independence, assertion and curiosity were male traits, inappropriate for women. Women's nature was emotional, powerless, passive and nurturant, and they were not expected to achieve in the public domain. Hysteria offered a solution to the onerous task of running a household, and of adjusting husband/wife or father/daughter relations, and it was one which did not challenge these core values.

The hysteric could opt out of her traditional duties and be relieved of responsibilities; as 'sick' she enjoyed sympathy and privileges while others assumed her tasks as a self-sacrificing wife, mother or daughter. The scope which this allowed for considerable, if ultimately limited, power in the household is superbly described by Proust in his characterization of Aunt Leonie. Proust himself, like Darwin and Nightingale, was personally familiar with how the same role could offer even the dominant male extensive and sophisticated scope for autonomy and influence.

The development from simple conversion symptoms to a recognized social position as 'a hysteric' seems to have provided a parody of some core values – women's expected dependency and restricted social role – an exaggeration of the politically extruded female. The hysteric was characteristically female, the hysterical woman being perceived as the very embodiment of perverse femininity, an inversion of dominant male behaviour.[74] Hysteria was a conventionally available alternative behaviour pattern for certain women, which permitted them to express some dissatisfaction. Many of Freud's patients with hysterical symptoms were women who had been forced to sacrifice their public lives in nursing a sick relative. Employing this model, they might themselves take to their bed because of pain, paralysis or weakness, and remain there for months or years. What Freud was to term the 'secondary gain' conferred by the hysterical role allowed a limited adjustment of wife/husband power relations in the family: 'Ill health will be her one weapon for maintaining her position. It will procure for her the care she longs for ... It will compel him to treat her with solicitude if she recovers; otherwise a relapse will threaten.'[75] Hysterical women were engaged in a struggle then, a battle fought with weapons from the armoury of men, double-voiced, a parody of male dominance but a strategic parody with certain very specific advantages: 'a form of logical resistance to a "kind and benevolent" enemy they are not permitted to openly fight'.[76] And yet, the general schema of power remained undisturbed; Bryan Turner argues that hysteria provided the Victorian bourgeoisie with a 'solution' for the perceived sexuality of their unmarried women in a period of delayed marriage.[77] The status of the 'hysteric' before Freud did not involve acceptance of individual responsibility for the illness. Male physicians, and men in general, employed biological arguments to rationalize this exaggeration of a traditional gender role as one immutably rooted in anatomy and pathophysiology.[78] Female problems were deemed to be problems of biology, and hysteria was only their logical extension. As Freud's colleague the gynaecologist Otto Weininger (in his *Sex and Character*) wrote: 'Man possesses sexual organs; her sexual organs possess woman'; this was to be expected if, according to the psychiatric opinion of Paul Moebius (*On the Physiological Imbecility of Women*), woman was an intermediate biological form between the child and the adult. Thus the nineteenth-century medical view of women, or at least of bourgeois women, was of frail and decorative creatures whose temperamental excesses were the result of a peculiar functioning of their sexual organs and whose very physical nature limited their activities to family roles. The fact that these hysterical women tended to be particularly sexually attractive for men[79] was regarded by the new psychoanalysts as a clue to the pattern only in that a sexual (rather than a gender) aetiology was still implicated; internalized repression rather than overt oppression. The pattern of symptoms of Charcot's hysterical patients has been replaced by a less dramatic pattern of diffuse somatic complaints.[80] Female identity vis-à-vis men is particularly reinforced in collective and passive settings such as nurses' training schools and boarding schools, and these are the contemporary settings in which doctors have continued to encounter hysteria.[81]

Agency, opposition, resistance

The contemporary reaction which offers close parallels with the doctor/ patient relation in hysteria is 'parasuicide' with medically prescribed drugs. As with hysteria, the normative situation of active male (husband, older doctor) and passive female (wife, younger patient) is reflected in the drama of the hospital casualty department. The unease and anger which the overdose evokes in the medical profession reflect its perverse transformation of the clinical paradigm. The official translation of the behaviour into symptoms takes place under socially prescribed conditions by the physician who alone has the power to legitimate exculpating circumstances. As with nineteenth-century hysteria or saka, the resolution of the reaction invokes a 'mystical pressure' which only replicates the social structure in which the reaction occurs;[81] like other 'culture-bound syndromes' it displays core structural antagonisms but shows they are 'soluble' within the existing political and symbolic framework. As with possession cults, overdoses can sometimes become collective with the possible development of an oppositional or strategic perspective.[82] The drama of the overdose scene in the casualty department replays the male doctor/female patient theme without questioning it, but it does afford a degree of negotiation for the principal, who induces a mixture of responses, but particularly guilt, in family and friends;[83] these women certainly act but hardly under conditions of their own choosing.

Ideas of 'structure' and 'function' are currently unfashionable in social anthropology because we now recognize them as simply external models independent of people's own meanings of their experience and possibilities. Structure is not an empirical, and seldom a subjective, reality (and perhaps a more appropriate term for my model would be a 'map'[84]). Certainly, a cybernetic schema of the sort I have outlined leaves individual motivation somewhat mysterious.[85] Actually how 'conscious' (and thus for us how 'responsible') is the principal? I would suggest that we can never answer such a question empirically for the local perception of agency, or lack of agency, is itself an essential element in the model itself. Ambiguity over conscious interest is built into the whole pattern, and may be found even in the spirit possession instances, as well as in those patterns, like Tikopian suicide trips and overdoses, which employ more internalized mystical pressure such as 'psychological illness' or 'pressure' or 'female personality', and which thus come somewhat closer to a recognition of the individual's agency (and only through which may our patterns then possibly emerge locally as explicit political resistance).

Nor am I arguing that my model represents a neat homeostatic system in which each extrusion is automatically followed by exaggeration and restitution. The principal may – perhaps generally – remain in the subdominant or extruded position, in a hopeless surrender to authority or in a perhaps more comfortable internalization of her position. For women who take overdoses which do not resolve their immediate situation may be left powerless and with 'internally directed hostility'.[86] The same phenomenon is susceptible of a variety of interpretations: reflection of social misogyny; hopeless identification with overwhelming 'stress'; an attempt to assert control over trauma by mimesis; social catharsis or homeostatis; cultural loophole; individual catharsis; role reversal; theatre; entertainment; ritual reaffirmation of gender relationships; rite of passage; genesis of sorority; standardized resistance;[87] revolutionary prototype; expression or resolution of symbolic ambiguity; calculated motivation; not to mention the enactment of such individual cognitions as distress, parody, play, adventure or revenge. And even, should we wish, biological sub-dominance. I suggest that overdoses may be understood in any of these ways, or indeed all of them. Claims to the primacy of a particular interpretation ultimately remain arbitrary, grounded not only in the immediate outcome but in the observer's own academic, professional and political assumptions. If my map suggests core cultural themes and practical possibilities implicitly and often explicitly 'recognised' by a culture, its workings out may invoke tentative attempts and aesthetic play within the theme, in microsituations and misinterpretations, toyed with, fantasized, presumed, hinted at, as well as in overt distress and disaster; unless the restitution occasionally fails, mystical pressure ceases to maintain its power. The overdose is socially compelling because, every now and then, we know that a woman dies.[88]

4. ... and the Nurse and Certain Others

What then of the immediate experience of the woman? A helpless identification with her struggles, with the opinion that places her immediately as without value? Or a conscious rebellion, howbeit not with weapons of her own choosing? To take another instance:

The housewives' disease

Perhaps 10 per cent of women develop the symptoms of *agoraphobia*,[1] the inability to go into public places alone or unaccompanied, particularly without a member of the family. Attempts to do so result in anxiety or other unpleasant symptoms, a fear of falling, fainting or otherwise losing control. Agoraphobics fear any situation in which escape to a safe place or dependable companion might be impeded. The majority are married women, hence the popular term 'housewives' disease'.[2] Physical space replicates our social space, and the home represents core social values:

> ... the framework within which the deference of wife to husband operates. Encouragement of ideologies of the home and home-centredness enables the identification of the wife with her husband's superordinate position to increase by emphasising a common adherence to territory, a solidarity of place. A woman's 'place' is therefore in the home, partly because to seek fulfilment outside the home could threaten to break down the ideological control which confinement within it promotes. The ideology of the 'home' ... is therefore a social control mechanism in the sense that escape from the home threatens access to alternative definition of the female role, as Ibsen brilliantly realised in *A Doll's House*.[3]

Agoraphobia reproduces such restrictions while denying any other motive except an inexplicable anxiety: it seems only to have become common when urban streets became physically safe for middle-class women, and thus when husbands became concerned about their wives' independence; agoraphobia acts as an 'internal chaperone' (as anorexia nervosa is perhaps an 'internalised corset') for it 'recreates ... the semblance of the nineteenth century bourgeois family'[4] where the wife is the 'angel in the home' in an opposition to the supposed 'whore in the street'.

Like drug overdoses, the agoraphobic reaction employs an exaggeration or caricature of the traditional female role with its lack of control or power, accurately mirroring the situation of Western European and American women in many areas of their lives with their extreme dependence on men.[5] Major decisions within families are usually made by the husband and the very decisions about the nature of the woman's 'place' (such as its location or whether to sell it) are taken by husbands. In one study, 16 out of 20 female agoraphobic patients had felt strong urges to escape from their marriage and home at the time of the onset of the phobia, but were unable to do so because of realistic fears of isolation, and the loss of economic support.[6] Agoraphobia is conceptualized by some behaviourist psychologists as avoidance behaviour in an insoluble conflict situation posed by the simultaneous desire to escape and fear of autonomy.[7] Symptoms may develop concurrently with a sense of dislocation: a wish to end the marriage or to 'violate' the marital contract.[8] The agoraphobic is often an unhappily married woman, low in self-sufficiency, in whom the fear evoked by physical isolation accompanies a persistent but unrealistic fantasy of liberation from the marriage – unrealistic because it is seen as leading to a social abyss.[9] It is not simply a reflection of an acceptable fear of the dangers of the street. A patient of mine who as a single parent successfully brought up three children in a ten-year stint of devoted and self-sacrificing denial allowed herself a relationship with a man when the children reached adolescence. Dramatically ensuing agoraphobia prevented this relationship from developing and she became housebound within a few weeks – which necessitated the children doing the shopping and going to the post office for her. Ironically, she had a half-realization of the situation: 'The illness seems to be a continuation of the demands of the children. It's as if I can never be me.'

While agoraphobic women can like this demonstrate in their situation allegiance to certain core social values, and express their sense of dislocation through them, the reaction like the overdose has been regarded as practically instrumental. Agoraphobia may serve as an alternative to overt marital conflict[10] and 'refusal to go out can draw attention to oneself, it can be used to control or punish others, it can protect from the dangers involved in living an independent social life, from having a social life, from having ... to face the possibility of failure'.[11] The agoraphobic married woman conforms even more to the stereotypic publicly extruded role, but she gains a strategy which, without open defiance of the husband,[12] requires him to make sacrifices and gives her a veto over proposed joint activities.[13] The very nature of a woman's household responsibility makes her illness the most potentially disturbing of all to family equilibrium, and agoraphobia is thus a particularly adaptive strategy.[14] On occasion it is able to severely restrict the husband's activities to the point where he is virtually unable to leave the home: 'Husband and wife are compelled to live together in mutual distress, consoling themselves for all their differences with the mutual idea that this thing has been imposed upon them, beyond their control, and they can do nothing about it.'[15]

Agoraphobia articulates the early socialization into the typical 'female' behaviour of helplessness and dependency; by the age of 13, girls have five times as many 'fears' as have boys.[16] The norms for appropriate male and female behaviour are learned and internalized very early in life. Socialization within the family and within the education system teaches children what women are like and what men are like, and how they should behave towards each other. Shirley Ardener notes that 'the nature of women affects the shape of the categories assigned for them, which in turn reflect back upon and reinforce and remould perceptions of the nature of women in a continuing process',[17] producing a complex set of shared images and conceptions which denote their general characteristics and appropriate behaviour in society. There is ample documentary evidence of the way girls and women are presented in the media, especially children's books, which points to a relationship between fearfulness and dependency in women's social roles, providing the basis for the later development of agoraphobia. In a study of sex roles in school textbooks, the illustrations portray girls and adult women as if agoraphobic, pictured behind fences or windows, immobolized, helpless and watching.[18] Durkheim only slightly exaggerated when he wrote: 'The two sexes do not share equally in social life. Man is actively involved in it, while woman does little more than look on from a distance.'[19]

Is the illness necessarily the exaggeration of a normal gender role? In the nineteenth century the *menopause* was associated with insanity.[20] Recent medical literature presents the menopausal woman as biologically depressed, irritable, tired and asexual, although the only well-documented menopausal experiences are hot flushes and night sweats.[21] The menopausal syndrome has become organized out of amorphous complaints and malaise which leads to a possibly functional illness role but also to physical (endocrinological) treatment. Townsend and Carbone have drawn attention to the devalued status of the post-menopausal woman who remains 'female' but deprived of her sexuality and thus the potential for developing such symptoms. In other societies, however, the loss of the role of reproducer (mother, wife) frequently signals access to an enhanced 'male' role: thus Rajput women in North India apparently enjoy a symptom-free menopause, reflecting a valued change of status with access to activities previously forbidden.[22]

The menopause is obviously less flexible than the model outlined in Chapter 3 in the way that it is 'once and for all'. I warned that we must take the Butterfly/Serpent as a map not as an invariable model of the psychopathology as gender-based power. The role of the nurse, for instance, as a characteristically female one, as a carer, poses certain contradictions within such a rigidly binary model. While nursing is a professionalization of aspects of women's traditional domestic tasks, an extension of her 'natural' nurturant and caring role, it is not totally at variance with the role of the doctors. Yet the nurse threatens to approximate in popular medical perception to the role of the patient. Some ambiguities are resolved during the socialization of the nurse into her professional role or later in various strategic ways. Particular problems arise for female doctors in traditionally male specialities such as gynaecology, for male nurses, and for female nurses who themselves have only partial access to the negotiating power afforded to other women by the neuroses. I shall consider here three patterns of 'abnormal illness behaviour' which the medical profession has perceived among nurses.

Is female to male as patient is to doctor?

One fundamental characteristic of Western therapies, self-help groups excepted, is that they take the form of a dialogue between a healer and a patient,[23] particularly the dialogue between doctor and patient. Till recently it has seemed as if this was the only form of serious therapeutic intervention. Doctor and patient. The doctor–patient relationship. There is a resonance about it. A salience. It seems the very essence of Western healing.[24] Medical textbooks include introductory chapters on it, and since Entralgo's pioneering book *Doctor and Patient*, much speculation has centred on its social and historical significance.[25]

The *doctor–patient* relationship then. By contrast the *nurse–patient* relationship does not sound so socially resonant, more a jargonized professional idiom. Whilst nursing textbooks certainly provide information on its practice, it always seems contingent on political and symbolic constructs external to the pair. The doctor–patient dyad by contrast seems to stand by itself, as if it were a part of our natural order of things. A preference for binary classifications may or may not be rooted in all human thought,[26] but here at least we cannot blame the structural anthropologist. A simple triad *patient–doctor–nurse* does not seem quite right, for the nurse's role seems less simple, comprising nurturance yet also a certain passivity. Indeed, as I shall propose, the pair which includes the nurse and which strikes the most powerful resonance in contemporary Western medical practice is that of doctor and nurse.

In all societies, illness is experienced and manifest through conceptual categories which encode aspects of the social order. What are the everyday contexts from which the patient's sick role is derived? I have suggested that there is a close approximation between the role of the patient vis-à-vis the doctor and that of women in relation to men. To be a patient is to be embedded in a web of beliefs, norms and interests which represent the political and personal relations between the sexes. The historical origin of the contemporary female role lies in the Industrial Revolution, with a radical division of work by gender and a physical separation between home and workplace which exaggerated the existing social and emotional segregation of women. Bryan Turner and Jacques Donzelot have suggested this produced a close relationship between the woman and the family doctor which, in many areas, replaced that of wife and husband.[27] The move away from the household as a focus for productive work also diminished its responsibilities for religion, education and recreation, reducing its social significance, contracting women's general responsibilities and isolating them from significant areas of public production.

Compared with men, contemporary Western women are permitted greater freedom to 'express feelings', enabling the woman to define her distresses within a medical framework and bring them to the attention of her doctor. The more women take on characteristically female responsibilities, the greater their reporting of medical symptoms.[28] The ambiguities of the 'lady doctor' are most manifest in the areas where the doctor–patient relationship closely replicates that of male–female: obstetrics and gynaecology. There are relatively few female gynaecologists compared with women in other medical specialities. If the codifications of distress produces many psychiatrized patterns – overdoses, agoraphobia, shoplifting, anorexia nervosa – through a ritual play on the male/female: doctor/patient set (p. 50), the mediator, the psychiatrist, is thus more 'feminine' than other physicians (see Figure 3, p. 61). There are many female psychiatrists and paediatricians, but these are areas of sickness where the male/female bipolarity is muted, where a mother/child opposition becomes appropriate. By contrast gynaecology permits no ambiguities or symbolic play – it is a simple manifestation of the biologically rooted set. Through childbearing every woman becomes a potential patient. Woman doctors are not allowed to be female through bearing children themselves: one questionnaire study reported that they 'were not taken seriously in their career intentions once they had become pregnant'.[29] The 'Wendy Savage affair' demonstrates how a female obstetrician who attempts to cut across the symbolic conceptualizations, no longer acting as a classificatory male, creates havoc in the whole system: clearly, natural childbirth and the women's health movements have to adopt an ethic which inverts the traditional relationship.[30]

And the nurse

Nurses in prisons and mental hospitals excepted, the nurse is quintessentially female. She is female both in popular perception and in actual statistics. Those occupational tasks with which women are now characteristically associated – hairdressing, cleaning, nursing, prostitution and to an extent infant teaching, catering and waiting at tables – are developments of women's traditional domestic tasks which have become split off and rationalized as separate professions.[31] Nursing is an extension and codification of woman's nurturant role as a mother. To 'nurse' is indeed to mother. These female professions have not developed simply as professions parallel to those of men, for men have now entered them and re-established themselves at the top of the hierarchy. As more men enter, the profession becomes divided into upper (male-dominated) and lower (predominantly female) sections. We have this distinction between cuisine and catering, between higher and primary education. The entry of men into general nursing from their traditional area of psychiatric nursing (with its role derived from that of the untrained and custodial mental hospital attendant) has now led to male domination of the Royal College of Nursing and a relative over-representation of men in the newer nursing administrative positions.[32] The nursing specialities most closely associated with a traditional female role, midwifery and health visiting, are the last to admit men. In a recent examination of the imagery of drug advertisements in the medical press, I found only one which portrayed a male nurse (with a female doctor). However, not only was it not concerned with medical treatment but rather insurance, but the structural 'imbalance' was rectified by the presence of a third figure, an older, and not surprisingly male, hospital consultant. By contrast, advertisements featuring male nurses are now commonplace in nursing magazines, but without a doctor.

Because of the association of nursing with 'care', with female nurturance and consolation, the male nurse has remained a particularly ambiguous figure: 'Men have always been a touchy topic in nursing.'[33] Like the hairdresser, who has also adopted female gender specific tasks, he takes on certain homosexual attributes.[34] The sexual orientation of the male nurse, like that of the female doctor, is a constant matter of interest, while the sexual interests of an engineer or an anthropologist appear irrelevant. A supplement on men carried by a nursing journal was entitled 'Man Appeal' and was principally concerned with the popular perception of the male nurse, weighing the images of 'tough' versus 'tender', 'macho' versus 'soft', of custodian versus carer.[35]

In some particulars then, the nurse–doctor relationship presents a standardized system of emotional attitudes in recapitulating professionally that of mother–father, but the immediate popular image of the nurse is, of course, one who is young, gauche and sexually attractive, as witness the endless newspaper cartoons and jokes hinting at (never consummated) physical intimacy between male patient and nurse.[36] A concerned *Nursing Times* wonders if 'the average male really does see general nurses as 18-year-old blondes who wear pretty caps'.[37] When nurses get older or enter administration the image changes dramatically to that of the well-known 'battle-axe sister' or 'dragon' matron, professional but thus defeminized and threatening, wielding bedpan or syringe. Senior nurses do indeed tend to be single, seldom have children, with little interest in life outside the hospital.[38] The situation recalls that noted in the magazine *The English-woman* in 1913: nurses who had not left to marry or had not become matrons were by the age of 40 virtually unemployable, for doctors preferred young nurses 'who are less likely than older women to interfere'.[39]

Patients and nurses then share certain female characteristics: socially ascribed characteristics of gender role, not directly of biological sex but, as we shall see, the 'natural facts' of biological sex from which they are derived, keep breaking in.

Relations with doctors

Nurses perform domestic tasks for doctors – making coffee, running errands, and for surgeons actually helping them wash and dress. If they make suggestions they are careful to do so in a way in which the suggestions can be perceived as actually coming from the doctor[40] – a lateral strategy which if it is detected in a patient would be termed in medical parlance 'manipulation'. Nurses remain defined by the doctor's tasks, mediating between biomedical and lay worlds. In spite of the attempt of nursing academics to establish a professional nursing ethic, a central core idiom which can stand alone, this falters on the question of what it might constitute. Care? Communication?[41]

If, as I have argued, the doctor–nurse–patient triad replicates that of the Western family, activity continues to be directed by the doctor who retains the prerogative of deep penetration and control of the body.[42] By contrast the nurse is an extension of the normal healing processes of the body itself.[43] The syringe, bedpan or enema (the popular instruments of the nurse) are, however, more obviously threatening – at least at the level of popular stereotype – for they seek to control the body in the visible sphere. The organization of the hospital replicates that of the domestic economy. The childbirth scene is represented in endless newspaper cartoons of the father, unshaven and smoking, pacing the hospital corridor, excluded and marginal. Inside the delivery suite his role is taken over by the doctor. Not

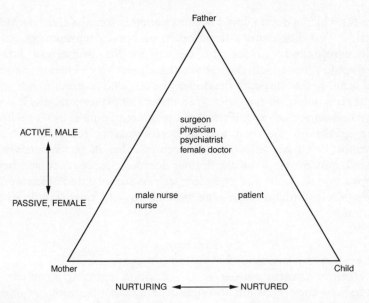

Figure 3

surprisingly, the radical midwife endeavours to supplant the doctor, and in this she reintroduces the biological father not as director of the proceedings but as caring assistant.[44]

The self-perception of the doctor, particularly the surgeon, is one of belonging to a confraternity of heroes. Like the gynaecologist, in Britain the surgeon takes the gender-specific title of 'Mr' rather than the gender-neutral 'Dr'. A recent academic paper describes the macho self-assurance of the ideal surgeon: 'The masculine society of surgeons admires cars, sports, speed, competence.'[45] Its author describes the embarrassment caused when one surgeon brings his wife to a hospital party where the other surgeons are busily engaged in sexual dalliance with their nurse mistresses. Whether at the level of fantasy, flirtation or actual physical sex (the quintessential embodiment of gender), relations between the doctor and 'his' nurse are heavily charged with sexual significance, a favourite theme of television soap operas or Mills and Boon hospital romances.[46] Doctors 'have' their nurses; nurses don't 'have' doctors. Indeed a doctor who fails to engage in at least the appearance of sexual flirtation with the nurse is a 'wimp', one who is professionally incompetent, slow, unable to act and thus clinically dangerous through his impotence.[47]

By contrast, the notion of a female doctor having sex with a male nurse is incredible and bizarre. If, as I have argued, the patient is quintessentially female, what of sexual relations between her and the male doctor? Again the possibility is abhorrent but not inconceivable, traditionally the worst offence for which a doctor could be summoned before the General Medical Council.[48] Too dangerous a situation to be openly represented, it is the dentist who stands in for the doctor in the numerous soft-core pornographic films which skirt about the issue.[49] By contrast the female patient is allowed to flirt with the doctor; he responds correctly with anxiety and embarrassment. In the official pre-history of psychoanalysis, it is when Freud's colleague Breuer realizes that his patient Anna is in love with him and he breaks off the treatment in horror leaving town for a 'second honeymoon' with his wife, that the central idea of psychoanalysis was generated: patients fall in love with their doctors, the idea that later became developed into the notion of 'transference'. As summarized in Figure 3, the doctor's perception emphasizes the vertical axis, the nurse emphasizes the horizontal.

Socialization

Until recently student nurses at the London teaching hospitals were inducted into their vocation through a period of segregated preliminary training. Throughout their career, the low salary constrained many to spend a considerable period of time in a hall of residence attached to the hospital. There they were treated as younger than their age, in need of protection and surveillance. In contrast with other student hostels, rules have traditionally been strict and male visitors segregated in a public space during specific visiting hours. Various authors have noted the tension in the development of nursing between offering the period of training as a type of finishing school for the less affluent young lady, with careful attention to chastity and deportment, and the attempt to train paid and skilled professionals.[50] In the 1970s when I was a medical student at St Bartholomew's Hospital in London, the annual Matron's Ball resembled a fashionable 'coming-out' event, the cloistered atmosphere of the Nurses Home (with its preoccupations with mislaid cap pins or dieting) enlivened with plans as to whom to invite, what fashionable dress to imitate, how much wine might decently be consumed: the whole recalling more the atmosphere of a girls' public school story than its reality as a rather tawdry piece of glamour punctuating a hot-house atmosphere centred exclusively around the hospital. Sexuality was constrained but highlighted through this constraint. The ideal was marriage to a young doctor and then departure from the hospital. One unfortunate nurse made no secret of her affections for one of the hospital porters and was warned by her ward sister that she would have to choose between her lover and her 'vocation'. Little wonder that so many nurses seemed to marry policemen, affections cultivated in the casualty department or in the nurses' canteen in which, by tradition, policemen in uniform whose work took them to the hospital were allowed to take a cup of tea. There were no male student nurses, whose likely ambitions would doubtless have threatened the notion of 'vocation'.[51]

Psychopathologies of the nurse

Given their position then firmly on one side of my patient–doctor paradigm, it is not surprising that doctors are believed (not least by themselves) to make poor patients, failing to accept a novel situation of passivity and obedience. The advantages of the public negotiating strategies of agoraphobia or overdoses – psycho-social distress modelled into clinical syndromes – are not available to them. Their pathologies are secret – alcoholism, completed suicide, marital violence and divorce – for all of which doctors have amongst the highest rate.[52] To an extent this is true for nurses – while overdoses are relatively common among student nurses, they are rare after they have qualified. In terms of our model they, like the doctors, are too much on the side of the Serpent in the Butterfly–Serpent pair to be able to express distress as such. Nor are the more 'transparent' strategies of neurotic patterns (employing a disease idiom for personal distress) available. Nevertheless, hospital doctors have perceived in nurses some characteristic psychopathologies: *loin pain haematuria*, *Munchausen's Syndrome by Proxy*, and *acute somatization*. Because they lack the transparency of agoraphobia, shoplifting and other patterns, and employ the biomedical idiom more closely and 'deceitfully', they occasion particular outrage in the doctor.

Loin pain haematuria: the rebellion of Edith Owens

The dismay of doctors faced with the patient who takes an overdose of prescribed drugs reflects a medical preoccupation with 'factitious illness' – apparent diseases induced deliberately by those seeking the advantages of the sick role. Prison doctors in the nineteenth century discovered 'Ganser psychosis' – the syndrome of approximate answers – a strategy of feigned madness, employing popular ideas of insanity, through which long-term convicts gained the more congenial circumstances of the prison hospital (pp. 4–5). Junior psychiatrists today are still taught to ask appropriate questions to detect it.[53] While a general acceptance of psychodynamic theories of 'psychosomatic illnesses' and the influences of life events and personality on physical disease are part of the currency of psychiatry, these are accepted only grudgingly by many general physicians and surgeons. If the signs and symptoms fail to add up to recognized pathophysiology or the laboratory tests do not concur, while the patient keeps returning with further episodes and cheerfully accepts hospital admission, then the physicians become suspicious of the possibility of 'factitious illnesses'. They divide them simply into *malingering* (a consciously motivated fabrication of symptoms) or *hysteria* (in which the patient is largely unaware of their production).[54] Malingerers are promptly discharged from hospital, while hysterics are referred to the psychiatrist.

Loin pain haematuria, like laxative abuse,[55] was described as a new syndrome in the 1970s – characterized by blood in the urine and pain in the lower abdomen for which no biomedical cause could be found. The initial studies showed a high proportion of doctors' wives and nurses among the patients and, in the absence of obvious disease of the kidneys, it was suggested to be a factitious illness.[56] Debate has continued as to whether there is a 'real' disease, the patients being nurses only by their proximity to other hospital personnel who have a readiness to investigate them more intensively.

'Edith Owens' is a nursing sister at a small clinic attached to a London teaching hospital, married with two young daughters. Of Welsh working-class origin, she was brought up by evangelical Christian parents, left school to enter nursing and later came to London. She was referred to the hospital renal department at the age of 33 complaining of loin pain and fresh blood when she urinated. Repeated hospital admission for investigations and blood transfusions occurred when her haemoglobin dropped to dangerously low levels. Petite and attractive, looking younger than her age, Edith sat passively in bed, her face dead white from her anaemia, apparently considering her situation with total equanimity and leaving her male physicians disconcerted by what they felt was, if not strictly flirtation, at any rate some type of heavily charged but implicit emotional communication. Concern was also expressed over the large doses of the potentially addictive morphine analogue, pethidine, she required for her pain. She was closely observed and encouraged to see a junior psychiatrist – myself.[57] Formal psychotherapy sessions with me three times a week continued rather fruitlessly for two years, interrupted by Edith's frequent admissions to hospital. I often thought 'something else' was going on but was always met with her bland indifference. Eventually she was detected by her nursing colleagues one night in her hospital bed removing blood from her arm with a syringe (which had been hidden in her handbag), removing the needle to then inject the blood into her urethra. She was confronted with the evidence at a specially convened meeting in the presence of her husband by the triumphant physicians while I sat rather uncomfortably at the side. She took up the offer of some time in a psychotherapy ward, during which she became considerably more animated and less bland. She recalled the stratagems she used to hide her syringes but said she was never consciously motivated to take her blood:[58] 'It just sort of happened in a dream.' Afterwards she had 'just felt – I don't know – well, good. I had done it, my own little thing'. Her hospital stay was suddenly cut short when it was discovered that her eldest daughter at home, aged 6, although on the surface comfortably adjusting to her mother's absence, was pulling out her own hair in handfuls.

Mrs Owen's parental home had been strict but not harsh. Her father was distant and cold while fair, her mother harassed and always worried about money. Disobedience by the seven children was not tolerated by the parents nor apparently ever offered. Edith as the oldest girl adopted enthusiastically the role of a 'little mother' from an early age, looking after the youngest children and at 10 was cooking for the family when her mother entered hospital for a few months. Her father celebrated her to the other children as their new mother. There were few family holidays for financial reasons and life centred around the local evangelical church to which all the children have continued to belong when grown up. Nursing seemed an obvious vocation for the 'little mother' and she left home to stay in the nurses' hostel. At a hospital dance she was introduced to, and soon married, her first boyfriend, a young businessman of similar background to her own. He was her first sexual encounter. Life now became transformed as his company prospered – a higher standard of living, two cars, detached house, not to mention sex which Edith suddenly discovered was rather more fun than might be expected. Although it was not financially necessary, she continued working as a staff nurse in the operating theatre and, while there, in a daze of opening opportunities had a brief affair with the anaesthetist who just happened to be a friend of her husband.

She discovered she was pregnant but whether by her husband or by her lover she was uncertain. Her father died suddenly at the same time and she became quite distressed: terrified it was not her husband's child, but unwilling to deliberately abort it, she started severe dieting and purging herself, and using hospital syringes to remove blood from her veins, miserably punishing herself but also hoping through this to lose the baby. Admission to hospital and blood transfusions were followed by the successful delivery of the child without any apparent ill effects. The couple moved to London; a second girl was born and Edith continued to work at nights, devoting the day to her husband and children. Her girls were 'perfect', well behaved and loving, and she spent all her spare time with them, a prosperous suburban life enlivened by teaching at the Sunday School, somewhat tiresome dinner parties and trips to the opera at Glyndebourne. Superficially all was successful but Edith herself no longer felt 'real', constantly getting preoccupying thoughts that both her children were not hers. In her job she was extremely hardworking, a good teacher and a loyal colleague. She was then offered a year's course to become a nursing tutor and accepted, her husband not very enthusiastically agreeing.

While waiting for the course to begin, she went to her doctor complaining of passing blood and pain in her lower abdomen. She was forced to take time off from work: her course had to be postponed but life continued its sedate public tenor.

Munchausen's Syndrome by Proxy

The most dramatic form of 'malingering' observed and classified by doctors is Munchausen's Syndrome (more recently called 'hospital addiction syndrome') in which convincing abdominal symptoms (typically) in men and women led to urgent hospital admission and operation. In the extreme form 'Munchausens', as they are called by hospital staff, spend their lives moving from one hospital to another, changing their names, passing an impressive proportion of their lives in hospital beds, sometimes to be operated on yet again, sometimes to be ejected by indignant doctors after consultation of the 'blacklist' in the casualty department (which records their pseudonyms, appearance and favourite symptoms). While it may be characterized as an extreme form of 'abnormal illness behaviour' as sociologically trained medical students now put it, British psychiatrists usually classify the patients as 'inadequate personalities', citing their incapacity to live any type of conventional life.

A proportion of Munchausen's patients have obtained jobs as hospital porters or orderlies and some studies suggest factitious illness is more common in women who have taken nursing training.[59] A recently studied related pattern is Munchausen's Syndrome by Proxy,[60] in which mothers produce factitious, sometimes real, diseases in their children. Techniques include placing menstrual blood in the child's orifices, contaminating specimens, altering hospital records or, more seriously, producing rashes on the child with abrasives or caustics, aspirating milk from the young child's stomach with a syringe and tube to produce weight loss, or producing fits through asphyxiation. In one study, out of 47 parents involved, all were women. Seventeen of the group were nurses and another four paramedicals; several claimed falsely to be related to a doctor. The children were admitted to hospital for now necessary investigation and operations, including in one case brain surgery.

A common feature of many of the mothers is that they are of a 'higher social and intellectual status' than their husbands, many of whom are absent from the home, working away for considerable periods as drivers or mechanics.[61] Reading the case histories it seems significant that a close personal relationship is built up through the child's illness between mother and doctor. In many cases the mother has previously induced or simulated physical illness in herself, and its discoverer, Meadows, suggests the pattern is related both to personal factitious illness and to child abuse. He emphasizes there can be considerable gains: as he puts it, 'A medical illness is one of the few available tickets to a source of help. Involve a child and that can be a first-class express ticket.'[62]

Whatever our conclusions as to how 'conscious' a mechanism is involved, how pragmatically it is motivated, in symbolic and political terms we again have a pattern in which the relationship doctor to nurse replicates that of father to mother, both united in care of the child. At the same time, the principal achieves for herself a role as patient/child/spouse. If we examine an individual instance, the symbolism is more complex and rich, reflecting intense personal affects and contradictions. My model merely sketches out the bare bones of the choreography: out of it the principal develops her own pattern of meanings and expression.[63]

Why do people become nurses? I'd argue that for many there is an attempt, Diana Princess of Wales style, to seek to transcend one's own distress. And this may be horribly misplaced. The most dramatic form was illustrated by the case of the nurse Beverley Allitt who was convicted of two murders of young children, and serious bodily harm of eight others. Ms Allitt was suffering from an eating disorder at the time of the trial:[64] as with many of the syndromes described in this chapter, there is a cross-cutting and elision between different patterns. Like Munchausen's by Proxy, her action allows the expression of ambivalent feelings: nursing is not only characterized by the need to care.

Gulf War Syndrome and Royal Free Disease

Sick days outnumber days on strike by a factor of 400. Physical illness may provide the model for acute physical symptoms which may occur in an epidemic form: each episode of illness may make the susceptible individual more likely to become ill. Whatever the outcome of clinical studies into *Gulf War Syndrome* – the situation of the private soldier in many respects parallels that of the nurse – it provides a good instance, similar to that of the *marching band illnesses* which affected pre-adolescent members of paramilitary instrument bands in the 1970s.

From September 1990 to June 1991, Britain deployed over 50,000 military personnel in the Gulf War. In the months after the conflict ended, reports of various medical problems began to appear among American soldiers: 60,000 (out of the 697,000 troops deployed) reported symptoms ranging from memory loss to cancer. After a television programme in June 1993, British troops reported similar complaints and by 2000, 1100 were seeking compensation or disability payments[65] for what was originally called Desert Fever and then Desert Storm Fever, now Gulf War

Syndrome. Complaints include chronic fatigue, diarrhoea, aches and pains, headaches, bleeding gums, hair loss, insomnia, irritability, muscle spasms and night sweats – and some claims by veterans that their vomit glows in the dark, and two cases of bodily shrinking.[66] Explanations advanced include exposure to chemical warfare agents, vaccinations, toxic fumes from burning oil wells, depleted uranium used in projectiles and tank armour and organophosphate insecticides.[67] Many believe it is contagious and can be passed through semen, sweat or through the air. Official military clinical investigations have revealed nothing and in a recent study, Kilshaw emphasizes the passivity of a disciplined soldier in a highly technological war, and current concerns with genetics, environmental toxicity, HIV and the immune system. A newspaper report describes a soldier whose 'immune system has vanished. He lives in a room lagged with this foil against the risk of infection with a blue plastic tube inserted into his nostrils'.[68] A striking feature is the way Gulf War Syndrome apparently affects wives and lovers: 'burning semen' causes open sores which bleed, and subsequently born children have birth defects and malformation.[69]

In July 1955, a different epidemic occurred among the staff of the Royal Free Hospital in London, the teaching hospital which first trained female doctors and had long been associated with women's medicine. Within two weeks the hospital had to be closed, to open three months later after over 300 people had been affected, the majority women; 198 staff needed in-patient treatment, of whom 5 were men (0.8 per cent of the male staff) and the rest women (11 per cent). The conclusions at the time were the illness – headache, malaise, dizziness, nausea, neck stiffness and limb pain – was caused by a virus; a year later a leading article in the *Lancet* entitled 'A New Clinical Entity?' proposed the name of 'benign myalgic encephalomyelitis' (ME). There the matter rested until 1970 when two papers appeared in the *British Medical Journal* suggesting that 'epidemic hysteria' was a more likely diagnosis and noting that 'the occurrence of a mass hysterical reaction shows not that the population is psychologically abnormal but merely that it is socially segregated and consists predominantly of young females'.[70] The authors detailed 15 similar epidemics, eight of them involving hospital nurses. An accompanying editorial noted 'the epidemic spread of panic-stricken and hysterical conduct has been more characteristic of women'. A lively storm of abusive correspondence followed.[71] Doctors wrote to say they were 'upset' by the article: 'I regard the conclusions ... as nonsense. Many of these girls were known to me. Illness was alien to their natures.' The editors of the journal were forced to justify having published the papers. One letter pointed out that hysteria had been considered initially at the Royal Free as a likely diagnosis: 'Later, as medical staff of various seniority succumbed, such a suggestion was silenced by unspoken agreement ... even now it is rarely applied except to girls of subnormal intelligence.'[72] Follow-up 30 years later found that six of the nurses had committed suicide.[73]

'Epidemic (or mass) hysteria' is frequently summoned as an explanation in the editorials of medical journals to characterize sudden mass movements of which they disapprove. (Indeed, one doctor wrote in disparaging the critical comments made by others on McEvedy and Beard's original paper to characterize such responses as a 'second wave of hysteria'. To doubt hysteria was hysteria.) This is not the place to recapitulate the many sociological studies on hysteria. Suffice to cite Ellenberger who describes it as 'a folie à deux ... a culture-bound syndrome emerging from the interaction between the professor and his clientele', or Chodoff and Lyon's famous description of hysterical personality as 'a picture of women in the words of men'.[74]

The notion of 'mass hysteria' has been examined in the same way.[75] Another nineteenth-century medical category, it emerged in the same sociological climate as Le Bon's study of *The Crowd* – in which a collectivity of people have a 'mental unity' analogous to a hypnotic trance, in which the individual 'having entirely lost his conscious personality, obeys all suggestions of the operator who has – deprived him of it ... His acts are far more under the influence of the spinal cord than of the brain.' Crowds are like savages and women; the psychological anthropology of Rivers and McDougall relied too on a notion of 'sympathy' or 'psychic contagion' and contemporary psychiatry still regards hysteria as the particular preserve of non-Europeans and women.[76] It continues to be reported in medical journals from closed communities of women and girls – boarding schools, convents and nursing training schools.[77]

Given its assumption of 'lower mental functioning' and 'psychic contagion', there is no surprise over the furore that McEvedy and Beard's papers generated. Not only had the nurses been affected but female medical students and doctors. And some men. The indignant medical correspondents quite rightly realized that to recognize an episode of mass hysteria in the only 'female medical school' had serious implications for the image of women doctors. Indeed, the Royal Free epidemic still remains part of the folklore of every male student who has never heard of the serious outbreak of poliomyelitis in Britain which preceded it and on which some suggested it had been modelled.

We do not have to follow the medical detectives in choosing between the two explanations – viral or psychological. The personal experience of illness does not directly reflect a disease process. The disease provides a ground on which personal life, social context and indigenous theories of sickness erect a pattern of experience, expression and behaviour. Illness, as I have argued, is embedded in social roles and expectations. Its form may be modelled on pathophysiological changes but be induced by social context, and it may subserve deep-seated personal needs as psychotherapists maintain.

A third of women admit to being 'always tired' and 20 per cent are 'currently tired'.[78] The imitation of illness entails an already recognized sickness. No wonder then, that the lassitude and loss of energy common in many physical sicknesses still provide the core symptoms of the inchoate diagnosis of *myalgic encephalomyelitis* (post-viral fatigue syndrome or as it is often called in the popular press *yuppie flu*).[79] Symptoms of episodic somatization include severe fatigue, weakness, fever, depression and sore throats, and difficulty in concentration and remembering.[80] The majority are aged 20 to 40 with a slight bias to women and to those in residential accommodation – like the Royal Free nurses' hostel. Militant self-help organizations have developed who stress the illness is 'real' and oppose doctors who question it ('the burden of proof of illness should not be borne by the sick and disabled'[81]). A recent television programme ended in a near riot as the studio audience, largely sufferers from ME, barracked a doctor who suggested that the majority of victims were depressed.

The majority of English sufferers have apparently had a virus infection before the onset of symptoms (hence 'post-viral fatigue syndrome'), unlike those in Third World schools: an epidemic in 1993 of fainting fits among girls occurred after 'smelling something distinctive . . .'. None of the boys was affected. A recent instance was the West Bank Epidemic of 1983 among Palestinian schoolgirls who developed sore throats, peripheral cyanosis and fainting (Palestinian doctors implicated poison, the Israelis, hysteria); and similarly among Albanian schoolchildren in Kosovo then part of Serbia.[82] All three instances were followed by political violence as if the tensions expressed were part of the wider social domain. In Malaysia, acute somatization in schools and factories largely affects Indians and Malays.[83] 'Marching bands sickness' was initially explained by parents as contamination from pesticides used by farmers, and in many episodes of mass illness among children the parents provide the explanation – such as exposure to toxic gas.[84] Gruenberg, in a review of 'psychic epidemics', restricts himself to consideration of the social psychological conditions necessary – status of initiator's group size and so on.[85] In the nineteenth century, J. F. C. Hecker had suggested the natural facility of sympathy or imitation became 'morbid' with an abnormal stimulus, and the German physician Rudolf Virchow even suggested cases were a pathologization of the thwarted political impulses of 1848.[86]

Elaine Showalter in her recent book on modern 'hysterias' – Gulf War Syndrome, multiple personality disorder and ME – describes them as folk panics spread by stories circulated through self-help books, articles in newspapers and magazines, TV talk shows and series, films, the Internet, and even literary criticism . . . As we approach our own millennium, the epidemic of hysterical disorders, imaginery illnesses, and hypnotically induced pseudomemories that have flooded the media seem to be reaching a high-water mark. These hysterics are merging with the more generalised paranoias, religious revival, and conspiracy theories that have always characterised American life, and the apocalyptic anxieties that always accompany the end of century.[87]

She notes that popular (and medical) aetiologies include 'a virus, sexual molestation, chemical warfare, satanic conspiracy [and] alien infiltration'. She has subsequently received death threats from illness activist groups.

Why, however, are only certain people vulnerable? Returning to the example of the nurse, the perception of her as a woman by male medicine coalesces with a notion of the nurse as a mother. While those not engaged in health care and treatment have relatively easy recourse to 'neurotic' patterns, employing an idiom of sick role behaviour but with a predominantly psychological idiom, the nurse as a self-sufficient carer has to have recourse to a variety of patterns more closely allied to the presentation of physical disease, patterns more elusive to symbolic analysis, lying congealed in the medical text.[88] Thus, a common measure of nursing 'morale' on a ward is the extent of sick leave.[89]

A common feature of all three patterns is the male doctor as investigator, constantly tracking, suspecting, testing new hypotheses, accusing, while the nurse, elusive behind her sickness, seeks to avoid being caught.[90] Doctors complain bitterly that these patients 'play games' with them, and the rhetoric of theatre or game would indeed be irresistible to them did not such play involve serious physical risk to the protagonists. To determine the extent to which the reactions are 'conscious' pragmatic attempts at adjustment is not possible; while to the theorist there is an element of parody in all of them, the irony is only rarely perceived by principal and audience. Participants certainly experience despair and self-hatred.

All the patterns I have described are likely to be found as part of an endogenous depressive illness; I think that the mediating factor is the sense of extrusion and isolation which is so characteristic of depression as well as other situations. The emphasis on cultural rather than psychological or physiological antecedents should thus not be taken to mean that individual personality or biology are irrelevant in the choice of reaction. It is not surprising that agoraphobic patients are anxious people or have 'phobic personalities' or that anorexics were overweight as children. The final path is polysemous and over-determined:

> The efficacy of ritual as a social mechanism depends on this very
> phenomenon of central and peripheral meanings and on their allusive
> and evocative powers ... All symbolic objects make it possible to
> combine fixity of form with multiple meanings of which some are
> standardised and some highly individualised.[91]

Our nurse–patient's venesection commenced after she had an extra-
marital affair (with an anaesthetist!) and an attempt to lose the subsequent
pregnancy by severe dieting coincided with the death of her father.
Nevertheless the individual reaction is socially embedded: the male who
takes an overdose or who develops anorexia is inevitably 'feminised'.
Another patient of mine shoplifted from a fashionable London store where
her domineering mother was well known as a customer, ostensibly to
purchase her own birthday present for the mother to give her later in the
week; in this setting the mother stood in a relationship to her analogous to
that of husband to wife. (We would be surprised to find a man engaging in
shoplifting in a similar relationship with his wife or even a son with his
mother.) Similarly Moroccan men with *ḥamadsha* possession are in a
'feminine' position with regard to their fathers.[92] Male reactions occur
typically when men are younger (*flashing*), displaced (*sieges*), or depressed
(following unemployment).

   I have previously outlined the interrelations between social, psychological and symbolic inversion.[93] Reversal theory suggests inversions of
everyday life occur in some universal non-rational and 'ludic' mode,[94]
while Chesler emphasizes that it is women who are 'conditioned to lose in
order to win'.[95] Devereux[96] characterized this passive 'appeal of helplessness'[97] as masochistic blackmail and illustrates it with an agoraphobic
case history and the 'psychology of cargo cults'. Rather than characterize
such life-threatening or constricting reactions as simply 'self-punitive' or
'manipulative' with all the psychodynamic baggage that implies, I would
prefer to see the powerless individual as enmeshed in a situation which she
cannot control, one which reflects neither her interests nor her perspective
but which does afford room for manoeuvre by employing the dominant
symbolism itself. If it was not a dangerous game it would not work:
physiological integrity is temporarily sacrificed to semiotics. 'The stakes are
high: they involve a real gamble with death.'[98]

   The dominant structures are only represented, possibly adjusted, but not
challenged; whether self-help groups or women's therapy groups can, like
women's groups in the Third World,[99] actually develop into alternative
political structures ('counter-cultures'[100]) is unlikely. It is interesting that
these reactions are often 'resolved' through psychiatry: the psychiatrist,
relative to other doctors, is more passive, more empathic, more 'feminine'.
The inversion can, however, be institutionalized, either just as a physical

illness (the various chronic fatigue and Gulf War groups), as an undesirable identity in relation to dominant norms (Open Door phobic groups) or as valued identities in their own right (the American Big Beautiful Woman (BBW) network). The irony of affirming a stigmatized minority identity is that this identity remains determined by the dominant culture.

5. The Instrumental Body in the Transition to Modernity

Disorders of civilization

As with any other social fact, one can interpret an illness like Gulf War Syndrome or Munchausen's by Proxy as somehow characteristic of the particular society in which it is found; whether as demonstrating shared sentiments refracted in individual situations, or as some expression of what observers recognize as the 'tensions' between constituent groups such as men and women (or civilians and military). As we have seen in Chapter 1, such specificity has been a continuing problem for comparative studies in psychiatry. Can those patterns recognized by doctors as 'culture-bound' be fully explained through an understanding of one particular society? Or should these patterns be subsumed under more universal categories? Or, more modestly if we seek classification, should these be placed in groups whose members demonstrate some family resemblances to each other? Can we argue both – local specification and superordinate category – when a 'behavioural syndrome appearing in widely differing cultures takes on local meaning so completely that it appears uniquely suited to articulate important dimensions of each local culture, as though it had sprung naturally from that environment'?[1]

Whether some general category we allocate adequately subsumes a characteristic local experience is fundamental for any human science. The case of medicine is complicated by its claim to demonstrate biological reality – so that individual illnesses can be identified as instances of some natural category which exists 'out there' independently of any local interests in which it appears embedded, our own included. The question recalls anthropology's debates, less as to whether *tabu* or segmentary alliance systems are categories which transcend local particularities, than whether sexual avoidance of close kin by non-human primates is homologous to incest prohibition or whether it is merely analogous, primate 'avoidance' then being an inappropriate extrapolation from our human concerns.

How culture-specific illnesses might stand for or reflect shared local experience remains controversial for the theorists, yet illnesses are commonly taken as emblematic of a group's predicaments by its own members. In 1734 the physician George Cheyne characterized *spleen* as 'the English malady'. In the next century 'American nervousness' was similarly identified: 'The chief and primary cause of the development and very rapid increase of nervousness is *modern civilisation*, which is distinguished from the ancient by these five characteristics: steam-power, the periodical press, the telegraph, the sciences, and the mental activity of women.'[2] Margaret Lock places the diagnosis of *bunmeibyo* ('disorders of civilisation') within contemporary Japanese uncertainties about Westernization, and Elaine Showalter proposes the hysterical woman as the Victorian exemplar through which changing gender relations were deployed and contested.[3] Nor are anthropologists themselves immune from proposing one or other medical drama as their own society's core dilemma: as Michael Kenny puts it, 'The current popularity of multiple personality is the product of the disorder of our times.'[4]

Perhaps the most developed arguments on the cultural specificity of psychopathology have concerned *latah*. In 1968 the anthropologist Hildred Geertz called attention to what she called the 'latah paradox': while this rich cultural phenomenon seemed 'tailor-made for the Javanese', she noted remarkably similar patterns in a variety of East Asian societies from Siberia to the Malay–Indonesian archipelago. How culturally specific was it then? Against medical explanations that latahs – women responding to minimal but conventionalized stimuli with exaggerated startles, passive obedience and obscenities, and with imitation of others' words and actions – were demonstrating a 'pre-psychological' (that is, a universal physiological) response, Geertz suggested it could be completely explained by Javanese concerns.[5] In reply, the cultural psychiatrist Ronald Simons argued from Malay instances that latah is a locally elicited expression of the mammalian capacity to startle, a potential on which a society can then elaborate additional features, out of which shared repertoire individual latahs, usually subdominant women, then develop their own characteristic pattern whether we take this as spontaneous or simulated. He noted similarities between obscenities in different societies and hypothesized that these were 'neurologically coded in some special way'.[6] Simons has been criticized in turn by psychodynamic commentators for ignoring the significance of teasing in Malay childrearing, while Kenny, arguing latah represents an inversion of the symbolic code, distinguishes his own emphasis on the 'culture-specific explanation of a meaning potential implicit in a limited human repertoire of concepts pertaining to order, disorder and self-identity' from Simons' 'culture-specific exploitation of a neurophysiological potential'.[7] Simons ripostes with a critique of the unverifiable nature of psychodynamic interpretations, and of the anthropological tendency to over-interpretation.[8] Against Kenny he quotes informants that almost anybody can be turned into a latah provided they are adequately teased, and argues that the pattern once established can then be elicited by a neutral stimulus quite independent of its situational meaning; and that anyway symbolic truths are more often elaborations of locally identified biological phenomena than anthropologists are prepared to admit.

As with other patterns of psychiatric interest, the latah question seems to me to be one of arguing how much the sensorimotor properties of an embodied 'natural symbol' such as the startle reflex may be said to constrain its meaning and deployment.[9] In much of comparative psychiatry it is difficult to propose convincingly any universal pattern, leading us to circular debates on the appropriate multivariate analysis of lists of 'symptoms' obtained in different societies in order to determine a presumed biological specification of the identified experience. Further problems come when a pattern seems to disappear from a society altogether – sometimes as with the phenomenon of multiple personality to then appear again – or else to transform itself into what we as observers take as a rather different pattern, a particular difficulty when professional Western medicine, the analytical procedure, itself becomes part of the local circumstances through which the pattern is reproduced. Thus the well-known 'rituals of rebellion' of southern Africa have been said by Loudon to be replaced among Zulu women by neurotic illnesses presenting to the medical clinic which, although they demonstrate a quite different context, experience, local response and observer's description, may be interpreted as articulating similar opposition and complementarity between the sexes (p. 26). Amok, once a standardized demonstration of retributive justice, has now become recognized in South East Asia as a purely medical question. What then remains our identified pattern? What aspect of it is considered to change, and what are the determinants of such change?[10]

Rather than assume that a salient 'pathology' necessarily presents an image of its society, we can start more modestly from the idea that where some general category of illness (or other loss of personal agency as in witchcraft accusations or latah) is locally recognized, this category is then deployed through the practical interests of experts, victims and others.[11] Social anthropology has turned from its earlier emphasis on the 'total social fact' as a given, to a recognition that institutions are constructed through instrumental actions, and that rather than take these actions as logically coherent reflections of the mores, mentalities or political structures of society at large, we might examine in finer detail how power is pursued by competing individuals and groups at particular historical moments.[12] And these two very different modes of thought – what we may term the structural (or for our medical colleagues perhaps the naturalistic) and the personalistic (or instrumental) – are not easily reconciled.

That society's patterns of illness are changing is frequently attributed to widespread political and economic changes, both by social scientists and the people themselves. New illnesses become emblematic of the new conditions of everyday life, of the loss of traditional values, the individual now being torn from established modes of adaptation and meaning and thrust into novel and bewildering circumstances. Contemporary women are seen to be particularly vulnerable to such changes, particularly where their accepted identity as a mother becomes eroded by an emphasis on smaller families, with many domestic occupations – caring for the sick and aged, food preparation, livestock rearing and small-scale production – now being carried out away from the household, and when responsibilities for nurturance and childcare may be taken over by professionals. Whether this is associated with a recognition of emerging new occupational and professional opportunities, or else with a restriction to an increasing passive but still domestic role, the wider changes are reflected in the woman's vulnerable body. What might otherwise be discussed in terms of moral change, of national identity, of changing patterns of economic power, now becomes read as individual diseases. As I have argued, in perhaps all societies women are located by common opinion so much more in their bodily nature – in their physiology, in childbearing, menstruation and the menopause; and their body itself is now seen as protesting against social changes at variance with its natural functioning.

In Japan, 'disorders of civilisation' (*bunmeibyo*) are recognized as problems of women and children relinquishing traditional role-bound norms and family obligations in transition to the more assertive and individualized personal values of apartment-bound nuclear families, a recent pattern generally seen as undesirable and disordered, though perhaps inevitable.[13] The popular media and the government in their encouragement of specialized clinics or educational programmes both take these illnesses as directly representing something unbalanced about contemporary Japanese society – the increasing emphasis placed on competitive educational achievement resulting in child suicide, bullying, the school refusal syndrome, and an increase in such childhood psychosomatic illnesses as asthma; the isolation of women alone in the household during the working day with its attendant pathologies of apartment neurosis, climacterium syndrome, kitchen syndrome, moving-day depression; while children themselves now increasingly assault their parents and are referred for psychological guidance. 'A floating generation, without any sense of purpose,' as one Japanese newspaper puts it, 'and the real problem lies in the family.'[14]

Margaret Lock has described how the Ministry of Health and Welfare in Japan has collaborated with the medical profession in enlisting the media to popularize new educational and health programmes for 'neurosis and other stress-related problems'. Such new syndromes do not necessarily have an

accepted immediate precipitant – and the treatment for a particular
condition may variously include pharmaceutical drugs, personal counselling or group and family therapy – yet close links are invoked between the
individual illness and changes in the traditional extended family,
particularly a loss of contact with nature in a now heavily urbanized
society. Lock argues that there seems a doctors' uncertainty about whether
women should be seen as the victims of economic changes and the
resulting absence from the household of their work-obsessed husbands, or
whether they themselves are the perpetrators, reducing their men to the
status of children, compulsively shopping and watching television,
addicted to drinking and smoking, and generally treating their bodies as
a personal possession rather than as the communal vehicle for leaving
descendants. It is the middle-aged woman who is particularly vulnerable –
or guilty: her menopausal syndrome is the product of boredom and
selfishness, of her lack of willpower and of that capacity to endure which
was so characteristic of her mother: 'The roots of even a healthy plant will
rot if given too much water.'[15] Lock suggests that the family, always a
central element in Japanese identity, seems the most accessible place to
confront wider disputes about the Western contamination of Japanese
society, and the ambivalent relationship between the West and an
economically strong but culturally and politically non-assertive Japan.[16]
As she sardonically points out, the menopausal syndrome is indeed a
problem of unemployment, not perhaps among the married women
patients with grown-up children but for male gynaecologists: she notes that
50 per cent of Japanese women are in paid employment and these are as
likely to consult doctors for menopausal symptoms as any listless
housewife.

Eating disorders are a group of 'new' illnesses which are still rarely
recognized by psychiatrists in developing societies, but which are now
increasingly common in Western societies and have recently appeared in
Japan and among non-European migrants to the West. And 'modernity'
has been generally argued as a salient cause. Personal struggles to redefine
woman's identity in a changing world, as well as the background social and
economic changes themselves, have been argued as relevant to *bulimia*
(purging after bout eating) and *anorexia nervosa* (self-starvation). The first
argument is put forward by family therapists as one way of making sense of
eating disorders as an instrumental but not planned strategy available to
young women in certain family situations; the second, favoured by
academic psychiatrists, explains (or restates) historical and geographical
variation as causal. If any Western illness is recognized by clinical
psychiatrists as a culture-bound or a culture-change syndrome, it is
anorexia.[17] As psychiatry generally takes 'culture' as a cause of illness only
for 'other cultures', the wider aspects of 'Western culture' tend to be

neglected when looking at European patients, in favour of taking more easily measured 'risk factors' as significant and changeable: in the case of eating disorders, the focus is on the social pressures on contemporary European women to diet.[18] This makes sense if one is predicting variation (rather than determining aetiology) within one particular culture, but runs into difficulties when one attempts to compare cultures in a fuller picture of the background and possible cross-cultural universality of a biosocial pattern.

To take a particular society with its distinctive pattern of psychopathology – eating disorders – and then argue that 'the cause' is simply the most immediate aspect of everyday life to which it appears to have a formal relationship – dieting – is partial. Is dieting the ultimate cause or is it itself the symptom of something perhaps more socially fundamental? If eating disorders are simply one end of a Western norm – female dieting taken too far – then we would not expect to find anything like them in societies where there are no pressures on women to diet. And we would perhaps expect such patterns to be fairly self-limiting, reflexively dependent on shared assumptions about acceptable dieting and the means to achieve it.[19] Let us examine these questions in a little more detail.

Social causality or instrumental action?

Anorexia nervosa was first described in France, Britain and Russia in the nineteenth century, particularly among young women of the emerging middle class. Like bulimia nervosa, it has been commonly argued to be highly specific to Western and other industrialized societies where the incidence of both is still rising.[20] It differs from the other patterns I have considered in resulting in more obvious biological changes: in endocrine status, serum proteins, the cessation of menstrual periods and involuntary infertility, and an altered pattern of body hair. After some years of debate these are now usually agreed to be the consequence not the cause of a 'fear of fatness' (the subjective exaggeration of one's own weight and size with consequent self-starvation).

The incidence of the pattern parallels culture-bound (and indeed class-bound) ideals of female body imagery, and the major cause factor argued for both anorexia and bulimia is the contemporary social pressure on young women to be slimmer than women in other societies (and slimmer than Western women of an earlier period), whether the response takes the form of severe restriction of food intake and consequent loss of weight and cessation of menstrual periods (anorexia nervosa) or of keeping to a more conventional weight with episodes of binge eating followed soon after by vomiting and purging (bulimia). The pattern is taken less as an intended action than as a local norm taken too far, just as the *dhat* syndrome was taken as an over-enthusiasm for Hindu preoccupations with health and semen retention (p. 17). Against a background of an increasing average weight, particularly in women, and a nutritionally determined earlier sexual maturation in Western populations, social expectations on women to be slimmer than average have grown in the course of the twentieth century. The very word 'weight' is now no neutral measure but denotes 'too much weight'. Slimness in both men and women signifies beauty, youth, health and self-control: even young children have been found to dislike 'obese' body shapes, with girls having more concerns about their own shape and weight than do boys. Dieting in response to this is recognized as the route into eating disorders, yet it is virtually ubiquitous among young English and American women, and is now becoming increasingly common among girls below the age of puberty.[21]

By the mid-1980s, the top four British slimming magazines alone had a joint circulation of over 650,000. Dieting has been promoted by an industry that provides an extensive range of low-energy food products and vitamin supplements to facilitate slimming, reinforced by extensive medical publicity on the dangers of obesity.[22] Body morphology in all societies is deployed to reflect core social values, and in the West this has become medicalized, arguably to a greater extent in the last twenty years where for both sexes the trim body recalls entrepreneurial self-sufficiency and personal autonomy, and where the 'overweight' may be refused medical treatment.

Contemporary dietary management emerged from a medieval theology of the flesh which avoided indulgence, through moralistic medicine to an applied science of the 'efficient body' in which, with consumerism, desire is now to be promoted rather than regulated. In a Swedish survey,[23] 72 per cent of young women felt that they had been fat at some time, compared with 34 per cent of the men; and twice as many women as men attributed their own excess of weight to 'weak character'. In a similar study in the United States, twice as many girls as boys perceived themselves as overweight; the girls were dissatisfied with their weight because they equated slimness with beauty. Women's self-identity is more closely tied to their appearance than is men's.[24]

Eating disorders are commonly identified among women whose professional role directly employs conventional beauty (but not sexual activity) and thus slimness and dieting: particularly models, actresses and dancers, among whom the incidence of anorexia has been estimated at perhaps 10 per cent.[25] Contemporary Western women may 'possess' their bodies phenomenologically but they do not 'own' them. Ritenbaugh[26] argues that while female fatness (and thus fertility) have generally been associated for women as marketable assets, the image of personal control is now the commodifiable advantage.

There are immediate pragmatic reasons for striving to achieve slimness. Excess weight is more of a professional handicap to women than it is to men, and successful business women (and indeed the wives of successful men) are rarely 'overweight'.[27] Women are more harshly penalized for failing to achieve slenderness for they are more likely to be denied or granted access to social advantage on the basis of physical appearance: obese schoolgirls are less likely than their slender peers to be accepted for colleges despite comparable qualifications, and women in Britain have lost their jobs for being 'overweight'.[28] 'A woman increases her market value by being slender'; thinness is associated with upward social mobility, while fatness is the sign of 'ethnic minority status'.[29] The reverse transformation – from the pragmatic into the symbolic – is illustrated by the 'fairy tale wedding' of Diana, Princess of Wales, who as an ethereal young bride was hailed as a role model for British girls – in contrast to the average weight of another young woman marrying into the royal household soon afterwards who acquired a less important prince and was immediately criticized in the press as being too fat. In her period of popularity in the 1980s slimming contests featured 'look-alike Princess Di's' as the winners were dressed, coiffured and photographed like the princess: readers of the *Daily Mail* were challenged to tell the difference. If the princess herself was later revealed as clinically anorexic, the earlier message had been clear – self-starvation enabled a young woman with few other assets to become a real princess.[30]

It has been suggested that the contemporary ideal of female thinness is the consequence of various changes: economic and public health changes associated with industrialization in the nineteenth and twentieth centuries, leading to improved nutrition, earlier menstruation and lower mortality rates but reduced fertility[31] and thus less emphasis on women's maternal and domestic identity; an increase of women in the labour market competing against men; with the assumption of social equality – and perhaps identity – with men, and thus a different 'fit' between social role, class and body shape; and possibly a related shift in male preference for an infertile, androgynous and 'younger' morphology in sexual partners.[32] The currently preferred sex object for Western men is slender; a fuller figure can imply sexuality but only through pregnancy, and contemporary Western men appear to be less attracted to pregnant women than their forefathers even as traditional prohibitions on sex in pregnancy have faded away. Social and sexual maturity are not synchronous; and the ambiguities of adolescence mark contemporary schoolchildren as sexually but not socially 'mature'. If plumper girls are seen as more sexually mature, the male choice of sex object has become increasingly passive and infantile – baby-faced and long-legged with shaven armpits, a paedomorphous doll.[33] There are requirements for women to diet and otherwise modify the appearance of their body in order to gain access to employment and to educational and economic resources: as the Duchess of Windsor memorably remarked and embroidered on her cushions, 'One cannot be too rich or too thin.'

In contrast, for women in many non-industrialized societies, plumpness, whilst actually rarer than in the West, still connotes success, prosperity and health.[34] A common anthropological assumption is that in contexts where there is uncertainty about the survival of children and about continuing security of food resources, larger fat deposits in women become the index of family fertility, indeed its practical precondition, and are thus a general personal goal by themselves and their relatives, and a significant factor in the selection of marital partner by spouses and their families.[35] In societies where marriage is a major economic transaction between established groups of kin on both sides, and the principal mode of redistributing durable resources, the woman's body directly represents the wealth of her family and a guarantee of the survival of any future children, and perhaps of the group itself.[36] And thus of her own identity as a woman and mother. Certainly, accounts of eating disorders from non-Western cultures or less-industrialized European areas are relatively uncommon, and then typically among the daughters of the urban elite.[37]

Is severe personal restriction of food intake then simply a statistical reflection of economic roles with better health and reliable access to food threatening overpopulation, the preference by men for less fertile women being some sort of biosocial adaptation? Recently we have had access to personal accounts of self-starvation in medieval and early modern Europe which seem to describe struggles for empowerment and autonomy in a context where women were still valued as mothers and food providers, yet simultaneously devalued as physically and emotionally greedy, lacking in self-control and polluting. Self-starvation occurred in situations where some limited autonomy was possible, and where fasting and asceticism already provided circumscribed routes to an identity which was independent of the domestic sphere – in enclosed religious orders.[38] Such autonomy seems to have been sought (perhaps deliberately) by women taking control of the only thing over which they had immediate power – their bodies – and thus their sexuality, against the assumption of their usual physical embodiment. While we must interpret earlier parallels with care, not reading back into the past our current concerns, remarkably similar accounts come from contemporary rural Portugal.[39]

As with other patterns we cannot expect to find any neat one-to-one equivalence between expected norm and personal subjectivity, for societies are not homogeneous assemblies of identical assumptions, and everyday life is lived strategically. Anorexia itself seems to articulate a profound contemporary ambiguity about women's public roles and their sexuality in industrialized societies. *Working Woman*, a glossy magazine aimed at would-be professional women in the 1980s, was illustrated with photographs of elegant and young (but not that young) women in female versions of male business suits. It offered advice on how to succeed in the office through ambiguously coupled maxims: 'Forswear sex in the office' but 'Use sex all you can'; 'Don't be feminine' yet 'Be feminine'.[40] Recent feminist accounts of eating disorders postulate similar personal ambiguities, often over adolescent entry into an apparently more autonomous yet conflictual female identity;[41] anorexic girls are often described as having previously been 'tomboys'.

Boskind-Lodahl takes issue with the common psychoanalytic interpretation of anorexia – a rejection of adult femininity and sexuality, manifesting as fear of oral impregnation.[42] Rather than a rejection of femininity, she suggests that the determined pursuit of thinness by an adolescent girl constitutes an exaggerated striving to achieve femininity – but not physical sexuality. Attempts to control her physical appearance demonstrate a concern with pleasing others, particularly men. Boskind-Lodahl points out that anorexics devote their lives to fulfilling feminine ideals and that case histories of patients indicate that they had been rewarded by their families for their physical attractiveness and submissive 'goodness', whilst characteristics such as independence, self-reliance and assertiveness were generally devalued. A drive towards perfection in physical appearance was often matched by an attempt towards academic achievement with the aim of pleasing parents (and implicitly potential husbands and employers). For anorexics are correct in assuming that to have a fat body is to court male rejection – and thus loss of access to power.

What's in it for the family? That anorexics frequently come from all girl sibships and tend to start their menstrual periods early, and that their mothers are described as career-orientated and domineering, have been used to argue that the reaction can serve to maintain the existing sexual and generational structure of the family.[43] Functional aspects of anorexia have been discerned in the context of the family, particularly as a means of avoiding overt parental separation – where the adolescent girl is threatened with extrusion as a daughter. Family therapists describe a household pattern in which the parental couple appear united, the parents submerging their conflicts in jointly protecting or blaming the anorexic daughter whose illness is identified as the only problem:

> In several such families the parents required that the children reassured them that they were good parents, or join them in worrying about the family. In most cases parental concern absorbed the couple so that all signs of marital strife or even minor differences were suppressed or ignored.[44]

In a third of one series of families studied, parental separation had been openly threatened: 'The exclusion implied in refusal to eat is a threat to the parents' capacity as nutritional agents, a role which is always an important measure of a parental function and in many of these families, central to their value system.' Through the illness the young woman remains a child:

> Within the context of her mounting panic at the prospect of her parents' marriage breaking up, her dieting quickly escalated, seeming suddenly easy and relieving to her and, as anorexia nervosa supervened, her father and mother were reunited in their unwritten contract together to care for her until she 'grew up'.[45]

Given the ambivalent relationship between anorexia and contemporary female identity, it is perhaps not surprising that its apparent converse, obesity, has also been recently described as a culture-bound syndrome.[46] Half the adult population of the United States are medically obese: simultaneously physical ugliness and a moral failing (indulgence, lack of control, the consumption of limited world resources).[47] A study of the life experiences of fatter women suggests that both men and women see them as unfeminine, in flight from sexuality, or on occasion as sexual in some quite perverse way, as incestuous, erotically out of control or sexually dominant.[48] While obesity seems to represent a clear inversion of core values, any instrumental value for the individual is less clear. The women's movement has recognized the pressure on women to slim as an internalization of male dominance,[49] and it may well be that confronting male and parental demands for slimness affords wives and daughters a demonstration of autonomy:

> By this time I was eating steadily, doggedly, stubbornly, anything I could get. The war between myself and my mother was on in earnest; the disputed territory was my body ... I swelled visibly, relentlessly before her very eyes. I rose like dough, my body advanced inch by inch towards her across the dining room table, in this at least I was undefeated ... It was a sort of fashion show, in reverse.[50]

Obesity is often experienced as a sort of uncontrolled consumption, as 'unconscious stealing', an irrational loss of control, or else as a rebellion against parents and partners.[51] Indeed, obesity and anorexia nervosa are perhaps more similar than might appear. In different ways, both offer to dominant parents and to men the threat of a desexualized social caricature of woman's public role.[52] If male/female relations are articulated through an interest in female morphology, then weight is the one aspect which can be most easily negotiated. Women start by being regarded as 'out of control' by men; they accept that it is through a control over their body which often involves pain and elaborate discomfort, sometimes danger – through sleeping in curlers, depilation, ear-piercing, face lifts, liposuction, breast implants, corsets, high heels, self-painting, massage machines, the deployment of hair pieces, false eyelashes and nails, contact lenses – that they achieve relationships with men.[53]

And the choice becomes objectified, as their nature, the way women imagine themselves. If women 'possess' their bodies, they do not 'own' them; as John Berger puts it, 'Men look at women. Women watch themselves being looked at. This determines not only most relations between men and women but also the relation of women to themselves. The surveyor of woman in herself is male.'[54] The self-denying struggle against fatness becomes an achievement of will, of providing some subjective control,[55] while serving at the same time as an instrumental strategy in negotiating autonomy with others: a strategy which, when successful, is likely to reinforce the original self-denial. Unlike the descriptive psychiatric perspective which emphasizes social expectations like dieting as causal (the 'push' factor),[56] these interpretations, like those of other feminist critiques of psychiatry[57] argue for individual moral agency and hence some albeit limited personal responsibility (the 'pull' factor); political *action for* rather than the clinical *as a consequence*; the illness is then to be regarded less as the simple manifestation of shared ideal norms than as a discrete instrumentality which both acts within them and generates them. Leslie Swartz suggests that the medical emphasis on 'push' factors in eating disorders is in part because these can be more easily quantified scientifically.[58]

It is not then that psychiatric theories of eating disorders are more or less accurate external descriptions: medicine itself is part of the context in which they occur.[59] Indeed psychiatry articulates in immediate situations of power precisely those ambiguities about women's bodies and autonomy which as a treatment it attempts to resolve. Western societies have always offered a model of female self-denial and extreme asceticism which only became medicalized in the nineteenth century.[60] From interpretation of the subjective understandings of contemporary anorexics, Banks suggests that the characteristic 'fear of fatness' is actually the doctor's medical (and male) preoccupation; women have always sought pathways to self-definition which we might term ascetic, which refused domestic and maternal duties, but which eventually have become medicalized as an end in themselves through others' framing matters in terms of health and sickness. We might argue for a parallel with intense religious experience with its emphasis on ecstatic transcendence – both of one's increasingly ethereal body and others' demands – very similar to the sense of freedom and self-control which is experienced in eating disorders.[61] With changing valorization of the body since the nineteenth century as now 'self-sufficient', yet at the same time increasingly vulnerable through inappropriate personal choices of nutrition and health care in a situation of potentially unlimited consumption (and hence the historically unlikely possibility of motivated restriction of food intake), eating disorders may be said to offer an alternative to other bodily patterns of communicating distress and redefining personal identities among Western women such as religious ascetism, possession states and hysteria.[62]

Modernity: culture or culture change?

How much can we distinguish practically individual subjectivity and intention from the social meanings and constraints which make them possible? Indeed can the principal actors themselves? Those societies which do have high rates of eating disorders may be characterized through their relative wealth, industrialization, urbanization, literacy, lower fertility and mortality rates, later age of marriage, the absence of prescriptive marriage patterns,[63] often a recent development of nationalism,[64] and a more immediate relationship with the world economic and cultural system than do non-industrialized societies. One rather generalized characteristic which has attracted particular attention, given the Western emphasis on the role of autonomy and self-control in eating disorders, has been what may be termed 'modernity'. 'Modernization' theorists argue that there has been a distinct historical shift, driven by technological developments, in social organization and in marriage and family life: away from personal status determined by kinship or other group membership to more universalized and individualized roles, and thus to an earlier and more complete independence of children from their parents; to greater geographical and social mobility; to less ascription of social position through caste, kinship or gender; together with literacy, tolerance, secularization and cultural pluralism, and with greater subjective self-determination and self-awareness; and with the separation and decontextualization of what we may distinguish as the once enmeshed domains of economics, politics and religion.[65]

Crude distinctions such as 'social-centred' versus 'ego-centred' cultures (or *gemeinschaft* versus *gesellschaft*, or earlier 'primitive' versus 'European') have continued to dog the human sciences since their nineteenth-century origins, and any such distinction has to be used with care, so as not to distinguish societies as homogeneously one or the other but to characterize a general individual shift from social norms to personal goals, to an acknowledgement of personal self-interest and self-reliance, and to a greater experience of personal choice over actions through a plurality of values (or indeed the absence of them), with the body as the self-sufficient locus of personal experience.[66] Again we have to be careful with distinguishing internal experience from external analysis: we cannot determine that in one society people objectively act in their self-interest *more* than in another, particularly in the case of illness, for personal choice and social values always reciprocally interact. While human experience is as biosocially constrained as it is instrumentally chosen, people's own conceptualizations may variously develop such notions as 'self-sufficiency' or the 'vulnerabilities of women'. All actions take place within the possible cultural worlds. What we can say, however, is that in some societies it is accepted that individuals seem to choose from a wider variety of fundamentally different alternatives than in others, in important aspects of their life. This is not to argue that the people we identify as at one or other end of our spectrum always do the same; for in an increasingly pluralistic world, individuals may seem to move, in different situations and at different speeds, towards the 'modern' without assuming all its characteristics are inherently interrelated.[67] Certain religious movements excepted, we might argue that the contemporary shift tends to be in this direction, one which is closely correlated with the flexible roles demanded by industrial capitalism.[68]

The obvious way to examine the relative balance of cultural subjectivity against causal modernization in eating disorders is to look at individual women from developing countries who are migrating to Western societies or women in societies which are rapidly undergoing industrialization and urbanization. Rather than compare one society with another rather different one (with all the usual problems of ensuring that terms in quite different languages have some sort of equivalence of meaning), we can look at the experience of those who can be said to participate in two different but not altogether unrelated societies as in the situation of Hasmat (page ix in the Preface).[69] I recall another young woman from Bangladesh in whose mother's line there was a tradition of spirit possession. In one still rather vague episode, she had become possessed after a sexual advance from an uncle. Two years later, at the age of 18, after migration to Britain, she was admitted to hospital with a 'hysterical crisis' after being accused of having a lover. Change in any pattern of illness towards that found in another society may be due to direct adoption of a distinct and recognized pattern, or through acculturation of the population during migration or increased cultural contact, or it may be a parallel development as part of similar underlying political and socio-economic changes. Earlier studies in the United States with non-European minorities, whether established communities or recently arrived immigrants, have found, relative to the European majority, a less negative conception of fatness,[70] less preoccupation with losing weight, and fewer eating disorders.[71] There is, however, some evidence that these differences may now be disappearing, perhaps with acculturation to the majority culture and thus to the dominant values of women's shapes.[72]

Given the variation in the occurrence of eating disorders, are these comparative studies talking about the same thing, some reasonably coherent pattern? Two studies which used Western questionnaires to look at personal accounts of eating and weight loss suggest that the pattern of 'illness' in the Third World is very similar to that found in European populations.[73] By contrast, doctors in Hong Kong and India report that the characteristic Western 'fear of fatness' and distorted image of one's body are absent among people whose self-starvation would otherwise be categorized as anorexic,[74] and it has been suggested that Western diagnostic terms can only be applied across cultures if we recognize that eating disorders have no such core features.[75] 'Self-starvation' is then perhaps a more appropriate term than anorexia nervosa. However, a study from Pakistan has argued that eating disorders can be considered 'culture-bound' only in that they specifically follow a concern with dieting, and that any other associated factors of 'Westernisation' are incidental.[76]

Studies of immigrant populations in Europe suggest that eating disorders are no longer limited to those of European origin. An even higher proportion of Egyptian women students in London have positive scores on a questionnaire which looks at abnormal attitudes to eating than do comparable Europeans, and they also have more symptoms, while British women of South Asian origin attending a family planning clinic have more 'disturbed eating attitudes' than do European women, and British Asian schoolgirls are more likely to have bulimia than are White schoolgirls.[77] Among British Asians, high scores on the usual questionnaires have been said to be associated with 'traditional', pre-modern cultural notions of female autonomy which lead to greater conflict between Westernized girls and their more traditional families, a conclusion which others have found unjustified.[78] Thus anorexia nervosa may be less some culture-specific pattern directly reflecting 'modern' dilemmas for women than a move towards them – a 'culture-change syndrome of modernising societies' as it has been called.[79] While any culture, and thus any culture-change, allows access to new patterns of distress for a group as a whole, it is in immediate personal contexts that individuals select, consciously or otherwise, these patterns.[80] If established and publically recognized restrictions on young women's autonomy were essential to eating disorders irrespective of the possibility of challenge, we would expect a lower incidence in 'modern' contexts, the reverse of the epidemiological evidence.

The 'culture-change' argument diminishes the value of using migration to look at the cultural context of eating disorders. Not only do we have a transition from one available pattern of expressing distress to another, but the very availability of the second itself may become the occasion for expressing distress. 'Intergenerational conflict' is of course hardly culture-specific but we might expect that if close-knit family groups are moving as a whole to values characterized by greater personal autonomy, then their children educated in Britain are more likely to define themselves sooner through these values than are their parents, and the family is the most likely place for disagreements about their acceptability. Again, it is important to distinguish this analytical argument from the popular stereotype of the South Asian family *as one* which stifles the individual, although that may well be how it is seen by some within it when contrasting two reified sets of values;[81] it is certainly described by individuals themselves as the immediate precipitant of overdoses, thence to be assumed by doctors as causal.[82]

When a pathology identified by doctors closely follows everyday cultural imagery, as seems true for eating disorders, there are problems of definition and comparison. Identification of patients and pathologies is dependent on local recognition and selection, and patterns considered pathological from the medical perspective may be locally incorporated into shared values, as in licensed ascetism or extended periods of fasting in South Asia or in dietary restriction among dancers and models in Britain. Ulrike Schmidt, Neelam Bakshi and I attempted to examine the contours of the pattern in the general population: in particular any associations between a complex of 'modernisation' and the conceptions of the body in a group of young Indians in Jaipur, Asian Britons, and White Britons in London, both male and female. We used a Western questionnaire which rates 'bulimic symptoms' and also asked questions about family choice between 'traditional' and 'modern' activities and concepts of family relationships, particularly about women's autonomy.[83] At a high level of generality, Europeans and South Asians (particularly in North India) can be said to have once shared a similar Eurasian social order and family organization,[84] and 'Westernisation' – the commonly used term may be a misnomer, for certain 'Western' groups from rural Southern Europe are less 'modern' than the urban bourgeoisie of developing countries. The average body mass index – the conventional measure of 'fatness' – was highest among Jaipur men, then Jaipur women, Asian British men, Asian British women, White British men, and least among White British women. The proportion who said they were actually unhappy with this – around 20 per cent – did not differ significantly across the groups. As in other studies, White women were significantly less satisfied with their body shape than were their male counterparts, but Jaipur women estimated themselves as less fat than they were compared with the other women. Symptoms of eating disorders were most common among Asian women in Britain, closely followed by White British women, Jaipur men and women, with Asian British men and White

British men having least. As might be expected, families in India were
significantly 'less modern' than their Asian British counterparts, and there
was an association between symptoms and personal modernization for the
Asian Britons.

Such questionnaire studies are easy to do but rather limited: the sample
size is usually fairly small, and students – the most accessible experimental
subjects for academics – are hardly the best group to demonstrate local
'cultural' norms: higher education facilitates the confronting of cultural
differences from a more distanced perspective, including the very notion of
'culture'.[85] Yet the measures used, both in general design and in specific
questions – such as about 'body shape' – could hardly have the same
meaning in all three groups; this cannot be avoided in any cross-cultural
comparison.[86] One item conventionally used in Western questionnaires as
a measure of pathology – fasting for a day – might reasonably be considered
to have quite a different local meaning in India.

Nonetheless, this study certainly shows no inevitable association across
cultures between the ideals of personal shape and what doctors would
recognize as eating disorders. Young Indians, who were generally thinner
than British Asians and British Whites, would actually have liked to weigh
more than they did. Thus, the attempt to lose weight, the major
determinant argued by doctors for eating disorders in Western populations,
was absent, yet their 'symptomatology' was similar; in Jaipur men and
women both had more bulimic tendencies than did White men in London.
Thus the urge to purge or vomit after eating seems not uncommon in
North India, but it appears distinct from any concern with body image.[87]
This might suggest that we might regard vomiting and purging in South
Asia as an action motivated by something other than an avoidance of
fatness.[88]

In broader terms, the study is consistent with the idea that eating
disorders are indeed available to women in Western contexts in part
through shared assumptions of morphological norms, whatever their own
cultural origin. While British Asians as a whole appear more 'modern' than
their middle-class Indian counterparts, the extent of family modernization
as determined by questionnaires does not, however, fit neatly with bulimic
eating patterns; although the bulimic inventory did demonstrate high
scores for those with 'non-traditional' personal norms.[89] Given the
increasing frequency of bulimia in Asian Britons, as reported from clinics,
can we particularize any social or cultural associations apart from a concern
with personal 'body shape'? A recent British study which compared people
who developed bulimia when young with those who developed it later
found that they were more often from minority cultural backgrounds – of
many different sorts,[90] suggesting that being 'culturally different' in the
West, irrespective of the particular culture of origin or of modernization,

may be significant. According to the culture change model of eating disorders, it is simply migrant populations undergoing rapid social transitions who may be particularly vulnerable to developing eating disorders when coming to the West. However, the social and personal processes leading to the development of an eating disorder may be quite different in recent immigrants and in their children: that there is some biosocial 'final common path' which is culturally available, in part through popular values represented in medical practice, is not to say that the preceding cultural constraints are necessarily invariant.[91]

Self-renunciation without modernization

To what extent can we argue for the instrumentality of eating restriction as a pragmatic way of self-determination? Declining food is a common sign of being unwell in any society and thus a culturally meaningful mode of expressing immediate distress and constraining others, particularly parents, especially in contexts where past nurturance and current family solidarity are demonstrated through the consumption of shared food prepared and distributed by women. And these actions become increasingly routinized and less flexible in part through the physiological consequences of self-starvation. However, we might consider the extent to which the cultural pre-conditions for 'non-modern ascetic self-starvation' outlined above (p. 82) hold for North Indian societies.[92]

Among North Indian Hindus, higher status for both men and women is traditionally associated with early marriage, hypergamy (marriage 'up' the social ladder) for women, differential female infant survival, larger dowries, infrequent divorce, with less female autonomy for women, and with chastity in marriage and rigorous religious observance, with frequent individual fasting and a vegetarian diet.[93] All these are arguably 'non-modern' characteristics. As in China, plumpness in women is valued, and food, health and sexuality are associated together through a number of popular medical understandings.[94] Cooking for others is a valued service, and while avoidance of particular foods is a measure of caste and status, it is also associated more informally with celibacy, religious asceticism and studying; fasting is recognized as a discreet way of avoiding associations with others, particularly if personal ritual or physical 'impurity' is suspected in oneself or in one's family by others.[95] 'Bodily purity' and 'spirituality' are associated together, both dependent on the readiness to accept family values and obligations;[96] the greater the presumed risk of women losing such purity, the greater the demands for bodily purification including self-denial and asceticism.[97] Related groups of women may fast together often, taking on and discharging impurity on behalf of their joint family; decisions to do this are determined by current relationships within the family. In a wider secular context, the use of public fasting to coerce others is an established political manoeuvre in India.

Despite modernization, local paradigms of experience and self-identity for Hindu women draw on powerful mythological images which in turn 'reflect the nature of an individual's interpersonal bonds within [her] family'.[98] Assumptions of 'devotion, forbearance and passivity' are manifest through shared images of renunciation and self-denial, often of retribution against others through self-immolation.[99] Suspected betrayal of family or group values through seeking inappropriate independence may be redeemed by young women through bodily trials to demonstrate female purity – as in the familiar instance of Sita in the Ramayana.[100] In the patrilineal joint family, these images of women are enacted in an accepted social and physical inferiority and thus dependence. Adult women recognize themselves as prone to pollution, a situation which can be mitigated in part through seclusion, continued virginity or asceticism, or more conventionally through maternity.[101] While no simple equivalence between rural and urban India can be argued, these ambivalent images and expectations persist and are reframed in secularized professional families, even in the context of overseas study or migration.[102] Indeed, it has been suggested that in India restrictions on women's autonomy may actually increase with the family's affluence, as these same families seek higher education for their daughters[103] as a dowry-equivalent. The experience of the self in North India, particularly for women, has been described by Indian psychoanalysts as one of overt passivity in relation to others.[104] The Hindu self, Bharati argues, is not the primary basis for existence and its practical autonomy is devalued.[105] (By contrast, we might take the Muslim self as somewhat more 'referential', universalized and individualized through monotheism.) Parallels may thus be argued with possession states, suicide and parasuicide as attempts to constrain others, whether practically or as fantasized retribution, and which closely follow the accepted models of self-renunciation. Actual suicide is reportedly seven times more common among Indian Hindus than Muslims and, compared with Europe, is more common among women and among young adults. It is more frequent in joint than in nuclear families and is locally attributed by doctors to 'the monster of family tensions'.[106] It is perhaps this pattern of constraining others through dramatic self-renunciation rather than specific attitudes to the ideal body which seems to continue in female South Asian emigrants.[107]

Without detailed studies of Indian ethnopsychologies, gender power, female sexuality, body symbolism and eating patterns, and their transformations, of the type we have developed over the last few years in the West, and in the absence of information on the expression, recognition and consequences of personal distress, it would be inappropriate to draw any general conclusions, but a common theme appears that, as in Europe, it is through bodily renunciation that South Asian women (particularly Hindus) can achieve relative autonomy, or at least resolve ambivalent demands. We cannot presume that the final common path of self-starvation with its biological consequences is reached in India or in Britain by the identical antecedents. At a high level of generality we might argue for analogous attempts at subjective and objective renunciations, and thus a form of limited 'power of the weak' through extreme personal self-denial. And that it is precisely in the ambiguous shift to 'modernisation' with the loss of other strategies of personal resistance and with the ubiquity of unlimited but personally restricted consumption, and in the context of a medicalized emphasis on the self-sufficient body as the locus of personal identity, that these become heightened.

6. Mimesis: The Perverse Masculinity of the Domestic Siege

> When a man injures his enemy, there is nothing to be pitied either in his act or in his intention, except that suffering is inflicted on another person. Nor is there when each person is indifferent to the other. But if the suffering involves those who are already close to one another, when for example a brother kills his brother, a son his father, a mother her son, or a son his mother – whether such an action is imagined or performed – then we have a situation of the kind [which especially arouses pity in others].
>
> Aristotle, *Poetics*

I noted earlier that the Butterfly/Serpent model is most applicable to situations where a permanently disadvantaged group – women, young men – are even further extruded from demonstrating agency. It was proposed then that the individual patterns are institutionalized, representing certain core antagonisms in a society. Clearly this does not meet all the instances where individuals are diagnosed as mentally ill or psychopathic in Western societies. In the next two chapters I consider the case of men, particularly how their recourse to violence or threatened violence may become standardized as a 'pathology'.

At a high level of generality, close parallels obtain between certain non-European culture-specific patterns (such as involuntary spirit possession) and such Euro-American patterns as drug overdoses, shoplifting, baby-snatching, hysterical conversion, multiple personality disorder, Munchausen's Syndrome by Proxy, post-traumatic stress disorder, loin pain haematuria or other idioms of distress which employ acute pain, agoraphobic crises and, more typically among men, threatened violence including sexual exhibitionism, public threats to kill oneself or to injure one's children. I have emphasized in Chapter 3 the time-limited quality of these patterns as dramatic demonstrations of local understandings of everyday distress and sickness, but such 'staging' is less relevant to chronic pain and such disability syndromes as Gulf War Syndrome, myalgic encephalomyelitis (post-viral fatigue syndrome) or to eating disorders and depression, although these, just like food refusal by young adults, may perform a similar instrumental function (Chapter 5). Grouping together in this way such disparate patterns does not argue for an over-extended and psychiatric reading of all standardized expressive behaviours (for any socially disturbing pattern may be interpreted through a medical focus); rather it endeavours to situate these patterns within an analytical framework in which medical, jural or religious meanings themselves variously allow local recognition of moral agency to be affirmed and contested in immediate situations.

The overwhelming majority of the classical 'culture-bound syndromes' in small-scale non-literate societies describe women as the usual protagonists, and in urbanized societies the majority of psychological distress is reported by women. As a number of commentators on gender and mental health have observed, in situations of socially disruptive action, European women may be identified as subdominant and sick, and hence not responsible, while under analogous circumstances adult men are taken as malicious and responsible; and this distinction is often codified in various medico-legal categories such as infanticide in Britain, where presumptions of altered physiology allow the distressed woman exculpation and restitution. Except in the limited number of instances where we can standardize both pattern and response, it is, however, difficult to define these 'analogous circumstances', for it is generally women who shoplift or threaten to kill themselves, men who housebreak or threaten to kill others. Gender disparities are located not just in social response (as in the concept of infanticide) but in people's own self-ascription and in the potential actions they find available – and perhaps ultimately in their genetics.[1] My very general model allows a number of patterns to be compared, within which gender or other such ascriptions already play a part, without criminalizing men or medicalizing women. Such an explanatory framework incorporates both the local ambiguities of 'intention' and the immediate consequences for others.

Many of the male patterns described as culture-specific syndromes certainly do involve threatened or actual violence to others, such as *negi-negi* and *amok*, so that Simons and Hughes in their book on culture-specific syndromes[2] argue these patterns should be placed together as a single 'sudden mass assault taxon'. While psychiatric interest in amok has focused on completed violence (in part because of its exotic salience, in part because in colonial societies it was these instances which were likely to come to the notice of the legal and medical authorities), its adaptive potential for the individual probably lies in the negotiation of sometimes only implicit violence as a potential sanction. In other words, any instrumentality of amok lies in threat not in completion, for the death of the principal and others in a completed amok makes it rather unlikely as a means of everyday social 'functioning': except, as sometimes in completed suicide in Western countries, as posthumous redemption or retributive fantasy,[3] similar to the not dissimilar Rajput *jauhar* when defeated men killed their women and children to deny them to an enemy and save them from rape or torture.[4]

Yet it is only through the occasional recourse to actual violence that threatened amok can attain any social power as a strategy of everyday negotiation. 'Successful' reactions thus only work through the occurrence of the rarer ones which 'failed' (from an everyday adaptive perspective), but, as we have argued above, it is not possible to determine empirically the extent to which a particular negotiation *is* strategically anticipated by the protagonist (say, denying resources to competitors) as opposed to the extent to which he simply identifies with a course of action to which he experiences himself as enacting external contingencies regardless of any consequences (as in a code of honour).[5] Observers will not necessarily be in agreement in a particular case. In those reactions more characteristic of women, it is the likelihood of self-destruction or the intrusion of some malevolent spiritual power into her body that generally compels others. Yet violence by men does not necessarily result in a local recognition of deliberate intent, for individuals initiating amok or negi-negi may, like possessed women, generally experience their actions as determined by some overwhelming impulse or malevolent power. And this may be locally agreed. Similar debates have occurred recently in Britain where the homicide defences of 'irresistible impulse' and 'provocation' have been argued to be biased in favour of men, the limited physical power of women making strategically delayed retribution – and thus the local ascription of greater responsibility – more necessary.[6]

Individual patterns involving potential violence would, however, appear a priori to be recognized as more motivated than those recalling illness. A common pattern in London for a brief period in the late 1960s and early 1970s was *baby-snatching*, when a young woman kidnapped a young child from a public place, cared for it secretly over a week or so, until after public appeals she made contact with its family or the police, and the child was returned.[7] Unlike shoplifting, where considerable emphasis had been placed by courts on medical evidence of diminished accountability due to psychological problems, British courts responded to baby-snatching with custodial sentences and the practice became less common, (as with amok[8]), although in the last decade there have been three well-publicized instances of women kidnapping babies from hospital maternity wards.

The moral economy of hostage-taking: public politics and personal mimesis

Where does a new syndrome come from? Standardized patterns of action are hardly immutable, and individual access to them fluctuates not only with shared crises and major shifts of the local understandings of agency and role, but through more restricted coalitions of expert or public interest as with post-traumatic stress disorder and multiple personality disorder (Chapter 10). The frequency of parasuicide has often been linked with exposure to media representations, fictional and real.[9] Indiscriminate mass homicide in Western societies (the so-called 'Whitman Syndrome' named for an earlier American protagonist) has been proposed as a contagious epidemic[10] following from certain well-publicized instances with firearms in Laos and North America which provided accessible public models;[11] so far there have been three British instances, in the streets of Hungerford and in schools in Holywood and Dunblane. (The first later became the site of a self-inflicted injury in which a police constable squirted 'super glue' into his own eyes and reported he had been assaulted and left to drown some hundred yards from where another police officer had been shot previously in the Hungerford killings.) The popular and psychiatric perception of such sequences as 'fashion' or 'imitation' recognizes their contagiousness but fails to explain the particular identification of the protagonist with antecedent examples or even with what may be regarded analytically as a cultural institution (the so-called 'Werther effect' named from a character in Goethe's novel which precipitated an epidemic of suicide among young males in the late eighteenth century). The notion of mimesis, once pejoratively used as an explanation of social contagion in those considered temporarily irrational (urban crowds and cargo-cults) has, through its recent deployment in literary criticism, been recognized again in the social sciences as a legitimate interpretation of any individual action and a necessary process of cultural continuity and transformation, which may for the sociologist evoke notions of iteration and play.[12] Any 'cultural psychopathology' is of necessity *mimetic*, both as a mirroring (in the Aristotelian sense of the term) and as a development (in the Platonic). Suicide and parasuicide, like amok, refer back to standardized heroic models,[13] just as the structuring of multiple personality disorder develops new identities from sources available in popular evangelism, computer games, soap opera and media concerns over child sexual abuse.[14]

This is hardly surprising: the possibilities of identity and agency are culturally limited. What a 'mimetic' model of epidemiology has to demonstrate is how an individual identifies with and transforms a pre-existing public model for personal action, and how in turn a series of such pragmatic actions become translated into a cultural symbolization. In this chapter, I look at an apparently increasing phenomenon in Britain, domestic sieges. The few psychiatric accounts of the protagonists of domestic sieges – the potentially violent men who hold members of their families hostage – do not examine the motivations and meanings of their actions which these individuals hold.[15] To what extent do these differ from the existing public understandings of the motivations of political or criminal sieges, and how does the average citizen identify with such available models? Anthropologists and cultural psychiatrists have argued that not only do such culture-specific patterns provide some personal adjustment for individuals, but that in their exaggeration and dramatic deployment of social norms (for instance, women as self-punitive, men as aggressive), they serve as standardized rituals, personalizing, commenting on and replaying core social conflicts on behalf of the community, constraining them within acceptable bounds.[16] If so, dramaturgical idioms such as ritual, theatre and catharsis, or even carnival, become appropriate. In small-scale non-industrialized societies as well as in the urban West, debate on whether the principal is to be considered as a justified agent is a necessary part of the uncertainty which all such patterns necessarily articulate.

To be instrumental in compelling the active intercession of others, individual patterns must articulate shared concerns. The practice of hijacking moveable property and of hostage-taking by nationalist and politico-religious groups since the 1960s has provided a standardized model for criminal, and later domestic, hostage-taking in Britain and other industrialized countries. The taking of hostages is, of course, deprecated by the various Geneva and Hague Conventions on the conduct of warfare but it has continued in civil wars, military occupation, 'low-intensity insurgencies', and thence among marginal revolutionary groups. It is not limited to particular countries: the taking of civilian and military hostages occurred in the Second World War in the European and Pacific theatres, in the Spanish and Greek civil wars and, more recently, in Vietnam, Afghanistan, Israel, Lebanon, Northern Ireland, Iraq and Bosnia. Hostages may be held by kidnappers in locations known to military or civil authorities in close proximity who intervene, and these situations we designate here as *sieges*. There is a considerable practical and moral ambiguity over what constitutes a 'hostage': prisoners of war, civilian as well as military, may be redeemed after certain concessions are made – whether cessation of conflict or access to material resources such as territory, armaments, food or transport. In societies which institutionalize feuding between groups, kidnapping people or livestock for ransom is not altogether a morally unacceptable activity, and a national government can find it difficult to distinguish resulting 'criminal' sieges from 'political' sieges, civilian hostages from military hostages. Hostages themselves may negotiate demands for their own release with the kidnappers, but the *raison d'être* is generally that there is a distinct third party from whom demands are made because it has an interest in the safety and liberty of the hostages. And this third party is often constrained by a fourth – the relatives of the hostages and the wider public. Closely allied to hostage-taking is the 'official' arrest and imprisonment for relatively minor offences (or even plain abduction) of civilians whose release is then contingent on concessions by a fourth party which has an interest in the prisoners, such as a political organization or foreign government.

Besides using hostages to negotiate certain ends or to prevent particular government actions, hostages may be taken for revenge and killed immediately or after limited attempts at making contact; depending on the practical exigencies at the time, hostage-taking can shade into the massacre of civilians. The threat to the captive, stated or implicit, may be death or mutilation, or simply continued imprisonment. Despite its international illegality, political hostage-taking seems to have developed tacit ground rules with assumptions of good faith, legitimate demands, negotiation through an honest broker as to the value of the hostages relative to the hostage-takers' demands, recognized procedures of guaranteeing the safety of the hostages during their release, and so forth. Unsuccessful negotiation of demands or attempts at rescue may be presumed to seriously endanger the hostages, while too ready a concession to the hostage-takers' demands may be argued by those not immediately involved as encouraging the practice. At the same time, hostage-takers themselves may be ambivalent or divided about their goals, and these may shift in the course of negotiations either to increasing or reducing demands depending on the perceived position of the other. In the course of negotiations, the hostage-takers can settle for less than the original demands (sometimes simply for publicity or legitimation of their political aspirations), or they can increase their demands if it seems advantageous.[17] National governments often publicly deny either that they take hostages themselves or that they will negotiate to release those held by others (for instance, the East German government in the 1980s variously rounded down the agreed figure for releasing individuals to the Federal Republic lest it seem a standardized ransom); and there can be one set of messages inside the negotiations and another for the general public and news media (the fourth party). Sieges only 'work' as an instrumental procedure if the party against which they are directed has an interest in securing the well-being of the hostages, whether through personal conviction or through the wider public response. Like threatened self-immolation to coerce concessions (in which the hostage-taker and the hostage are the same person as in threatened suicide or political hunger strikes in Britain and India), they are not generally effective against an authoritarian third party which controls the media unless releasing the hostages has some particular advantage, public or private. Hijackings and hostage-taking both receive extensive media publicity and are in turn structured by this publicity.[18]

Sieges have been of interest to psychologists not only because of the dynamics of negotiation and the consequent training of police psychologists and potential hostages in 'mock siege incidents',[19] but because of the so-called Stockholm syndrome: the close relationship of hostage to hostage-taker confined together through which the former may begin to identify with the latter against some external power which appears indifferent to their fate or may even take sides in support of the hostage-takers' original grievance. Public opinion too may side with the hostage-takers. To enhance the negotiating power of the 'third party', psychologists trained as negotiators for police, military or prison authorities will frequently distance themselves tactically from the judicial authorities to identify their own interests as brokers in seeking a peaceful resolution of the hostage-takers' demands. To justify their course of action to themselves, to the hostages and to public opinion, the kidnappers may identify the hostages as the actual oppressors or at least as representatives of this disorder: cognitive dissonance as well as duplicity and practical suspicion may explain why businessmen who unwisely stray over a border become translated into spies. In a sequence of reverberating violence it can be difficult to distinguish victim from perpetrator.

The popular image of political hostage-taking, however, is that of a relatively powerless individual or group, whose legitimate demands have been persistently ignored, leaving them with no option but to take hostage people who are not directly responsible.[20] Blame and causality may thus be attributed by hostage-taker and hostage on to the third person who is doubly blamed for causing otherwise reasonable and decent people to take such an outrageous action.[21] And it is this shift of responsibility – and thus causality – to an external agency that allows otherwise unremarkable civilians to have access to the pattern. To characterize hostage-taking simply as a crime misses its moral economy and the assumption of reciprocity; it would not be inappropriate to regard political hostage-taking as a standardized and dramatic public negotiation, a simple representation of the value of individual life and action, of relating ignoble means to justifiable ends, and as a demonstration of the power of the weak and of the magnanimity of the powerful, and of the moral ambiguity of a world where the hostage-taker is impelled to consider murder yet seeks to avoid it, sieges oscillating between brutalization and sympathy as negotiations drag on. Well-known episodes of hostage-taking which end dramatically have been made into films (e.g. *Entebbe*) and even an opera (*The Death of Klinghoffer*). Surviving hostages may become heroic or tragic figures, frequently publishing their memoirs, with their imprisonment a personal test of confronting adversity or even the realization of the meaning of their life. Patterns closely related to hostage-taking – kidnapping, rustling, threatened self-immolation and threatened amok, jauhar and its analogues, hostage-taking for 'surety' – may demonstrate existing moral and economic assumptions in a particular society. Through such notions as sacrifice, self-sacrifice and redemption they may be elaborated into wider theodicies as in Christianity and the Hellenistic mystery religions.[22]

What I have termed here 'political' hostage-taking shades into the 'criminal', depending on the public recognition of its explicit motivation and the advantages to be gained by the taker, whether monetary gain and escape (usually seen as 'criminal') or some more extensive social change or release of other hostages or prisoners held by the authorities (usually 'political'). The term 'kidnapping' generally refers to the former, although here there may be no appeal to a fourth party, the motivation of the kidnapping being closely related to the particular status or resources of the hostages who may themselves have to provide access for crime or to release money, and who are the potential focus for torture or rape.

Domestic versus criminal sieges

I examine next some characteristics of actual or suspected hostage-taking followed by sieges which occurred in Britain. While domestic sieges may plausibly be argued to be modelled on well-publicized political and criminal sieges in that they have become common later,[23] we may anticipate some distinguishing characteristics. To what extent can one claim these patterns as 'functional' for the individual, or indeed for society?

Sieges may be defined as situations where the place in which the hostages are presumed to be detained is known to the police. I do not consider siege situations without the presumption of hostages as when individuals threatened with eviction barricade themselves in their house. Sieges involve police as the immediate 'third party' in the negotiations and take place in private households or other generally accessible places: I have excluded prison sieges. By *domestic sieges* I refer to situations where the stated demands of the principal appear to be redress within a family conflict or to demonstrate personal wishes within a domestic context, rather than to gain financial or political advantage, or to avoid the consequences of criminal actions; these I term criminal or *non-domestic sieges*. I have excluded kidnapping which did not involve a siege. I use the neutral term *principal* to refer to the presumed hostage-taker whose actions initiate the siege. While my colleague, Maurice Lipsedge, obtained police permission to attend a number of sieges in London and to interview accused domestic hostage-takers, I have restricted myself here to a number of sieges consecutively reported in the local and national press. This is inevitably a restricted sample of sieges, and one which almost certainly exaggerates the proportion which end in dramatic violence or which occur in close proximity to the local media. Because domestic hostage-takers who are apprehended may be charged with a variety of quite diverse crimes (in

England, assault, actual bodily harm, grievous bodily harm or false imprisonment) or released without charge, it is difficult to derive estimates of the approximate incidence and whether, as public and police believe, they have indeed been increasing in frequency over the last 20 years.[24]

National and local newspaper reports of 58 siege situations where hostage-taking was presumed and which had occurred in Great Britain from April 1983 to August 1988 are considered. Four national newspapers, two broadsheet and two tabloid, were scanned; identified cases were then supplemented by television news reports and local newspaper reports. The number of media reports accessed per siege ranged from one to four. As this is somewhat new data, I include the actual figures.

Fifty-six of the 58 sieges were carried out by adult men, and all but three occurred in urban areas. The age of the principal was reported in 38 cases: 53 per cent were aged under 30, just under a quarter were aged 30 to 39 and the same proportion between 40 and 59. The average age was 32 (domestic) and 34 (non-domestic). Nineteen of the sieges were domestic; 20 of the remaining 39 developed in the course of a robbery. In 36 of the 51 cases where information was available, real or imitation firearms were used. Hostages were actually taken in only 65 per cent (31 out of 58) of sieges, generally the domestic sieges, but there were no significant associations between domestic versus criminal sieges. In four domestic sieges and 17 criminal sieges, there was no hostage; it is not clear in most of these instances whether a hostage had been presumed to have been taken or simply whether a threat of violence was recognized against police, bystanders or principal. All hostages taken in domestic sieges were previously known to the principal and in ten cases they were related to the hostage-taker (three were spouse or partner, four were the hostage-taker's children, and in one case the hostage-taker imprisoned both his own spouse and children). In 18 sieges the hostages were complete strangers; all of these were non-domestic.

Contrary to my initial assumption on sieges as a negotiation, domestic sieges were more likely to end in injury. Eight of the 19 domestic principals died, none of the 39 criminal principals. Hostages were twice as likely to be injured or killed in domestic sieges, other people were one and a half times more likely to be injured or killed. The deployment of firearms or other weapons was not associated significantly with injury or death, or with either type of siege. Domestic sieges were of an average length of 17 hours (with a range of a few hours to six days) and were more likely to last 13 hours or more; they were less likely to end in custody for a surviving principal.

Towards a dramaturgy

Quantifiable data inevitably simplifies what is often a very complex situation. To take one example for which I have personal knowledge and a detailed police report: Thomas White (a pseudonym) had a criminal record and a long-standing resentment against the local police in an English provincial town. Abandoned by Mrs White and their 5-year-old son, he was waiting to appear in court for stealing money from his wife and assaulting her. Together with a male friend, he entered the women's hostel where she was staying, struck another woman, took his son and left. Two weeks later the police received a letter, forwarded by the tabloid newspaper to whom it had been sent, in which Mr White pleaded his innocence. Following the letter, the police traced him to a 'squat' where he had obtained a shotgun. The house was surrounded by armed police and a team of police negotiators while the neighbourhood was evacuated. Mr White then also took hostage one of the adult occupants of the house who apparently was previously unknown to him. The others were able to leave. From the police report: 'Representatives of the press were allowed onto the Green, within a separately cordoned-off area, and under supervision, but nevertheless were within sight and voice range of [White] in his barricaded bedroom. It became clear, as the siege progressed and through his conversation with the negotiating team, that [the] reason for instigating the siege was to publicise his [domestic] grievance.' Five days later, after his adult hostage was exchanged by mutual agreement with the police for the friend who had previously assisted in the abduction of his child, he 'threw two knives and an air rifle out of the bedroom window. The following day he was persuaded to surrender the child [and] gave himself up on the afternoon of the sixth day of the siege without violence.' In the Crown Court some months later he was found guilty of theft, actual bodily harm and possession of a firearm with intent to endanger life. He was not accused of abducting his son for his wife had not yet secured the court order giving her sole custody.

Can one argue for a common pattern? In domestic sieges the principal is characteristically a young man, often estranged from his wife or partner and deprived of custody of his children. After a series of domestic altercations and threats, sometimes physical violence, he seizes one or more of his children or another close relative, removes them from the proximity of others, and then threatens, explicitly or implicitly, to harm them if the authorities attempt to remove them. A siege then develops, in the reported instances generally in a council estate, and is often publicly enacted on the balcony of a housing block. The actors include the principal, his hostage, the police and the media. Negotiations include the principal's protestations of innocence and appeals for justice. At a distance is typically a crowd of spectators, an ambulance and sometimes the estranged wife supported by women police officers, all of whom are photographed for the local newspapers. In many cases, if the siege continues for more than a few hours, this audience is itself extended via television. If the principal is not shot by the police or himself, the siege ends under police instructions, first in surrender of the child, then of the weapon, then the principal himself. In about half of domestic sieges, the principal is disarmed and arrested without being injured and without injury to hostage or others. The press photographs which are printed typically show him surrendering in a heroic pose, hands held high, facing the camera alone, defeated but unbowed.

At times, the spectators appear to be so involved by the spectacle that they participate in the event by shouting encouragement or advice to the hostage-taker, or by protesting against the police.[25] Frequently they are already aware of domestic tensions in the family, and their sympathies generally lie with the hostage or hostage-taker, seldom with the police. In one instance, as a televised siege in a housing estate was approaching its climax with the police moving in from the stairway on either side of a balcony to enter a flat and seize the hostage-taker, a spectator violently assaulted a policeman who was holding back the jeering crowd in the courtyard below.

The moral economy of ritual

The increasing frequency of domestic altercations developing into sieges appears to reflect increased access to real or imitation firearms (and thus a new spatial and temporal participation by the police), but also personal identification with the protagonists of spectacular political and criminal sieges or hijackings. The simultaneously increasing occurrence of 'hoax' hostage-taking reflects recognition of the domestic siege as a standardized public event; for it can only occur if both instigator and public have a definite notion of the 'real thing'.[26] I have been informed of an instance in 1996, not included in my series above, where the hostage-taker telephoned the police during his siege to find out the record length of a siege which he proposed to better! Yet we cannot assume that what often results in a lengthy process is anticipated as such by the principal. The siege may start from him simply denying an estranged spouse previously agreed access to the children[27] or perhaps an initially anticipated strategy but one that develops increasingly out of his control. In a society where the police pay less regard to the physical safety of presumed law-breakers and are more ready to gun down the hostage-taker, the waiting time and negotiations would be truncated and the hostage-taker would be routinely wounded or killed, presumably deterring other would-be hostage-takers.

In Chapter 3, I have argued that, at a high level of generality, many Euro-American patterns recognized as psychopathologies can be interpreted along with the so-called culture-bound syndromes in a standardized three-stage schema in which the principal's actions and the response of others are interdependent. Individuals who are in a subdominant or marginal social position (through their age, gender, character, adversarial circumstances or other restricted access to public power) may in a particular situation (i) recognize themselves extruded even further; (ii) then demonstrate what is identified as the illness in a further development of this extrusion in a way which evokes familiar recognitions of personal distress and agency by their immediate social network by whom they are not recognized as fully responsible, which now compels others to (iii) reintegrate them back into their everyday social position. Similar social schemata have been described by Devereux as 'masochistic blackmail' and by Scott as 'everyday resistance' among the disadvantaged;[28] they recall the situations described by psychiatrists as 'attention seeking', 'acting out' and 'hysteria'.

To what extent do domestic sieges fit this three-stage model which was elaborated for patterns more characteristic of women? Only imperfectly. Like the protagonist in the other dramatic syndromes, the estranged father/husband is certainly dislocated from his usual parental/marital role, and then enacts this extrusion as a public performance. Presenting a heightened image of the dominant and possessive father and husband, his personal predicament is reproduced before an audience of neighbours, police and spectators, poignantly articulating domestic conflicts which are familiar to all. As in other standardized forms of threatened violence (p. 41), there is some discrepancy between the potential injury and the enactment, and the recognized victim seems to be the hostage-taker not the hostage. But restitution – the third phase of the sequence – is absent since the hostage-taker is killed or, if taken into custody, does not later gain increased access to his child or estranged spouse. Sieges thus follow our earlier suggestion that men generally appear more likely to be regarded as responsible agents, women as ill. My limited follow-up material suggests that the High Court appears even less likely to award custody to a surviving father who has demonstrated his reckless disregard for the well-being of his child by exposing it to psychological, if not physical, trauma.[29] He is unlikely to have a diagnosis of psychiatric or physical illness accepted by a court. Nevertheless, his actions are argued by his lawyer as attributable to underlying 'stress', illness or toxic state; if this argument was accepted in court the hostage-taker might be exonerated.[30]

Yet displacement of personal agency from principal to some abstract notion of 'justice' or onto others, including the hostages, seems to allow some exculpation and justification similar to that of political hostage-taking

– at least from the principal's and spectators' (and press readers') points of view. Domestic hostage-taking certainly serves an expressive function in that it demonstrates the father's intense attachment to his child or partner. In a biosocial model of psychiatric disorders which has certain affinities with our three-stage schema, Gardner[31] has proposed that 'kidnapping without financial aims' is a contextual development of the biosocial goal of attachment in nurturance. The recourse to spectacle in the absence of any anticipated pragmatic outcome is illustrated by the common phenomenon of the publicly threatened suicide-leap.[32]

Domestic sieges articulate a number of shared assumptions. If the attachment of male parent to child is accepted as legitimate, it is the safety of that child which mobilizes police, public and the media. The centrality of the parent–child bond is attested to in Judaeo-Christian cultures by the well-known story of Abraham. The ultimate test of Abraham's commitment to his god was his willingness to sacrifice his son; as Kierkegaard put it, to destroy the only being whose value could come anywhere near that of a just deity. Is the notion of a 'ritual' – conventionally a periodic, formalized and collective action, both verbal and non-verbal, which represents a society's core values – appropriate then for what may be becoming a standardized institution in an industrialized society? (The popular British use of the term 'ritual' of course implies it is non-meaningful and does not really alter reality, and that it only recurs through tradition or atavistic inertia.) For social anthropologists, rituals are regarded not only as symbolically satisfying, as an expressive aesthetic – and they are that – but also as established procedures which maintain or transform social relations beyond themselves, and which may develop to negotiate new situations, contesting and playing out new ambiguities. Rituals may memorialize preceding actions yet they become the site for pragmatic replayings of novel and immediate relevance. They may be modified by individuals for immediate purposes from an existing pattern, yet they may deny the empirical reality of the event they signal: thus Christian funerals are, in a sense, 'anti-death' in that they articulate a notion of life beyond the grave. In the anthropological literature, rituals are often understood as passages between statuses, as expressive statements as well as instrumental actions,[33] and which embody local assumptions of self and psychological agency. Thus the frequency of indiscriminate mass homicide in the United States refers to and contributes to American notions of 'stress' and the 'cathartic release of strong affects'.[34]

In Euro-American societies, what are still regarded explicitly as 'rituals' are our remaining ceremonies of aggregation (thus marriage but not divorce). If even aggregation is increasingly seen as individualized, as tenuous and psychologized, divorce is especially simplified and deritualized as a social event. Like the classic rites of passage described by Van Gennep, domestic sieges as ritual may be said, however, to mark dramatically the separation of the man (from his married and parental role) and his re-aggregation to society (as single again).[35] If practical instrumentality appears absent, one might expect these sieges to become less frequent, yet their precondition and the cultural dilemma they articulate – resistance to the estrangement of adult men from partner or child – are likely to become more frequent. Men in Western Europe and North America increasingly describe themselves as beleaguered by unfair legal decisions which favour women's supposed natural capacity for nurturance, the overwhelming majority of women gaining custody of the children after marital break-down, while men's own parenting contribution is regarded as purely financial with close physical affection for their children becoming dangerous to display.[36] 'I am on the verge of a nervous breakdown because of the way my 3-year-old daughter was taken from me at 15 months and I was denied all access to her ... There are no more legal steps I can take and my anger is such that I'm thinking of illegal ones – like bashing down the door and snatching my child.'[37] 'I think every man in Families Need Fathers [a group for fathers denied access to or custody of their children] has been on the brink of either abducting a child or taking drastic action against either his ex or his ex's solicitor.'[38]

This attitude is reflected in the recent pattern of *stalking*; a high proportion of incidents are carried out by jealous ex-partners. While erotic jealousy and infatuation have long been recognized (fictionally in *Othello*, *The Kreutzer Sonata*, *Carmen*), there appears to have recently been an increase among men – for this is predominantly a male pattern. British newspaper reporting reflects an increase after a period when 'celebrity' stalking was regarded as an American phenomenon: from no mention in 1991 to 45 in 1996 (in the *Guardian* and *Observer*), from two in 1991 to 59 (*Daily Mirror*).[39] 'They will send blood, body parts, hair samples, body fluids, mutilated photographs: they will follow you and follow you around everywhere you go during the day and night; they will telephone you fifty to one hundred times a day with strange and threatening messages.'[40] Frequently excused by the man as 'old-fashioned love' inconsistent with a more callous modern view of sexuality,[41] there appears to be a complete absence of commiseration for the woman subject to sudden appearances, unwanted gifts and letters, which will strike the observer as fatuous. Although some instances of stalking overlap with long-recognized paranoid psychotic disorders (Othello Syndrome, De Clerambault's Syndrome), there is widespread popular concern about the lack of protection the police afford. A typical example is the police handing yet another stalker's note to the terrified victim with a comment that 'he just says he needs to see you to get things straightened out'.[42] Like exhibitionism (see the next chapter), stalking can end in violence to the victim. That it (or indeed love) is

somehow connected to men's desire for power over women is suggested by
the comment of one stalker: 'I knew I had such power over people's lives
and that is a tremendous feeling.'[43] The current 1997 Protection from
Harassment Law has been of debatable utility.

That domestic sieges too frequently end in violence suggests that as
standardized patterns they simply exemplify the social or domestic violence
of men against women. Yet one of the most difficult things to understand is
the readiness of the father to sacrifice his own children. If agency for the
threatened death of his child is transferred to some other power, the
principal has identified closely with his child, and still does. From a
psychodynamic perspective, a useful approach to this willingness to
conserve through sacrifice what is conventionally most dear would appear
to be found in object relations theory. Here we will refer briefly to
anthropological considerations of sacrifice as a common standardized
model. In sacrificial ritual, the victim is typically identified closely with the
sacrificer through some shared vitality or action; a common nineteenth-
century (and thence Freudian) account of Abraham's thwarted sacrifice
was that the biblical story recalled the moment in Western history when
once conventionalized sacrifice of children was displaced onto male
circumcision and animal sacrifice.[44] The Athenian killing of the human
pharmakos ('scapegoat') persisted into the historical period. The sacrificial
victim, human or animal, remained a public substitute for the ever-present
danger of killing one's children as demonstrated by animals and recalled in
the state-sponsored Greek tragedies of *Medea*, *Heracles*, *Ajax* and *Iphigenia*.

While this sort of conjectural psychohistory is no longer compelling, and
anthropologists generally emphasize the contemporary place of sacrifice in
the social order rather than its ultimate psychobiological motivations,[45] the
idea of the substitution of one victim or object for another which it closely
recalls remains a common ethnographic finding: thus an appropriate plant
may serve as the usual sacrificial animal if the latter is not available. The
earlier idea of the sacrifice as an exchange, in a moral economy in which
something is lost in order to gain some other good, is currently
unfashionable in anthropology, yet contemporary analogues may be
argued in serious illness when some personal renunciation is proposed
mentally to a deity, to fate or justice in exchange for life and health, in
votive transactions or in the 'superstitious' mental bargains of exchange by
prisoners, gamblers and sportsmen, as in those popular aphorisms which
argue that success will necessarily be followed by misfortune. The
principles of substitution and exchange interpenetrate in a moral economy
in which a gain must always be offset by a loss which is avoided by
transferring agency to a higher moral order; and the sacrificial victim serves
as a renunciation of some valued object or person whether in expiation or
reciprocity.

Girard has proposed that sacrifice serves to avert reverberating cycles of violence in a society when perceived injury or injustice threaten escalating disorder.[46] Sacrifice and ritual scapegoating, like their successors – dramatic tragedy and civic justice – circumscribe violence and unite the community.[47] In these standardized rituals, sacrifice as well as legal process, individual agency is transferred to a higher power, fate or justice; and in a close identification with the sacrificial victim the individual becomes absolved as a tragic hero. The sacrificial victim must be innocent yet must represent our social obligations and conflicts. As Aristotle noted (p. 94), the powerful effect of mimetic 'pity' in classical tragic drama is because, just like sacrifice, it has to involve close relatives; the 'pity' of the audience is an active recreation on their part. Girard argues that sacrifice, drama and law remain precariously close to indiscriminate violence and may on occasion exacerbate conflict or threaten to revert to more widespread disorder.[48]

If this suggests an overambitious general model for domestic sieges, in any social pattern normative values must be manifest in the subjectivities of individuals; and, as with suicide, the individual who dramatically renounces self and family may transcend their own death and failure in what Grottanelli has termed 'retributive fantasy'.[49] While cultural models for individual reassertion and resistance may attain their validity through approximation to existing patterns which, like political sieges, appear instrumentally successful in the everyday world, they may serve as a means of extreme self-expression which we might not inappropriately regard as 'aesthetic'. A dramaturgical approach is thus one possible reading. Whether we take domestic sieges as a mimetic pathology, a crime or an adaptive strategy, as fantasized expiation or retributive justice, as a carnivalesque theatre or even an ambivalent sacrifice remains arbitrary, dependent on our interpretation of local representations of illness, agency and power.

7. Soldierly Rape

Given revived anthropological interest in armed conflict,[1] and more generally in the human body as the phenomenological locus of agency and experience (and not just as a symbol available to represent collective interests), and the attention to aggressive sexuality raised by the women's movement, together with fashionable cultural studies into the history of transgressive sexualities, it is perhaps surprising that there is little anthropological interest in the sexuality of war. Sexuality, that is, as lived experience, not as iconography. We may wonder if the subject is too horrific and shameful for Europeans to consider, for it is in the former Yugoslavia that the International Criminal Tribunal at The Hague has again brought mass rape by militia and armed civilians before the liberal conscience. Military rape is, however, hardly restricted to European societies.

A deliberately empirical stance is adopted in this chapter, through my own uncertainty as to what sort of understanding is going to make most sense in limiting a phenomenon which is generally ignored by social scientists; and second through my responses to it: revulsion at actions found in the anthropologist's own society and sex is no reason for exculpation through claims that atrocity transcends analysis, or for adhering to an objectivizing or pathologizing position. Such revulsion may be less a 'cultural' response to such a pattern than intrinsic to its maintenance.

To introduce ethological and psychophysiological explanation as an understanding of human actions which we saw as primarily voluntaristic, motivated strategies manifest in competing interests, not altogether surprisingly arouses a sense of vertigo or indeed nausea. Particularly so when we attempt to deal with standardized sexual violence in societies including the European: not just individual rape and sexual killing (we have learned to pathologize those as socially aberrant) but with what frequently appears as an instrument of public policy. Surely men choose to engage it? Military rape may be more evidently a pathology for Euro-American societies but it is hardly limited to them. African Rights' powerful indictment of terror against the Tutsi in Rwanda frequently uses an idiom of deviance and abnormality, such as the 'pathology of genocide'.[2]

I do not intend to propose here any sort of unitary theory, but rather to sketch out some of the problems with what appear to be our available interpretations. It is not just that sexuality and violence may be manifest together in troubled times, but that the mass rape and sexual killing of women appear standardized in certain ways. Their frequency argues rape in wartime to be a normal part of what it is to be human; yet any attempt to consider it outside of an immediate outrage or ascription of chaos and pathology threatens to become independent of compelling human concerns. For there is a perhaps welcome relief in referring men's sexual violence to something other than their choices, as when we relegate it to the workings of a masculine ideology, a psycho-physiological contingency, or evolutionary adaptation. Our choice of terms is immediately problematic: do we talk here of pleasure or of gratification? Of agents, principals or perpetrators? Of performance, act or atrocity? And should an account of 'rape' restrict itself to the current English sense of forced sexual intercourse, as I do here, or should it take in local connotations which might include an abduction or a failure to pay bride price? Or the use of the idiom of rape as an analytical trope – such that 'flirting is rape'? Real sexual violence has been argued to be the 'depersonalisation' of women, 'a conscious process of intimidation by which all men keep all women in a state of fear', and as 'terror warfare'.[3] Given its particular associations with standardized and collective violence, can sexual aggression by men in situations of social conflict tell us any more about physical violence? Or men? Or sexuality?

Or indeed our human institutions? For something like war rape appears virtually ubiquitous, and it is even carried out or simulated by child soldiers.[4] To reduce military terror rather optimistically to the local 'culture' in which it is manifest[5] is perhaps equivalent to attributing male aggression to societal meanings alone. And some contrary notion of a common human (or male) nature is equally banal. The exact frequency of military rape is uncertain, for its recognition reflects badly not only on the principals – perpetrators if we will – but on the victim, for an explicit justification frequently made by the soldiers who rape women is that it is to degrade and humiliate them.[6] War rape is generally concealed, sometimes to remain as a popular rumour. (Were the American servicewomen captured in the Gulf War sexually tortured or not?) It is publically ignored on the supposition that it is both individual deviance, yet too common to be noteworthy.[7]

The issue of sexual violence by the military has been recalled to European awareness by estimates from the former Yugoslavia that up to 60,000 Bosnian women have been raped, many becoming pregnant and bearing the children engendered in that assault.[8] Some of them, instead of as in past conflicts remaining silent through their shame, have been persuaded to describe their experience to the international press.[9]

Following therapeutic practices and self-help support groups developed in Western Europe and America to assist the *survivors* (formerly the *victims*) of crimes and civil disasters, these women have attempted to attain something we might gloss as psychological healing. Centres such as Medica have been established for rape victims at Zenica and elsewhere, where women are encouraged to articulate a testimony beyond shame.

Military and paramilitary rape is hardly limited to Bosnia. As General Sherman protested to Union critics after his devastation of Georgia in the American Civil War, war is hell; it seldom recalls a game of chess between consenting males, the moves accepted in advance. It is estimated that tens of thousands of women were raped by the Allies in Germany at the end of the Second World War.[10] Rape was common among both sides in the Vietnam War. Between a quarter and half a million Tutsi women were raped in Rwanda in 1994.[11] Asia Watch reports that Indian soldiers in Kashmir currently rape 'to punish and humiliate the entire community',[12] apparently calculating that local response will hold the women responsible and disorientate the community, for shamed women will be reluctant to give evidence in public courts. Similarly in the former Yugoslavia.[13] Indian soldiers rape not in prisons or detention camps (the Bosnian situation), but during house-to-house searches and reprisal attacks; rape is often justified to their victims as punishment on the grounds that the woman has been harbouring terrorists.[14] Amnesty International suggests that army and police regularly engage in sexual violence towards the families of insurgents in Assam, and throughout India against low-caste and tribal communities.[15] And there are documented accounts of extensive sexual violence by soldiers during the partition of India, and against Tamil women during the Indian intervention in Sri Lanka in the 1980s.[16] Thousands of Somali refugees have been raped by Kenyan soldiers and police, frequently after the scarring of infibulation ('female circumcision') is cut through by knife or bayonet.[17] And there are documented accounts of extensive military and police rape in Central America, Haiti, Burma, Indonesia, Peru, Sri Lanka and elsewhere.[18] There is perhaps nothing so very European here.

Nor so new: Hebrew, Anglo-Saxon and Chinese chronicles recognized the rape of women as a consequence of defeat in war – as did Herodotus and Thucydides – not endorsing the horrors but certainly recognizing them as an inevitable part of military conflict. Medieval sieges frequently ended in sexual violence and mutilation directed against the defeated defenders, and surrenders were often negotiated with this in mind.[19] While 'war' was recognized by Europeans as fairly circumscribed physical violence between men in socially sanctioned contexts, it was accepted that women and children were likely to be caught up – in a sense naturally – within the conflict as deliberately targeted victims.[20] In the Roman apology, '*inter arma leges silent*'.[21] Not only violence to disarm or eliminate men then, but violence which seems to have a motive of sexual gratification or at least to use sexual idioms to establish domination.

It is difficult to distinguish these two: sexual gratification from physical sexuality as a representation of political interests. Indeed we might argue, at the risk of repeating the generally discredited 'psychological extension' theories of the nineteenth century (used to explain societal incest prohibitions) that these two are inherently associated in human action: the politics of sexuality and the sexuality of politics. As conventional representation, sexual violence in war is normally depicted as directed by men on to, or rather in to, women: from Titus Andronicus to Goya's *Disasters of War* to Godard's *Les Carabiniers*. A myth of origin, like incest, may take the breach of an everyday prohibition as the act which inaugurated human (or civil) society: the story of the abduction and rape of the Sabine women was once familiar to every British schoolchild. And popular ethology on territorial expansion and genetic hybridization may argue something remarkably similar.[22] But, as it is practised, rape in war moves beyond the male co-option or fertilization of alien women into insult and genital mutilation whose consequences cannot easily be seen as the pragmatic assimilation or impregnation of women, but rather as destructive male violence aimed at the body or society in its sexual aspect, directed against the sexual organs or in ways that have evident sexual connotations to victims, the men involved and others.

And which may be independent of the gender of the victim. The Zagreb Medical Centre for Human Rights estimates that 4,000 Croatian male prisoners were sexually tortured in Serb detention camps: 70 per cent of them remain with physical injuries, 11 per cent were castrated or partially castrated (sometimes by women), 20 per cent were forced to fellate their fellow prisoners.[23] In 1996, rebellious Iraqi officers were apparently forced to rape each other before 'execution by slow mutilation'.[24] Instruments of penetration are not only the erect penis but military weapons, blunt instruments, knives and so on. I am doubtful that the frequent reports from Bosnia of male prisoners (of all factions) having their testicles bitten off can be fully explained as it is by our journalists as a rather folkloric equivalence between sexual organs and the virility (and thus military capability) of the opposing side – or indeed as reversion to some peasant ethic of the mutilation of livestock and enemies in times of conflict.[25] Nor, I think, can we easily take the opposing view and see war as simply unleashing indiscriminate violence which, once provoked, seeks to engage or consume all residues of the opposition, and easily turns back onto neutrals or indeed one's own side. What could 'indiscriminate' violence be? Can physical violence have no object, no end (in either sense)? As Marshall Sahlins reminds us in a not dissimilar context, 'Cannibalism is symbolic, even when it is real.'[26]

Militarism

The standard view, such as it is, argues that collective sexual violence is only the frankest expression of men's desire for power over women of the sort we looked at when we considered stalking: sexual only in that the genitals are the emblems of the politics of gender. Given a natural aversion to the killing of other human beings, war is only made possible through its rituals, symbols and conditioning.[27] And killing of the raped woman is part of this process of cultural violence. I think it would not be unfair to identify this view with much American feminist arguments, such as the work of Andrea Dworkin and Susan Brownmiller. I would suggest that this view would be the most acceptable for social anthropologists: in other words, rape is primarily a question of political power. The use of gendered, even sexualized, representations of national or group identity, whether as a victorious armed maiden, or an innocent child facing a lascivious and anthropoid enemy (the Rape of Belgium, of Nanking, indeed of Nature) allows men ('our side') to represent their collectivity as something like a family, and thus as including the female, nurturant and asexual, as sister and daughter, perhaps as a mother (Warner, M. 1985). Asexual, defenceless and innocent, they have to be protected. And the soldier represents himself as quintessentially the active man: inducted American civilians are initially referred to in military training as 'girls'.[28] Take the twentieth-century war posters and cinema which represent European aggression as the protection and rescue of 'our women' – or 'our sort of women' – from the crude sexual interests of aliens: from Blacks (in Griffith's *Birth of a Nation*, Huston's *African Queen*), revolutionaries (Lang's *Metropolis*), Amerindians (Ford's *Stagecoach*) or whoever;[29] the liberated woman then yields herself freely to the male rescuer, her mate by nature and by choice (which here run together). And this ambivalent idealization of 'our' women may go together in a set of shared ethics and physiologies which deprecate their control of fertility, promoting our men as the active agents, the guarantors of our society's physical continuity: generation and regeneration through the individual male body.[30] Life from death.

At a less drastic level, *flashing* (exhibitionism), like anorexia nervosa, demonstrates such core cultural notions of body imagery and sexual identity in the West.[31] In a society which condemns the overt display of male sexual arousal and which is, at the same time, intensely preoccupied with avoidance of effeminacy, the flasher is frequently a young adult male, 'passive and lacking in self-assertion and with poor social skills, reflected in his conviction that he has a small penis.[32] As in *hamadsha* possession (p. 72) he fails to live up to cultural norms of male activity, here seduction and sexual activity. As with sieges, flashing is a dramatic time-limited public performance with a contravention of normative behaviour, but now a caricature of rape rather than of paternal authority with the female element no longer being an object of observation, for normally 'men act but women appear'.[33]

> A common theme is one of dominance and mastery: the exhibitionist, usually timid and unassertive with women, suddenly challenges one with his penis, briefly occupies her full attention and conjures up in her some powerful emotion, such as fear and disgust, or sexual curiosity and arousal. For a fleeting instant he experiences a moment of intense involvement in a situation where he is in control.[34]

The principal is frequently not held responsible by courts for his act for he has an illness; Magnan suggested in 1890 that the irresistible urge to exhibit one's erect penis 'annihilated the will' and should therefore carry exemption from legal sanction. If the dislocation is seen purely in terms of physical sex, flashing does not seem immediately adaptive: the performance only rarely ends in coitus and hence is regarded as a pathology. Taking the longer view (and exhibitionism as a syndrome has developed in relation to a biomedical as well as a judicial ethos), treatment involves encouragement and facilitation of more conventional sexual relationships. As with shoplifting, the immediate result of the drama is the ceding of control to others: 'Discretion is not always the rule' as the medical observer coyly remarks.[35]

The elevation of women to be degraded in this way requires some other site for the contrary representation of the women of men's everyday experience to rest upon.[36] So, in the conflict situation, 'their women' are the converse. Not chaste, not maternal, not offering themselves freely for men's use, they have to be taken. And thence the equation of enemy women with booty: urging on American troops in France in 1944 General Patton promised them Paris – as French women; a perhaps not atypical elision of defeated (emasculated) ally with enemy.

This established masculinism (if I can use such a word) as an established ethic of violence and security we might not unfairly characterize as *militarism*, at least in the modern period. Even in peacetime men as a group seem more likely to engage in sexual provocation than they do as individuals (take the 1990s US sexual assaults at the Tailhook naval convention and the Aberdeen Proving Ground). Compared with conscripts, professional soldiers engage in earlier and more frequent sexual activity.[37] Emblems of power are inscribed on the male body through heroic insignia and war paraphernalia: their converse on the enemy body – which may be already dead – by stripping off clothes, castration and other mutilation, body counts, displays and photography of corpses as trophies and so on. Raped and then 'wasted' Vietnamese girls were left dying with US military insignia placed between their open legs.[38] Compare the 'punishment' (significantly never sexual) of women who allowed the enemy voluntary access to their bodies: this is desexualizing, as in the shaven heads of the *tontes* in Cartier-Bresson's well-known photographs of the Liberation of Paris; German women who consorted with Polish slave workers in the Nazi period were sterilized or sent to the death camps.[39]

This perspective – the military as the embodiment of a sexualized masculine ethic – will perhaps not be implausible for anthropologists. Yet it is with the development since the seventeenth and eighteenth centuries[40] of bureaucratized standing armies with their professional codes of honour and hierarchical discipline that explicit rules for the conduct of European warfare first appeared, which advocated restraints which we hardly find before, notably the protection of non-combatants.[41] I might date such restraints to Grotius' *De Iure Belli ac Pacis* of 1625 (which specifically disallowed war rape), and by the twentieth century, with the development of the Red Cross, The Hague (from 1899) and Geneva (1907 onwards) Conventions on the conduct and limits of war, and the Nuremberg and Tokyo Trials, sexual violence against combatants and civilians is no longer an unfortunate but inevitable component of war (and of course a potential attraction of war) but prohibited as a war crime, as clearly specified in the 1949 Geneva Convention where rape is subsumed under 'any attack on [women's] honour'. The professionalization of national warfare – and its publicity through photography and cinema – has not involved training in sexual violence.[42] (Not at least publicly as we shall see.) After Frederick the Great, the professional European 'battle' approached something like our contemporary notion of 'a game' with, ideally, engagement on an open but delimited terrain, logistics, strategy, with clear markers between players and others,[43] recognized criteria for engagement, surrender, hot pursuit, and the identification and mutually accepted treatment of combatants, civilians and spies. In a clear-cut 'surgical' military engagement (the Falklands and Gulf Wars must approach the exemplary, at least from the victors' perspective), the direction of violence outside the field of engagement is clearly disallowed. (Limits, of course, remain contested in practice. Argentinian corpses were mutilated by British infantry to obtain jewellery; their ears were collected by some; those who 'surrendered late' were shot.)

Making and remaking boundaries on the woman's body

It is in those contemporary situations which do not recall a bounded battle – in treason, civil war, 'pacification', low-intensity conflicts and counter-insurgency[44] – that sexual violence seems particularly common; in decentred conflicts where a distinction between 'us' and 'them', between professional soldier and armed civilian, between civilian on the one side and on the other is less evident: encounters where, as Mao put it, the camouflaged guerrilla hides amongst the people 'like a fish in water'. And it is these situations, Goya's Peninsular War for instance,[45] that women more commonly became combatants and may themselves carry out sexual killing and mutilation: such as, in the Peninsular War, castration or cutting off the penis to be stuffed in the live or dead person's mouth (a pattern which has recurred in Bosnia and Rwanda where women have again been combatants). And with women recognized as fighters, or at least as supporters of an armed or rebellious male population whom they shelter and supply, they became the accepted victims of sexual violence (the Mexican and Spanish Civil Wars, the Japanese occupation of Shanghai, Turkish Armenia in 1915). I am not proposing that women bearing arms is the explanation of sexual violence directed against them, but it is commonly cited by men as a provocation.[46] As if their rape returned armed women to a female and hence non-combatant status; and male-on-male sexual violence is perhaps similar in its feminization – castration, sodomy and so on.

In these situations the male may be less a professional soldier than a recently armed civilian or member of a political militia, but I am not arguing that uniformed professional militarism necessarily guarantees the safety of women. The Eastern Front in the Second World War would be a salient counter-example. If the Americans supposedly hanged (not, significantly, shot) some of their own soldiers who raped European civilians in the same war, the French were accused of encouraging rape by their Moroccan[47] troops advancing north through Italy in 1943. I would suggest, however, that something akin to a 'military ethos' has the potential to see non-combatant women as in need of protection not rape. As if they were just too easy hunting targets (compare criticisms of the Gulf War 'turkey shoot'). It is in situations of actual or perceived subversion, with women as irregulars (a significant term), or where warfare is carried out by armed civilians on their own ground, that the game analogy collapses, tactical advantage being replaced by simple individual aggression with women raped as a more-or-less accepted technique. And I want to return to this common assumption that rape is a motivated instrument of terror – that is, that there is at some level of analysis something one can call a strategic intention in using sexual violence to achieve some other goal – terror, 'pacification' or whatever.[48] An often cited instance are the Argentinian military who in the 1970s genitally assaulted women prisoners in front of their children and partners in an instrumental action of terrorization.[49] (My continued use here of a term like 'assault' is a gross euphemism when we are talking not just of rape but of vaginal and anal penetration with sharp instruments and gun barrels, dismemberment, enucleation, cutting open pregnant women, dismemberment of the foetus, and so on; and the not uncommon posing and photography of the results as a warning or trophy, common in Vietnam and on the Eastern Front in the Second World War, which raises the significance of post-war memorialization and commemoration, whether as pornography, souvenir or necromantic catharsis.[50])

Sexual violence then seems less a standardized pattern of conflict enacted against a defining other across some accepted boundary than a way of clarifying, developing and affirming such boundaries;[51] less playing the accepted war game beyond the rules so much as working out boundaries on the woman's body, symbolically but also pragmatically (as destruction of the opponent's social institutions). The more a war is a war (on the board game or toy soldier analogy), with its declaration of hostilities, return of ambassadors, exchange of civilians and neutral inspection of prisoners, the more a professionalized military ethic is held in common by both sides, the greater potential for the physical safety of non-combatants. And rather than place responsibility for atrocities simply on militarism, we might perhaps pay some attention to those journalistic accounts which talk of 'reversion' to some earlier pattern of less bureaucratized conflict.[52] One can try to assess the contribution of military ideology without assuming it is solely responsible, at least in those wars which recall – to men – a game of chess.

Under the army's regime in Greece thirty years ago, military torturers abused and humiliated those assistants who were drafted in as – shall we say – trainee torturers:[53] physically assaulting and torturing them, a pattern perhaps 'spontaneous' (again we have to be careful of the instrumental 'they did it in order to . . .') but which injured their young colleagues to the brutalizing of others, and which recalls the hazing of military academies and schools, which frequently demonstrates sexual aggression and humiliation.[54] At times, it seems difficult to see sexual violence as goal-directed except as in expectation of immediate pleasure; for it approaches aimless violence, interconversions of perpetrator and victim, those cycles of atrocity and retribution which Girard has termed 'reverberating violence', and which can end only in total defeat or in the exhaustion of victory.[55]

'Reverberating violence'? Is atrocity to be matched by atrocity, as we might speculate from the militarism model (and as indeed proposed by the military themselves)[56] such that if the male understanding of woman is divided between the inviolate and the all-to-be-violated other, any insult to 'our womankind' has necessarily to be matched by further insults to 'theirs' in order to preserve the distinction between the two sides?[57] This would support the idea that, at some level, collective sexual violence is indeed a mode of dissolving or maintaining boundaries. A tragic idiom of escalation and reciprocation is common both to ethnohistories of feuding and to academic studies of contemporary warfare, sometimes as a pragmatic process in which each side seeks an immediate advantage which is then countered by the other side, as in the military history of weaponry and tactics, or else as a humiliated attainment of meaning and justice.[58] The first use of battle gas in the First World War was reciprocated; in the Second it was avoided by tacit agreement. Biological warfare currently appears avoided by the threat of 'non-conventional' reciprocation. McManners describes how in the Falklands War, British soldiers devised a pragmatic Kantian code of ethics, calculating the behaviour which would be expected from the enemy and thus which would be reciprocated: the shooting of a British officer negotiating the surrender of an Argentinian group led to an informal decision by other ranks that no prisoners would be taken. Does physical aggression tend to follow in a series of positions and counter-positions, as in Mutually Assumed Destruction during the Cold War with the agreement not to develop certain types of anti-missile-missiles? And thus a game theory model of 'deterrence' is valid?[59] And how is the pattern of communication and response on such issues maintained in times of conflict? Michael Walzer proposes that 'the purpose of soldiers is to escape reciprocity'.[60] Against the militarism argument, we might suggest that military institutions (or at least frequent and conventionalized warfare) actually facilitate the communication of messages along the lines of 'we are protecting your civilians here, please do likewise' standing for 'we won't rape your women if you don't rape ours': patterns of deterrence which require a certain reciprocally recognized soldierly culture on both sides.[61] And which cannot be easily agreed in colonial or mercenary war ('too different ethics') or in insurgency ('non-reciprocal ethics' for a nation should not be at war with itself). Without them, can we argue for some pattern of escalation, whether biosocial, psychodynamic or strategic, in which violence mounts through a series of stages from 'good war' to a 'total war' beyond Clauswitz's visions, ending only when the final dismemberment of the dead and the living can be considered adequate?[62]

The first two sets of understandings then which we find immediately available (and they are hardly mutually exclusive) are:

(1) The *militarism* (or reciprocal violation) argument. Collective sexual violence by men simply mirrors and exemplifies an ethic of male exceptionalism, violence as masculinity, requiring the simultaneous elevation of 'our' women in opposition to the degradation of theirs to dehumanized sexual objects, carried out and made real to men and women alike through charged national emblems of violation, rapine, arousal, assault, surrender, protection, penetration and the like. When a society incorporates images of women as valued or devalued ideals, sexual violence

in war is a practicable enactment by men of this everyday set of understandings. Their personal performance of what at other times would be recognized as atrocity is 'symbolic' in that its primary motivations are political, yet the close association of exceptional public concerns with men's everyday interests makes the exercise of this power congenial for men, and facilitates its adoption as a collective enterprise.[63] The militarism argument does not, however, easily deal with the increase in sexual violence at times of ambiguity and intra-state conflict, its association with 'other ranks' rather than officers, nor readily with male-on-male sexual violence nor the occasional participation of women in sexual violence. If, however, 'militarism' is simply local male interest consolidated at the level of the state, then the devaluing of enemy women and men as sexual objects may be enhanced in civil conflicts when in-group gender relations are perceived as threatened.

(2) What we can call the *transgressive* (or lack of restraint) argument: the unchaining of a generally disallowed biological imperative of absolute desire and destruction following an increase in individual power over others; male propensities and their realization usually being checked by social sanctions but now unleashed through the opportunities of war, initially by those who might otherwise be regarded as psychopathic (and who merely represent men in a strong form), but which are then enacted by others through suggestion, solidarity and imitation,[64] sexual caprice and opportunity. As one code ('do not kill') is officially transgressed against a dehumanized enemy,[65] other less formal transgressions may follow more easily; the sanctioned killing of armed civilians in civil war is already a greater transgression than the uniformed war game, for which, after all, every European male is prepared through childhood toys and organized sport. Like the militarism argument, lack of restraint proposes all men as inherent rapists, but here social values initially limit rather than encourage sexual violence. Once it occurs, rape becomes conventionalized as a local practice with its own rules as to appropriate practice[66] sometimes approaching local institutions of actual bride capture.[67] Despite its origins in government calls to physically eliminate a minority group, rape of the Rwanda Tutsi became locally regularized in various ways: captured girls as young as 5 were mutilated, then 'liberated' (the local euphemism for rape) and killed; older ones could be rescued by others who then proposed protection and sexual relations under the threat of abandonment in a hierarchy of emergent local power through which abused girls were handed down or sold for rape to less powerful men and allies (compare the perks for Indian and Nepali police protection of child prostitution[68]); rape as public humiliation in front of crowds at crossroads or road-blocks yet sometimes accompanied by a secret promise of later marriage; rape as interrogation, and the rape of corpses; ownership of women determined by

conflicts over which military sector they were captured in, military tribunals allocating these 'second wives'[69] as booty to men who were then sometimes accused by rivals of consorting with the enemy and were killed in their turn together with the women.[70]

If the loss of restraint explanation is satisfactory in itself, however, I would suggest that collective sexual violence would be more common in peacetime. Group rape is fairly unusual (compared with wartime) in civilian Euro-America except in contexts which parallel the military: typically motor-cycle and ethnic gangs (as among young American Whites during Reconstruction after the civil war) where it may be standardized as an initiation, the norms of the local grouping outweighing and deliberately inverting those of the wider society. In situations of insurgency and civil war, it is not, however, easy to hold to customary distinctions between professional and inducted soldiers, political and religious militias, local ad hoc groupings banding together for protection, and territorial or kin-based armed bands. Or indeed to local versus wider norms.

Why sexual violence? Biosocial and situational arguments

There are some questions which neither argument – militarism or loss of restraint – easily explain. Why *sexual* violence? Why this association of the erotic and the generative with the destructive? There can already be something like a 'Dionysian' sexual ecstasy in hunting humans not unlike that of competitive sport. If sexual violence generally presumes male genital penetration, it would seem to involve sexual arousal. Now, how does this occur if we assume – on the militarism reciprocity explanation – that individual motivations are in close correspondence with a gendered public ideology itself reliant on human morphology and physiology? How does a man become sexually aroused as a patriotic act of terror? (And this is an issue for those other, largely feminist, accounts of individual peacetime rape which take it as less a bodily indulgence than a preconceived means to accomplish something else – terrorization and humiliation.[71]) The phenomenon seems to presume a closer concordance between human physiology and the public symbolic order than we generally allow. Despite the recent Western popularity of sadistic pornography which employs a dehumanized image to facilitate masturbation, I would suggest that in everyday life violence and sexuality are not generally associated. Yet, in situations of collective terror against women, military and police presumably are sexually stimulated and presumably achieve something like their usual pleasure in penetration, coitus and ejaculation.

Perhaps we have to consider the counter-intuitive (and, for Brownmiller, apologetic) idea that it is not that conditions of war unleash an inherent but usually proscribed pattern of action, some innate potential for sexual violence, but rather that the circumstances of war might specifically *promote* such a potential, or else that sexual pleasure is the primary objective, with the not uncommon lethal penetration by a weapon as a frustrated or disgusted response to a failure to be aroused when power and the encouragement of comrades should confer opportunity, anonymity and impunity. War is less a continuous period of excitement than a time of new and rapidly changing social meanings and bonds, boredom and constraint, punctuated by fear.[72] And anxiety and fear are not the general conditions for men to become sexually aroused – as any sex therapist can tell us. Yet sexual assault, at least in popular perception, is not something that occurs in the heat of battle – when men have other, more pressing biological concerns – but in a reaction to the period of danger afterwards, as in the notion of the spoils of warfare which include the 'rewards' of alien women.

In psychophysiological studies, the period after sustained anxiety or exertion is frequently one of significantly decreased anxiety and loss of inhibition – and this is used in a number of psychological treatments for anxiety. Soldiers themselves view sexual relations as countering battle anxiety.[73] McManners suggests that rape as an effective 'coping style' was endorsed by American army chaplains and psychiatrists in Vietnam. Does sexual violence occur after military victory[74] or after defeat – or both? Robin Dunbar has described how, amongst other primates,[75] a male threatened by other males may engage in flight followed, when safe, by indiscriminate sexual relations with the first female he encounters. Rape of Bengali women by Pakistani soldiers followed their retreat not their advance. Can one propose that sexual violence makes a man less anxious? (Brownmiller notes that it is consistently second-line and support troops who are most likely to rape.) Is rape, like heavy consumption of alcohol,[76] particularly likely after one's own comrades' deaths? (Conversely, away from the war zone the sight of one's partner's naked body during sexual intercourse can awaken memories of stripped corpses with a decrease in immediate sexual arousal.[77])

There are, of course, counter-examples where sexual arousal is more evidently part of an established institution. Rape by police is not uncommon in situations quite devoid of any personal threat. Let me take one example (a particularly unpleasant one because of its elision of individual sexual violence with cultural meanings) which deals with something we might term standardized 'spoiling'. It is drawn from an unconfirmed statement submitted a few years ago to the British Parliamentary Human Rights Group by Sarmast Aklaq-Tabondeh, a former intelligence officer and Revolutionary Guard in Tehran:[78] 'Virgin women prisoners must as a rule be raped before execution. The prison officials would write down the names of guards on the firing squad and the names of officials present, and would then conduct a lottery draw. The night prior to execution the woman is injected with a tranquilliser and the "winner" conducts the rape. The next day, after execution, the religious judge would write out a marriage certificate and send it to the victim's family along with a box of sweets.'[79] Now, while this was related by the same soldier to the institution of *sigheh* (temporary marriage) and a religious court ruling that executed women if they were virgins could still go to paradise,[80] my question here is what is the immediate motivation of the military rapist? What are his notions of sexual pleasure, of his usual sexual pleasure, his expectations (here evidently impossible) of fatherhood through sexual intercourse, and so on? What does he think he is doing? I would argue – and in this clash of understandings, between a wish to condemn and a wish to comprehend, my suggestion is unlikely to be convincing – that we need to know much more about the soldier's view at the time of his act. How does he consider and deal with the conventional objections to rape? Perhaps by dehumanization which then justifies violence as a collective practice? But then how does he justify sexual intercourse with a non-human?[81]

Am I being too cognitive, pursuing meaning beyond the limits of its likely application? Our obvious reluctance to extrapolate from physiology or primate analogues but rather to emphasize human meanings follows the near impossibility of research in humans (any findings in this area from military medicine are not publicly available) and because of the post-conflict disgust, on the part of both principal and his surviving victim, which prevents any sort of detailed contextual study. War is sanitized in military memoirs, certainly on the part of the victors. T. E. Lawrence's hints of his having been sodomized by Turkish soldiers in Syria is unusual.[82] It has taken us 50 years to have any sort of open knowledge of the hundreds of thousands of Korean and Chinese 'comfort women' (sexual slaves) of the Japanese military, and that without any apology that atrocity was necessarily concealed because scientific knowledge gained from it was secretly appropriated by the eventual victors (as with the American data on Japanese medical executions of Chinese prisoners by hypothermia). Indeed, discussion of sex in war is avoided by military historians. At a more banal level, we know little about the military brothels organized by Allies and Axis in the Second World War apart from some sardonic comments on the introduction of penicillin in the memoirs of British military doctors stationed in Cairo.[83]

Even if 'innate' is not 'inevitable', any study of the motivations of men who carried out sexual violence, or of the particular contexts in which sexual violence becomes possible and is carried out, threatens to turn the men from perpetrators into something like victims, or at least to normalize the pattern as a 'social activity': understanding as exculpation rather than as explanation. (And thence recalling nineteenth-century explanations, such as those of Herbert Spencer, which took war as constitutive of social relations.) One is reminded of Allan Young's recent book where he shows how the novel category of *post-traumatic stress disorder* emerged in the 1980s out of arguments by psychiatrists in the Veteran Administration's hospitals in the United States.[84] The diagnosis of PTSD allowed those soldiers guilty of sexual massacre and rape in Vietnam to become victims in their turn, victims of the 'trauma' of war in general; atrocity becomes the natural act of the traumatized.[85] And it may be that public recognition of sexual violence by our contemporary military is too recent to allow moral outrage to be replaced by any sort of explanation. While social anthropologists might now be at ease with describing football gang violence as a 'performance', they are likely to have difficulty extending this idiom to standardized sexual violence which must remain deviant and exceptional – if not primitive.

I would, however, add two more general interpretations to those of militarism and lack of restraint.

Sexuality and violence are inherently (that is biosocially) associated or, if you prefer, aspects of the same male group interests. (Hutu rapists of Tutsi women persistently demonstrated a murderous curiosity about Tutsi sexuality and reproductive capacity.[86]) Each may lead to the other, for men's sexual relations are already in a sense aggressive, while violence may approach or facilitate sexual ecstasy. Prevention is thus an issue of restraints on war in general. We might term this the *psychoanalytic* or else *Stalinist* argument, Stalin having replied to muted Anglo-American protests as to the mass rape of German women in 1945 by arguing that sexual violence was inevitable in any war.[87] Indeed, the Soviet poet and novelist Ilya Ehrenburg urged his victorious compatriots to 'Kill. There is nothing that is innocent in the German ... Break by force the racial haughtiness of German women! Take them as your lawful prey!'[88]

Finally, both violence and sexuality are contingent and incremental, possibly in reaction to each other or related through psychophysiological (limbic) mechanisms of 'arousal'. War is an unusual biosocial situation which increases the possibility of sexual violence against women, perhaps because sexual activity reduces anxiety and confers a sense of necessary autonomy in conflictual and overwhelming situations. Like the restraint transgression argument, this might account for escalation to total terrorization, as sexual penetration by itself proves increasingly inadequate in a situation of escalating indiscriminate violence for its own sake.

The four arguments are partial and they are complementary to each other (militarism, for instance, being the value of male group interests), and I would argue that perhaps they are all valid within certain limits which as yet we do not know. They are not only my attempts at interpretation but presumably similar to those used by the men concerned, both at the time and afterwards as legitimation or (rarely) apology. There must be more than a million men alive who have carried out collective sexual violence against women in war, insurgency, riots or gang activism. And on these acts (with the exception of 'The Winter Soldier Investigation' of the Vietnam Veterans Against the War) they have remained silent. How they make sense of them – forgetting, excusing, memorializing – we do not know. Nor whether their exculpations are all of a piece when talking to, say, their current sexual partner, their priest, doctor or former comrades.

Men in a group

Consolidation of male interest groups appears cross-culturally (and across species) linked to lesser consideration for female interests.[89] I do not propose to detail here the psychoanalysts' biosocial arguments as to the inevitable association of sexuality and death – or, as they generally put it, on sexuality and aggression.[90] Certainly they are the most detailed of any discipline. Their notion of 'sadism' as frustrated or displaced sexuality does provide a model whereby sexuality as the primary impulse may be transformed into violence, why the fetishized weapon rather than the male genital organ becomes the physical power of penetration, and why anxiety may be a mediating agent.[91] That war *is* primarily a rape is now hardly current as an explanation of warfare in general beyond some commentators in the women's movement, but if I am right in maintaining that rape in war is all but ubiquitous, we might wonder if the sanitization of war into a military history of decision-making (such that even to describe warfare as 'collective violence' appears rhetorical) does avoid some essential concomitants, perhaps even material causes, of collective violence. Judicial castration of violent civilian sex offenders in Scandinavia has some effect in reducing the sexual focus of their actions, but not their violence.

Psychoanalysts offer interesting, but I think unlikely, suggestions as to the relationship between men participating in collective sexual relations with women. Sexual violence in war is generally a collective action which suggests the association between the men may be significant. Serial rape involves each successive male penetrating and ejaculating where another male has just done the same, a pattern of inter-male intimacy[92] generally unusual outside war situations and which psychoanalysis proposes as primarily a sexual relationship between the men themselves. Implausible, yet I think the complicity of every male present (recalling that of the members of the execution squad) is not to be explained simply by a decision of the instigators to spread the responsibility and reduce the number of potential witnesses later,[93] but that it is generating or affirming some particular relationship between the men. But what? Quasi-affinity? Whether there is any psychological or ethological evidence for males in a group that has been exposed to violence to then seek sexual activity as anxiolytic more than each would individually I do not know. Nor do we know much of those men who do not join in rape yet who are complicit through their witnessing. A surprisingly common account by a surviving woman in both Rwanda and Bosnia is of the low-status soldier who does not join in the collective rape, who apologizes and helps her dress and escape, sometimes to later demand sexual access in the name of protection in contrast to the brutality of his comrades. He appears so frequently that I am almost persuaded that he is an integral part of the whole business.

Genes, territory and resources

Based on a systems theory comparison of non-state polities, Otterbein has argued that the frequency of warfare can be predicted better from social structure than from ecological or environmental causes: where a political subsystem mobilizes localized groups of agnatic males, rape is also common and warfare is more likely to resemble a feud in its killing of male captives and valuing of prestige and booty in a practical emphasis on reciprocity rather than deterrence.[94] And we might argue that the collapse of central authority together with the tactics demanded by contemporary weaponry in 'small wars' now promote something recalling such groupings.

Assumptions of male solidarity may for anthropologists be a more congenial implicit psychology than more evidently psychophysiological proposals yet they are equally tenuous. Biosocial theorists have emphasized a sexual potential – if not imperative – behind war, citing its ubiquity and primate analogues, its pragmatic irrationality but ability to fascinate, the enthusiasm it arouses in both men and women and its capacity for uniting the group which organizes it, that wars are waged primarily by men against men, that fighting and subsequent reproduction are temporally associated among many mammals, that females preferentially select powerful mates, that 'dominance' in other primates (gorillas) may involve mounting and even ejaculation, the quality of female vocalizations during orgasm, and that rape of the enemy results in genetic hybridization – or if you prefer it, exogamy.[95] In this sense, war between men goes inherently with the rape of women, and their proximal meanings and sufferings are irrelevant. As with other biosocial models, those of war may or may not be plausible but they are unprovable,[96] yet aggressive sexuality is certainly associated with human reproduction, and the consequences of military rape frequently include pregnancy: 25,000 Bengali women became pregnant in rapes by Pakistani soldiers in 1971;[97] 5,000 newborn babies were abandoned by their mothers after the Rwanda massacres.[98]

Since the Nazi Holocaust, an explicit 'eugenic' motivation (the opposite of the implicit hybridization argument) has been of academic interest in explaining massacre and genocide, whether in immediately displacing or eliminating another human group so that material resources and territory may be acquired, or else as some elaborated or implicit notion of denying reproductive advantage related to local notions of 'race' or the biological integrity of a 'nation'.[99] In the former Yugoslavia, General Mladic claimed that Serbs were being outbred by Bosnia's Muslims – 'a demographic bomb'. In Rwanda, the violence was sparked in part by planted rumours that family planning policies were targeted specifically on the Hutu, and that Tutsi women's sexuality was a political threat,[100] while argument as to the reproductive capacities of minority groups and their future electoral significance have surfaced in Northern Ireland and in Israel. It may be significant that the Bosnian Serbs were led by a doctor, and local medical professionals have been implicated in the mass killings in Bosnia; whether this is simply because doctors are prominent among the local elite – like clergy and teachers in Rwanda[101] – is uncertain.

One of the Serb rapists was a doctor who, as his victim later reported, shouted as he entered her: 'Now you know how strong we are, Croatian utasha [fascist]; you should be raped, killed, destroyed.'[102] This argues sexual violence as simply the violence of war, but other accounts by survivors record that Bosnian women were told as they were raped that they would 'make a Serb baby', and were kept in custody to be raped continually until they became pregnant, and then secluded until too late in their pregnancy to make an abortion feasible.[103] Croatian male prisoners in a Serb camp were beaten on the testicles: 'As they were beating us, they were shouting "Now you will not be able to make any more Utasha babies."'[104] However, in another Bosnian instance, the rapist who impregnated a fellow villager, sent her a message later to say that after the child was born he would come and kill it.[105] These may, of course, be less two contradictory motivations than two stages: a desire for the enemy woman to bear one's child (denial of reproductive advantage to the enemy), followed after the conflict by shame and a wish to blame the woman and destroy the human evidence of what only now is recognized as a crime.

The term employed in the former Yugoslavia, 'ethnic cleansing', though not elaborated as a eugenic theory, uses familiar clinical imagery of purification, excision and integrity in favour of the *lebensraum* and unity of the social order which will emerge, while the Rwandan impregnation of enemy women as 'second wives' after the killing of their men returns us to the bride capture justification of social foundation. Whether we can claim here any biosocial potentiality is doubtful: there are few obvious primate analogues, nor are there historical data of any consistent military preference for the co-option rather than the physical elimination of women. But we can certainly regard sexual violence in terms of the local meanings – whether or not we take these as materially causal – for displaced populations in situations of contested boundaries, where idioms of fecundity (reproductive advantage), kinship, locality and physical appearance intersect and constitute each other in recreated local ethnohistories. In the case of the Holocaust, extermination was, of course, explicitly linked with the medical profession's existing racial genetics which was murderously fascinated with the enigma of twins, and which attempted to co-opt 'Germanic' women among the conquered Slav nations to breed with chosen German soldiers and police.

The slippage between my own suggestions as to the relevance of biosocial models (generally of a 'fraternal interest group' or 'late palaeolithic genes in the twentieth-century three-part brain' sort) and those explanations offered by war criminals themselves must, I imagine, cause concern. The objection to primate analogues (which we shall consider more in the next chapter) is whether a particular identified pattern is equivalent in humans and animals, that it is a discrete process, and that its occurrence always has the same antecedents. The not unreasonable objection to any interpretation which is not couched in terms of cultural meanings and motivations is of course the 'Darwinian' anthropology of the nineteenth century which provided a scientific legitimation of Nazi terror, the responsibility for human action cast onto a natural process which, seen as inevitable, removed consideration of morality from actions we would now regard as political strategies. And despite the denials by contemporary biosocial theorists, postulated genetic mechanisms for complex institutions offer less hope of human alleviation than purely 'cultural' interpretations. Despite ascribing them to local meanings (and thence they might be susceptible of change), social anthropologists assume that extensive rape and violence among Europeans are essentially 'irrational' and inevitably destructive of human institutions.[106] And in doing so they perhaps have difficulty avoiding recourse to tropes evoking something like 'underlying primitivism'; and thence their preference for immediate political and instrumental motivations.

Eric Hobsbawm has recently described the Great War's blurring of the distinction between combatant and civilian as initiating what he terms our 'age of catastrophe'.[107] Similarly, Omer Bartov has argued that this war of attrition became a paradigm for industrialized mass killing by civilians in arms, lowering the threshold of what was permissible, and thus allowing the Holocaust.[108] It may be that the professionalization of European warfare in the early modern period which I have perhaps unfairly characterized as 'militarism', with its board game idioms of a clear field with boundaries between civilians and combatants, has been a brief and geographically limited phenomenon. If so, the current 'privatisation' and deritualization of war by armed civilians as a cheap proxy for a professional army, the shift from battle to attrition, the uncoupling of bodily strength from lethal capability, the transformation of conventionalized and limited feuding into religio-political total war, together with increasing global potentials for making, remaking and unmaking communal identities, do not auger well.

Whether rules of war were accepted by professional armies in the early modern period through a pure transformation of ethical values, through the risks of unprecedented military technologies, or simply through fear of escalation beyond civilian ethics of human conduct, is debatable. Despite global publicity, the attempt to hold to account those we now recognize as 'war criminals', whether in Bosnia or East Timor, appear limited. There *are* no sanctions. Perhaps, as the historian John Keegan observes, 'There is no substitute for honour as a medium of enforcing decency on the battlefield . . .'[109]

8. Genetic Sexual Attraction and the Theory of Incest

My suggestion of what are humanly meaningless naturalistic models in the last chapter might have given rise to some discomfort: am I arguing for sociobiology? The Butterfly/Serpent relationship (Chapter 3) can certainly be on some inherent as well as cultural tendency of women to surrender to men. Let me offer an instance of another 'new illness' – or at least of a non-adaptive pattern of action – which illustrates the contingency of human action rather than the inevitability of 'biology'. And which incidentally tells us much about a once favourite theme of anthropological theorizing.

This pattern only became possible recently. Following Britain's Access to Birth Records Act of 1975, which enabled anyone over 18 who had been adopted to trace their parents, an increasing number of reunions of the adopted have been possible with their biological relatives. In anticipation that personal difficulties might follow tracing, a counselling clause was included under Section 26 (now 51) of the Act. A number of counselling agencies then developed, initially intending to focus on the problems faced by the adoptive parents, but increasingly responding to the adoptees, the biological parents and other relatives.[1] As the number of successful traces has increased, the focus of counselling includes problems that arise following reunions. Among these complications is a problem referred to by counsellors as 'genetic sexual attraction' (GSA): powerful erotic feelings developing between reunited relatives.[2] Estimates of the frequency of GSA vary;[3] its recognition and resolution have proved difficult in conventional counselling because both clients and therapists recognize that acting on these feelings is illegal. Counsellors are torn between maintaining the conventional psychotherapeutic distance, and a wish to actively prevent dangerous sexual attachments which they recognize as unusually powerful.

The prohibition of 'incest' – sexual relations between closely related kin – remains a major issue for biosocial theories of human culture.[4] Nineteenth-century biologists and evolutionary anthropologists argued that the essential step which differentiated human societies from earlier hominid groups had been the injunction against sexual relations between siblings, and between parent and child. Psychoanalytical reconstructions of early human history linked this schema to a continuing social repression of innate incestuous desires. Whilst contemporary ethological theorists similarly argue for genetically determined erotic interests, they perceive these as reinforced or redirected by demographic and ecological constraints which social injunctions against incest then simply reproduce.[5] Contemporary social anthropologists also argue for the universality of the avoidance of incest in their analysis of kinship, but they have generally emphasized a clear opposition of nature (biological promiscuity among primates, and potentially among humans) to culture (incest avoidance and by extension marriage rules in human societies).[6]

Assuming that societies actually do successfully prohibit incest, these reconstructions of the origin of incest prohibitions have deflected interest away from their not infrequent breach.[7] The actual incidence of intra-familial sexual relations in contemporary Western societies is unknown. Estimates range from 3 to 62 per cent of children for adult–child sexual relations (with rather different sample populations and definitions of incest or other sexual abuse including that of non-relatives.[8]) Figures for sibling incest are even less certain: over 60 per cent of the population in some studies have reported some sort of early sexual experimentation with other children, but physical relations between siblings after sexual maturity seem much rarer. Regarded as uncommon and relatively trivial until recently, father–daughter incest is now identified as a predisposing factor in a number of psychopathologies, resulting in a critique of psychoanalytical assumptions that incest is personal fantasy rather than actual occurrence,[9] and in the argument that father–daughter incest should be regarded as physical and emotional abuse. Cross-generational incest, particularly the most common, father–daughter, is now pathologized through television programmes, support groups and telephone crisis lines, yet in the United States there have been a number of legal challenges to the prohibition of consensual sexual relations and marriage between adult siblings, and between parents and their adult children.[10]

Both the earlier historical reconstructions and our contemporary concerns argue psychological processes as a mediating biosocial variable: in the former, that human psychology is itself engendered in the conflict between biological drives and social demands; in the latter, that individual psychological development and identity are damaged through a contradiction between generational role and personal gratification. Little interest has been paid to the adult motivation which is regarded popularly as perverse recreational sex; by feminists as a standardized manifestation of men's coercive power over women;[11] or simply as male sexual desire in situations where parenting responsibilities and constraints are undervalued.[12]

Why is incest avoided?

A number of arguments have attempted to explain the rule against sexual relations between closely related kin. Social anthropologists, for whom indigenous conceptions of kinship are of major theoretical importance, argue that any functioning society must organize itself around fundamental distinctions between the generations, and that depending on local understandings of reproduction, procreation between family members would seriously confuse this.[13] And also that it may be appreciated by societies themselves that continuing incest would decrease the availability of young women for marriage with potential allies:[14] 'Marry out or die out' as the anthropological aphorism puts it. In other words, incest is simply 'good to think with', and incest prohibition and exogamy (marriage outside the group) are closely related.

In the contemporary West, by contrast, incest is now regarded primarily as an assault on the dependence and trust justified by biological relatedness. When incest involves a child it negates the 'natural' generational relationships which seem essential to the nurturing of young primates with their extended period of immaturity.[15] While small-scale and non-industrialized societies have complex systems of kinship and descent, most contemporary biosocial theorists maintain that these are symbolic manifestations of certain core biological imperatives;[16] or at least that any continuing cultural pattern must be consistent with the biological survival of the group.[17] Evolutionary explanations for the infrequency of mating between individuals where relatedness by direct descent r is at least 25 per cent argue for a sharply increased risk of recessive genetic diseases in the offspring who may also be infertile;[18] and that this may somehow be culturally recognized. There is certainly evidence that repeated in-group mating lowers the genetic heterogeneity of a population, thus perhaps rendering it less adaptive,[19] but alternation between inbreeding and outbreeding can be an effective way of promoting and dispersing advantageous genetic characteristics,[20] and only in highly outbred populations are deleterious recessive alleles likely to accumulate significantly. Inbreeding is not disadvantageous if the costs of trying to find a less closely related mate are high, such as might be imposed by high rates of predation during movement to another group. From the perspective of the child's inclusive fitness, an incestuous attraction might even be in its interests, diverting the father from further reproduction in favour of continued involvement and nurturance.[21]

The genetic arguments against close inbreeding are variable and inconclusive: evolutionary explanations are concerned with statistical tendencies not absolutes. Nor do non-Western kinship systems explicitly argue anything like this although other sicknesses, notably leprosy, are often regarded as a consequence of breaching incest prohibitions. Historical exceptions have been described where sibling marriage (but not parent–child marriage) was enjoined over considerable periods between elite members of stratified societies in order to consolidate power and property.[22] The current law against incestuous sexual relations (as opposed to the existing proscription of incestuous marriage) was introduced in England only in 1908, and under circumstances which suggest less widespread popular concern than lobbying by the eugenics movement. That cultures have necessarily recognized and incorporated biological justifications into their institutions, whether explicitly (as pragmatic knowledge) or implicitly (through the natural selection of advantageous cultural traits), is controversial and by no means accepted.[23] Certainly cultures consider incest avoidance as itself 'natural'. In the West popular justifications invoke genetic interpretations however inaccurate; incest in Britain is incorrectly regarded as both rarer than it actually is, yet particularly prevalent in certain deviant groups, among isolated rural communities, and those who are less educated or less intelligent.[24]

How is incest avoided?

The universality of incest prohibitions of various types has led most authors to conclude that they continue to be inherently associated with individual psychological development and socialization. Two rather different 'proximate mechanisms'[25] have been suggested. The first assumes that the focus of early erotic inclinations is indiscriminate and thus directed to immediately available individuals, including family members, but that these interests then diminish through boredom and thence indifference. (In ethological terminology, co-rearing in co-residential families leads to outmating.) That 'familiarity breeds contempt' has long been popularly recognized,[26] and was first proposed theoretically by Westermarck who argued that sanctions against incest are redundant since 'custom and law' simply restate natural human behaviour.[27] Contemporary evidence includes the lack of erotic attachments, indeed actual sexual aversion, between non-related children reared together on kibbutzim.[28] In societies where endogamous marriage is encouraged between individuals who have been brought up together, lack of sexual interest, low birth rates and marital breakdown are common, as in Lebanese patrilateral parallel cousin marriage or one form of Chinese marriage where the young girl is adopted into her future husband's family.[29]

The second approach, exemplified by psychoanalysis and social anthropology, argues that the prohibition of something already unlikely is implausible. Cultural rules are always necessary to prevent expression of incestuous inclinations which are universal from early infancy and closely associated with affiliative affects, and which remain powerfully associated with anger and guilt.[30] Successfully resolved, they are the basis for the child establishing appropriate self-identity and interpersonal relationships.[31] Support for this comes from psychoanalytical and ethnographic descriptions of early child development, from the identification of incestuous themes in myths and in the course of adult therapy; from the cultural associations between sex and violence, and from the ambivalent literary and popular interest in incest – the very idea of which occasions horror or hilarity (or indeed both). And also, paradoxically, from the recent recognition that parent–child sexual relations are actually more common in Western nuclear families than psychoanalysis once assumed; according to Westermarck's model they would not be likely.

Empirical evidence for arguing either position is uncertain, as in any attempt to distinguish biological (potential) from cultural (meanings) in a given biosocial pattern: the distinction may be argued to be an instance of the erroneous Western opposition between nature and culture as essential categories.[32] There is considerable debate in the human sciences as to whether human sexuality can be taken as some fixed universal ground which cultural patterns represent or whether it is dialectically related to social action.[33] As with parenting, there are always ambiguities as to where 'natural' competence may be said to end, and where the cultural institutions apparently based on reinforcing, or exemplifying, these potentials begin.[34] Primate studies are of uncertain relevance, for apparently similar proximate mechanisms in different species may evolve for rather different functional reasons, while neither indiscriminate nor fixed species-specific mating patterns are observed in non-human primates.[35] Primates generally do not have sex with close relatives, both by dispersion of the population, and thus relative lack of opportunity, and by apparent direct 'avoidance';[36] but such 'avoidance' is variable, a statistical outcome contingent on ecological and demographic constraints.[37] It is not clear whether such a sexual preference for strangers and reduced sexual activity in the presence of opposite-sex relatives requires some sort of phenotypic kin 'recognition' learned through early proximity.[38] And whether this is recognition of the other as an individual or of some shared features of a common site such as the nest. Rodents avoid sex with those who are not related but with whom they have been experimentally reared together, but not with phenotypically related but unfamiliar siblings.[39]

A common objection to sociobiological arguments is to question whether particular patterns such as 'avoidance' and 'recognition' are equivalent in human and primate. Should we use in both instances some functional definition of 'recognition' as simply the differential treatment of conspecifics as a function of their genetic relatedness? Or for humans (and perhaps animals) invoke some sort of identification of particular individuals through self-reference? Any identified 'erotic' sentiment among humans towards close relatives can be distinguished only with difficulty from: the affective attachment by the young to their care givers; the converse, parental nurturance; affiliative sentiments to kin; mutual teasing; sexual 'play' and experimentation; the socially prescribed (or biological) attachment of younger females to dominant older males; or – in the case of the adult male – from a generalized erotic interest in young females among whom relatives just happen to be more 'accessible'. And it is their plasticity of affiliative affects which characterizes humans. [40]

The continuing symbolic power of incest and the frequency of actual incestuous relationships in many societies argue against the Westermarck hypothesis in its original form. Robin Fox deals with the weaknesses of both proximate ('how') theories by arguing that it is the cultural impetus for marrying out that is biologically selected. [41] While incest and exogamy do not run neatly together, they are closely related. In the general run of things, he suggests, early hominids had no strong aversion to incest, or particular inclination to it; it was just unlikely because at a gatherer–hunter level of social organization, the parent was likely to be dead before the child became sexually active, and male sexual interests would be directed to the younger mature females in preference to a surviving mother, while high rates of infant mortality and thus wide spacing of births made sibling incest unlikely. [42] As with the prohibition of homicide, some societies happened to reinforce this general infrequency of incest by encouraging something like exogamy and incest prohibition, and these societies then proved more successful in cultivating alliances and expanding their numbers. And thus while the cultural institutions and rules selected by biological survival are generally opposed to incest, and boost its initial unlikeliness, there is considerable variation in the institutions which are adopted, depending on local ecological and demographic needs, and on the later development of state-level organization. It is the cultural recognition of incest, then, not its random genetic consequences, that is biologically significant: in practice men can engage in 'incest' with young female relatives by reclassifying them as non-relatives. [43]

According to Fox's model, the possibility of intrafamilial sexual relations has continued even when the cultural prohibition has been established but generally they still do not happen for demographic reasons. [44] In modern Western societies, however, while the cultural prohibition remains, incest is now perhaps more likely because earlier sexual maturation, longer life-spans and better nutrition result in longer periods of potential sexual activity, which overlap with those of another generation; and individuals in an industrialized society have less economic interest in establishing marriage alliances with their fellows. Increased domestic privacy (and thus reduced proximity) may also contribute.[45] To which one might add a concomitant individualization and eroticization of the young, with the notion of 'adolescence' ambiguously marking the recognition of sexually mature but socially immature young adults.[46] That there has been a related Western shift in male sexual interest towards less mature young females is also possible.

Post-adoption incest

Current research is largely concerned with intergenerational incest as the sexual abuse of a child. There is little information on the psychological antecedents and consequences of sexual relationships between consenting adults who are related biologically or through adoption. Recently the Western media has reported a number of such cases (notably Eric Gill, Anaïs Nin and Woody Allen) which assume, with debatable evidence, personally harmful outcomes; the outrage these attract argues for a continuing Western antipathy to parent–child incest (and a fascination with it), despite the loosening of the nuclear family as an enduring and cohesive social unit, and the untying of moral norms from race, age, parenthood, gender, sexual choice or other 'biological' attributes.[47]

Evidence to support both Westermarck and Freud comes from ethnographic studies of various cultures, primatology, social psychological and judicial investigations into the reported frequency of incestuous activity, and psychiatric studies focusing on its consequences, together with literary and anecdotal sources. All these, however, look at incestuous relationships as they occur involving children and where some degree of close association in co-residential families already occurs at the same time as any incestuous interests, whether fantasized or otherwise. They cannot be said to test the familiarity hypothesis, since they do not include situations where first-degree relatives who are unfamiliar with each other later have sexual access to each other. One needs to find situations where it is common for close relatives to be separated at, or soon after, birth, and then become reunited in adulthood. Whilst such situations do occur during migration or widespread civil and military disruptions (and were a common theme of nineteenth-century Romantic literature), it is difficult to standardize the experiences or to allow for confounding psychological traumata.

It is precisely under such conditions that genetic sexual attraction appears. In order to clarify some of the issues, my colleague Maurice Greenberg and I set up a project at a London post-adoption agency both to discuss GSA with the counsellors and to interview clients who had personal experience of it.[48] These people were self-selected in that they had requested counselling for their 'illness' and were also willing to be interviewed for research purposes, or who had responded to a notice placed in a post-adoption newsletter briefly describing the issues and inviting responses. In addition, many individuals phoned or wrote (sometimes anonymously) describing experiences of GSA; unlike those formally interviewed, many of these were the adoptive parents.

The instances summarized here are derived from an interview with informants. The data collected included: social and demographic background and personal relationships including marriage; a birth history with details of the biological parent and siblings; similar data about the adoptive family, the circumstances of the adoption and how much information had been provided and when; a developmental history which included any earlier medical or psychological problems, together with informants' description of their personality; details of the reunion, how it was organized, by whom, and feelings at the time. Informants were asked about any erotic interests – when they emerged, their quality and consequences. Details of any sexual relationship were recorded: informants were asked to comment on the outcome, how they made sense of it, whether any particular complications had arisen, and whether they had wished, or found it possible, to continue the relationship in a non-sexual way.

Experience and personal meanings

The social background of the informants varied from higher professional to unskilled. All nine were White. Three had degrees; all were articulate. Adopted before 6 months of age, all except one were brought up knowing they had been adopted; the exception was a family in which 'everybody knew but nobody talked about it'. The adoptive milieu seems to have varied from happy to one where the young girl was repeatedly told she had 'bad blood coming out'. There were two instances of suggestions having been made by the adoptive families about previous incestuous relationships in the child's biological family. Individual mental health before the reunion varied: there were two resolved instances of eating disorders (one with a continuing alcohol problem), one of intermittent agoraphobia, and one informant recalled what might have been a behavioural disorder in early childhood. None had had sexual relationships inside their adoptive family, or as a child with other adults. The average age on contacting the biological family was 37. All had previously had heterosexual relationships, one also a lesbian relationship; five were in a marriage or stable partnership at the time of tracing. Informants often represented themselves as lacking in confidence yet as what might be glossed as 'vital and nervy'; they had anticipated that their biological families would be livelier than their adoptive families who were often considered staid or even cold. Some examples follow:

Case 2 [Married professional woman with three children who traces her biological family when she is 40, and meets her sister.] Jane knew I was my mother's daughter just by looking at me. I took my shoes off to show my feet, my hands and knuckles, photographs of me from the back. It began with fascination with similarities and differences. We needed to be together and still do. Last year Jane and her husband were apart while selling a house and we spent increasing times together. I liked feeling her against me, her hands, leaning. It was part of belonging – what I wanted from my mum because I never belonged anywhere. [She visits the post-adoption centre and discusses the situation; they warn her of the possible consequences which she denies: 'All we want is a cuddle!'] It just felt like falling in love. It was someone I'd belong to, it's my sister, it's nice, I'm lucky. We couldn't get enough time together. A goodbye kiss on the cheek, then the lips. No resistance. It seemed right, though it seems awful now. [The two families go on holiday together.] That's where it went below the waist, I never thought it would happen. I just wanted to be close. [The genital relationship has continued sporadically. She says that if it were not for her own children the two sisters would live together, but does not see herself or Jane as lesbian. She feels both the attraction and sex are mutual.]

Case 4 [A 22-year-old civil servant in a long-standing relationship with his girlfriend traces his mother; he 'knows' already from his birth certificate that she will be very pretty.] It made me feel good. It built up my expectation. I kind of knew I'd be attracted to her. [He phones. They speak a few times and feel increasingly comfortable. They 'love each other's voices'. She comes to visit and is advised by the counselling agency, already concerned about GSA, to bring her husband: she doesn't.] Neither of us wanted that, we wanted to go away and be alone on our own. I saw her – she waved. My immediate thought was that can't be my mother, she's really attractive! We meet, smile, kiss. [They have lunch together.] I notice her nose, brow, deep-set eyes; I am constantly looking for similarities – a happy smile, bits that were cheeky. She said, 'I've got to touch you' and touched my face with her hand. I shook. It felt nice. There was an increase in touching and hugs. I felt really odd, buzzing over the top. [He has an erection.] She said there's nothing between us as we walked the next day. I pointed out she kept her handbag between us. She looked coy and apprehensive, I felt the same. On the Saturday we sat on a bench in the park for hours, we talked about our feelings for each other. She played on my face with her hands and I began to kiss her fingers. When it got too strong we drew back. On the Monday we dressed up for each other and went out for the evening. She put her hand on the inside of my leg – I picked it up and put it on the seat. I said, 'What are we doing?' She looked gorgeous, I felt teased, and she admitted she was teasing me. We tried to avoid situations where we would get too close. However, we finished up in Camden in a dark passage. We kissed, tinkering on the edge. [She returns home and he now begins to feel increasingly irritated with her teasing telephone calls. He doesn't know how to address her. Mum? Susan?] When we talk on the phone I end up gibbering, saying Mummy. It feels like fainting. It's like being back in the womb. I imagine sucking her breasts. [The counselling agency suggests he introduces her to his adoptive parents; he cannot decide at present.]

Case 5 [A 35-year-old nurse who in her teens 'had a crush' on her adoptive father now traces her biological father.] It developed very quickly, we hugged and kissed a lot that first weekend. His skin felt like mine and he smelled like me. I had a sexual dream about him, wanting it. I just thought it was crazy, but discovered he was open to it. [Her father admitted he had wanted to abort her. She felt strangely relieved: this was the confirmation of earlier feelings in her adoptive family of never having been wanted.] I asked him if he had had other affairs: he got angry and initially denied it. We both knew we were going to get involved with each other. I suspected he was willing to – he'd had a vasectomy – but I definitely felt it was my decision. [They have intercourse frequently over the next year and then the sexual side gradually fades into a 'parent–child relationship'. On balance she reflects she would rather they had not had sex but] I got it out of my system.

The sentiments which all informants describe recall a romantic 'falling in love', intense and explosive, sudden and almost irresistible. They satisfy yearning expectations present before contact is established of a need to discover a particular form of 'closeness'. Some describe themselves as 'in love' with their relative before they meet them. (Another client has written a highly erotic five-page letter to the agency about her son whom she has not yet met and only talked with once on the telephone.) And informants suggest that the response of their relative is similar, both becoming jealous of other relationships, and only with difficulty allowing for the feelings of their existing partners and families. Each finds that they are somehow discovering themselves in the other, deliberately seeking out both physical similarities and emotional affinities: 'There was an immediate sense of recognition; he looked like me, as I had hoped, the face, the gestures. There was a very strong sense of having found each other at last'; 'He seemed familiar, not a stranger; he was me in a male body.' Four informants remark on their recognition of the other's odour, and two women note that they had previously had affairs with men who resembled their biological relative (one father, one brother). Sexual intimacy is felt to be an appropriate, almost inevitable, way of expressing these sentiments: 'It was something to do with recognition; it was like kinship, the proof you're finding each other. It was just mutual, unspoken.' Informants often seem to search for arguments to prevent full sexual intercourse taking place, focusing on the discrepancy in age or the possible impact upon their current family. However, when sexual relations develop, they are experienced as the appropriate consummation of an overwhelming necessity, as something happening naturally, and are seldom felt to be reprehensible: 'It gives me a completeness, it's as if I am trying to get as near to my natural family as I can.' Informants, like counsellors commenting on these accounts, argue that such relationships should not carry the opprobrium of the sexual abuse of 'children': it is as if the family as a natural parenting unit is dissolved when individuals became adults, but can then be reconstituted in new forms. But none of the relationships involve a wish for children to be born from them.

Although these attachments are experienced as complicated by other emotions recognized as inevitable – apprehension, responsibility, affiliation, dependency, fondness, excitement and fear – they are not altogether inhibited by them. With time, those respondents who avoid sexual intercourse, like those who engage in it as an isolated episode, see the relationship as having changed in other ways. One young man now regards his biological mother simply as an older woman to whom he is no longer so attracted. A daughter now recognizes that her father is not particularly likeable, and certainly no longer feels sexually attracted to him. In the one tragic case known to the centre, a mother sought out her criminal son, had a year-long sexual relationship with him as 'the only way to keep him'; he eventually rejected her brutally and she killed herself. In her last letter to the centre shortly before she died she comments, 'The Act of 1975 was the act of a moronic MP. [My son] despises me, the pure love of last year has turned into pure acrimony.'

Where a sexual relationship does continue, the individual wants to maintain close contact as frequently as possible. This led one woman seen at our centre to divorce her husband after she was traced by her adult son. The husband remains bitter: 'They were more like two lovers than mother and child. My wife would spend three hours on the phone to him every night. Then, when he came to stay, I'd walk into a room and find them embracing – they would break off when they saw me. The atmosphere was awful. I felt immense loneliness. I was totally superfluous: I was particularly hurt when I saw her showing him affection which I felt I'd never received from her. When I put my foot down, he moved out. But then she just fretted until she saw him. She couldn't bear being separated from him'.[49] The son too divorced.

Westermarck or Freud?

Post-adoption incestuous attachments are described by our informants as embodying a passionate need to identify themselves in someone whom they resemble, physically or in personality, as a return to some lost unity. One must be wary of generalizing from a small number of self-selected instances, particularly in a situation where the personal rediscovery of a lost family may evoke many kinds of overwhelming emotional responses. And where new attachments may be sought to counter a profound and remembered (or imagined) childhood loss; for the experience of adoption may lead to unusual representations of romantic love and personal identity.[50] Those who choose to seek out their parents may be unusual in some way, either because of some tendencies inherited from their mother (or father) who gave them up for adoption; or because early manifestations of a significant trait made the baby more likely to be adopted; or because of a less satisfactory relationship with their adoptive family.[51] Those who agreed to be interviewed may have had especially intense experiences. Nor do we know much about the other side – the experiences of the parent or sibling whose 'lost child' becomes a lover.

Yet these instances and those described to me by the counsellors offer some support for Westermarck's indifference theory (and for Fox's and Erickson's modifications of it): as Erickson predicted,[52] adults are likely to find themselves sexually attracted to people they meet in intimate situations and who happen to be close relatives but with whom they have not spent long periods of early intimacy which would have diminished erotic interest or differentiated it out from more general sentiments of 'attachment'.[53] Westermarck's theory in its original form would not, however, predict that relatives find themselves powerfully attracted *because* they recognize themselves in the other. The reverse. Yet there is a common popular assumption that people who are physically similar to each other are mutually attracted, contrary to the phenotypic avoidance argument (p. 134), and there is some empirical evidence that this is so;[54] Israeli studies suggest identical twins reared apart are later attracted to each other, and Twitchell cites a colourful example of post-adoptive incest.[55] The psychodynamic interest in 'mirroring' as a representation of personal identity (from Freud's account of narcissism to Lacan's delineation of the mirror phase, Kohut's introduction of mirroring into object relations theory, and Yalom's use of it in group analysis) resonates with this popular recognition of mutual identification as one aspect of romantic love, described by social psychologists as the 'self-matching hypothesis'.[56]

Are sexual and affiliative sentiments incompatible? Against the argument that 'incest' is too loaded and essentialized a category to describe both early inter-sibling sexual experimentation and the rather different parental sexual attraction to the child, we can note that here the subjective experiences seem similar whatever the type of relationship: child/parent and sibling/sibling, heterosexual and homosexual. Sexual and affiliative interests here seem enmeshed, as psychoanalysts and some ethologists argue. Post-adoption 'incest' then may be taken as akin to general attachment[57] which becomes eroticized, whether because the only recognized physical intimacy between adults who have not grown up together is sexual, or because no close parenting or sibling relationship had developed.[58] Comparison of biological fathers and stepfathers with differing degrees of early contact with a child suggests that biological relatedness (and thus recognition of phenotypic similarity) seems less significant in avoiding incest than a close parenting relationship with the child in its early years.[59] This is the same 'sensitive' period of development during which close sibling contact seems associated with later sexual aversion in humans and primates, a type of 'negative imprinting' as Shepher calls it, Fox's 'intensive tactile interaction'.[60] When in contact with their young children parents usually learn a parental role which is incompatible with an overt sexual relationship; incestuous fathers often claim that they had not been able to differentiate sexual from parental attachments.[61] Erickson and Roscoe argue similarly from the primate evidence that there generally seems an inverse relationship between 'familial attraction' (intense physical interaction, parental bonding and nurturance) and 'sexual attraction'.[62] But again in co-residential households it is impossible to distinguish either contingent proximity or bonding from the cultural meanings of paternity for both fathers and stepfathers. Mothers are generally in close parenting contact with their children yet there has been a continued debate as to the 'erotic' quality of both breastfeeding and maternal play with young children's genitals.[63] One mother seen at our post-adoption agency said of the reunion with her adult son: 'It reminded me of how I felt towards my [other] son when he was a baby – it was so sexual.' (And a virtually pornographic but apparently authentic telephone call recorded at the same centre detailed a young man's excitement at tracing his mother and then, on having sex with her, discovering she was lactating.)

From the perspective of the child, our informants' subjective reports are consistent with the Freudian and ethnographic arguments for the plasticity of libinal/affiliative sentiments, and with connectionist models of cognition and affect.[64] On the psychoanalytical model, in the post-adoption reunion any repressed incestuous desire for the adoptive parent could be later displaced onto a recognized biological relative for whom erotic attachments have never been repressed, and thus the incestuous desire for the adoptive parent satisfied in fantasy. One informant told us she had previously experienced not dissimilar feelings for her adoptive father which 'I repressed as incestuous'; while recognizing that similar feelings for her newly discovered biological father were conventionally regarded as incestuous, they did not occasion quite the same intense moral imperative to be resisted.

At a high level of generality, what is described by Freud as 'repression' is equivalent in social outcome to Westermarck's and Fox's 'indifference'. Adults are more likely to pursue their sexual interests with people who have been brought up outside their family unit: actual incest is usually avoided. Common factors include the social expectations for the young adult to develop a widening social experience with opportunities to experiment in other areas of social development. One essential difference between the theories is whether one views the change in the attachments of an individual as due to a necessary repression and transformation, or simply as biologically redirected into a widening area of interest irrespective of social prohibition. From the Freudian perspective, the original incestuous attachments are, in a sense, still there, transformed but potentially accessible and contributing to adult sexual attachments, although his emphasis on the child underestimated the continuing plasticity of affiliative attachments in the adult. From the Westermarck position, any early incestuous attachments have presumably dissipated. Such individualistic models (even Freud's) share a rather 'hydraulic' model, in which affect is considered as a fairly discrete need–drive biological imperative which acts in an on-off mode in different directions, an approach which continues in the ethologically derived psychodynamic bonding theories where cultural motivations are largely irrelevant.[65] The major existing theories all assume some unitary biosocial motivation fairly independent of the cultural meanings of incest for the individuals concerned; and this does seem to fit our informants' accounts of finding themselves 'swept away' by an overwhelming emotion beyond their conscious intentions. Yet one of the more puzzling aspects of their experiences is that they were half in love with their relative before they met – as if they already identified with some schema of an incestuous love, with some as yet unexplicated cultural representation of how to fall in love with someone who resembled them. And our representations of romantic love assume it is neither explicitly motivated nor strategic.[66] Fox's argument that incest avoidance in human adults is contextual, remaining dependent on variable identification with cultural models of parenthood, childhood and 'natural' romantic love, fits better with its actual occurrence, and with current ethological arguments for the importance of probable outcomes rather than fixed behaviours.

A parsimonious model

Post-adoption incest or 'genetic sexual attraction' should not be taken as the manifestation of some inherent promiscuity which argues for the universality of incest in the absence of social restraints; it is a contingent biosocial pattern like any other pattern of human or primate life. In the most sophisticated attempt to reconcile the anthropological, ethological and psychodynamic evidence, the French anthropologist Jean-Marie Vidal, like Fox, argues that our acceptance of ethological correspondences between primate and human does not entail a common genetic inheritance of incest avoidance.[67] He postulates continuity between primate and human in primates generally avoiding incest through proximity and some type of recognition of resemblance: in humans these persist in that they are 'rewritten' through cultural symbolization, becoming reinforced or perhaps even replaced by rules and institutions.[68] And, we might add, such symbolizations and resultant exogamy will themselves be biologically selected as Fox argues. Against earlier assumptions of invariant phenotypic avoidance in mammals, Vidal and Erickson cite evidence that it may be only very close relatives who are sexually 'avoided' and that there is often an actual preference for more distant kin (cousins) rather than strangers.[69] Such 'optimal out-breeding' or 'optimal non-resemblance' involves potential sexual partners being recognized as phenotypically recalling (in appearance or smell[70]) those with whom very early bonding had previously been successfully achieved. Particularly in humans the phenotypic markers of biological kinship might include self-referencing.

If 'optimal out-breeding' is an appropriate evolutionary model, I would suggest a two-stage interpretation of post-adoption incest: fitting (i) with the importance of recognition of physical similarity in motivating sexual interest, both in romantic love between strangers and in the post-adoption situation, (ii) while in the latter, the lack of early bonding has not diminished this interest towards close biological relatives, despite continuing cultural rules against 'incest' in general. Extrapolating from his own experimental work, Vidal argues that later sexual attraction may actually be especially common towards those with whom established attachments had been suddenly interrupted; primate observations suggest that disturbances in bonding with the mother may be associated later with the mature male preferentially seeking sexual relations with her:[71] a pattern which does not otherwise occur and which, as in humans, is often associated with physical aggression.[72]

Does the post-adoption evidence argue for regarding cross-generational incest as a 'maladaptive' pathology in Western (or other) societies? When incestuous behaviour does occur in spite of cultural proscription, it is either a manifestation of some atypical ('abnormal' in the moral context) personal development or social relationship, or both. When adult/child sexual actions are incestuous, they are likely to reflect family environment in which the customary care-giving relationship between powerful parent and subdominant child has already been eroded; and the consequences will be similar, whether the individuals are biologically related as within a nuclear family, or not as within a reconstituted stepfamily or foster family, or a children's home.[73] That incestuous activity is more common between young siblings, and is then less culturally abhorrent (or even recognized), suggests it is accepted in the contemporary West as part of the experimental repertoire of developing individuals, and is less likely to result in long-term transformations of socially ascribed generational identity and sexuality, power relations and role modelling being fairly symmetrical.[74] Post-adoption incest is regarded by our informants and their counsellors as less inappropriate than parent–child incest, and as akin to symmetrical sibling incest, supporting La Fontaine's point that it is not 'incest' in general which now arouses discomfort so much as the sexualization of cross-generational power.[75] On Vidal's model, such discomfort is one possible cultural 'rewriting' of what were once biological contingencies, and which now lessens social restriction on one type of 'incest' – consensual relations between adults.

An intriguing question remains. If human society is predicated on a culturally reinforced avoidance of cross-generational sexual relations, yet incest of different types is increasingly recognized in the breakdown of the Western nuclear family, then perhaps at some level of biosocial adaptation we no longer 'need' to avoid it. On biosocial reconstructions of the historical origin of human society through the incest taboo, and its recapitulation in contemporary individuals, it would be unwise to speculate given current ignorance of early hominid patterns of attachment and rearing; except perhaps to emphasize that a unitary explanation for both origin and continuance is likely to remain elusive, given the new impossibility of distinguishing 'natural' competence from 'cultural' action whether in human history or in the developing individual.

9. A Disorder of the Victorian Self

The idea of the individual

To the Mahanubhav healing temples of western India, women bring their seriously mentally ill relatives, after local hospital treatment has proved unavailing. Through a local understanding that women are in some sense responsible for the health of their family, the ill relatives are then effectively ignored whilst the women go into trance on their behalf.[1] Such trance is seen as a penance for the women; they explain that they themselves have been affected by the possessing powers which have caused madness in the family. To an extent, their seeking possession is an attempt to draw the affliction away from the psychotic individual further onto themselves. Such a model of sickness would appear very much at variance with the assumptions of biomedicine, with the possible exception of psychiatry where, for a number of years, family interventions have been used in psychosomatic illness and alcoholism and, as with the Mahanubhav temple, more recently in schizophrenia. Family and group therapies themselves are now often modelled explicitly on the classic anthropological accounts of healing in tribal societies such as those of Victor Turner, part of a Western trend against what is felt to be biomedical reductionism and in favour of a rather romantically conceived 'holistic' healing supposedly practised in small-scale communities – Senoi dream therapy, Naikan fire-walking.[2] The choice in these between (synchronic) structural theory or (diachronic) developmental models is demonstrated in their new terminology – 'enmeshment' or alternatively 'regression'.

Any conceptualization of sickness, but particularly psychiatric illness (or its analogues in non-Western societies), involves certain assumptions about the individual self and its relationship to shared values and perceptions and to others. Our rather Cartesian notion of a bounded individual self coterminous with the physical individual which informs both our understanding of the core symptoms of schizophrenia[3] and the form/content model of the older 'cultural psychiatry' has been examined by anthropologists and philosophers, following Marcel Mauss's suggestion that such a notion is as socially constructed as any other 'indigenous psychology'.[4]

The locus of the Western self is quintessentially the individual physical body. While the understanding of the body is a function of wider cultural

ideas within a society, its morphology and functioning reciprocally provide
certain root metaphors to describe society itself – homeostasis, periodicity,
genesis, structure and conflict (Chapter 2). The body presents us with a
'cornucopia of highly charged symbols – fluids, scents, tissues, different
surfaces, movements, feelings, cycles of changes constituting birth,
growing old, sleeping and working',[5] none of which can be understood
in independence of the meanings we ascribe to them. Classical Western
social science assumes that society comprises a number of similar and
essentially replaceable selves for each of which personhood is distinct from
social role.[6] The locus of psychopathology is thus within the individual
body, in its constitution, personality and history, and this is then the
appropriate focus for psychiatric intervention.

By contrast, the essential unit for Indian or Chinese society from the
point of view of the attribution and resolution of disease is not the body but
the community, particularly the family.[7] Not only is the family the locus for
what we might term 'psychopathology', but physical symptoms too can
only be understood through the individual's relations with others; a
disturbed body reflects disharmony in the social order and appropriate
treatment is less psychological than somatic and moral.[8] This understanding is far from the old colonial assumption that non-Western societies
have undifferentiated selves: it is rather that the self may be differentiated
according to quite different criteria, frequently 'moral' rather than
'psychological'.[9] Familiar psychodynamic distinctions between 'inside'
and 'outside' with their assumption that autonomy is in opposition to
collective values are inadequate for considering disturbances in *amae*, the
Japanese value, one both psychological and moral, in which the individual
gains selfhood through reciprocal obligations with others.[10] The usual
English gloss of amae is 'dependency', inevitably pejorative in a context
where selfhood is regarded as something achieved against others, as
something individual and psychological rather than social and moral. The
Western individual *is* a psychological entity which *has* independently moral
values and this is reflected in attitudes to mental illness. Not necessarily so
elsewhere. In India critical comments about a mentally ill family member
are still associated with 'warmth': not in Britain.[11]

We cannot, however, still make simple distinctions between 'Western'
and 'non-Western' systems. Popular Indian understanding of minor
psychological distress is often physiological while the traditional Hindu
self, the *atman*, is not something embodied in situational behaviour, as in
China, so much as imperfectly reflecting a transcendental self, close to
something English speakers might term the soul.[12] Even within a relatively
restricted group, American psychiatrists, a variety of different notions of
personhood are simultaneously employed.[13] A common idiom in the West
is that of development: the individual gains an identity through situations

and choices in the course of their life. In psychiatric emergencies patient and doctor together construct a 'narrative' of the events which have led up to the consultation which serves as the rationale for admission or other treatment.[14] One recent theme in social anthropology, particularly in studies of Western societies, is how the individual (and others) constructs their selfhood through a personal narrative of events in their lives. In a subject relatively neglected by cultural psychiatrists, Langness and Levine examine how people defined as mentally handicapped see their difficulties through various explanatory models which interpret their personal relationships with doctors, social workers and other agencies.[15] It is perhaps surprising that they sometimes prefer to offer to others the image of madness rather than 'slowness'. In a recent book Arthur Kleinman shows how the theoretical assumptions of Western psychiatry can be revealed through the clinical 'life histories' of patients; the biographical approach reveals certain strategies which patients may together use to shape and deal with illnesses such as strokes, epilepsy or chronic schizophrenia, or how relatives recognize 'senility'.[16]

If psychologies are regarded not as value free descriptions of how people actually function so much as a part of Western societies' (in particular) definition of the person and of moral agency, the psychological theories we use should tell us much about how abnormal experience and behaviour are caused and responded to. The emotions which are recognized and classified may be less an attempt to account for how people feel than what society believes they should feel.[17] While biology does appear to provide a discrete basis for patterns which develop in the adult as anger and fear,[18] the same is not true for such 'emotional' distinctions as that between envy and jealousy. The boundaries of such an explicit set of understandings which we can term 'a psychology' differ greatly;[19] as with the *atman*, the concepts employed may involve what to the Western-trained psychiatrist appear 'supernatural'. The 'multiple souls' of West African systems of understanding can, however, be read as psychologies, as ways of dealing with the relationship between thought and society, human agency and natural processes; with increasing Westernization they are likely to become more psychologized and personalized.[20] Similarly the Sora, a tribal people of Central India, engage through a shamanic medium with the *sonum*, the dead person, to discover the cause of their death, but a sonum is not just a rather personified spirit but something we might better gloss as 'memory', as a set of forces and values perceived as external but which affect the living individual through actually constituting part of their own experiences and personality.[21] The psychiatric understanding of the so-called 'possession states' places them as pathologies, in which a discrete bounded individual self is experienced as replaced by another 'spirit' regarded as a disembodied personage rather than as the operation of a psychological faculty or moral value. Medical interactions in the West have developed an equivalent which I shall consider in my final chapters – *multiple personality disorder*.

Double consciousness

The diagnosis of double consciousness – in which two different human personalities apparently coexist in association with a single physical body – became current in France and the United States (and to a lesser extent Britain) between 1880 and 1900. It collected together in a single clinical category a multitude of earlier phenomena: hysteria (which we have briefly considered in Chapters 3 and 4), catalepsy, somnambulism, fugue and trance states, mediumship and spiritism, demonic possession, visions and dreams, telepathy and telekinesis, automatic writing, crystal-ball gazing and other types of clairvoyance and second sight, *amour fou*, automatic obedience and the automatism of urban crowds and conscripted soldiers, crime and revolutionary acts, religious conversion and its stigmata, together with revivalism and folk panics and, as its core, the mechanism of hypnotism and its earlier manifestations, mesmerism and animal magnetism.

Popular periodicals attested to widespread medico-legal interest in the possibility that murder could be committed by a sleeping or hypnotic double under the influence of some malevolent mastermind. Indeed, by the 1880s, says the historian Henri Ellenberger, the 'medical world had become infatuated with hypnotism', a rather doubtful therapy popular among country doctors which was now taken up in the university clinic to provide an experimental model for the phenomenon of the double.[22] Nineteenth-century magnetizers had discovered that their subjects could be placed in a state akin to sleep and then induced to perform actions of which they had no memory when they later 'awoke'. Physical pains, blindness and paralyses could be induced and removed, as could amnesia for events during or preceding the hypnosis. Was this perhaps a bodily manifestation of planetary magnetism? Was it simply charlatanism, the suggestible subject acquiescing in the suggestions of the charismatic magnetizer?[23] Or, as the established churches still argued, an unwise tampering with demonic powers?

The medical explanations of double consciousness (*conscience double*) referred back to earlier accounts of what appeared to have been the same pattern. In his *Confessions*, Augustine had puzzled at how, long after his conversion, his earlier pagan self still appeared in his dreams, and whether his waking and now Christian self was accountable for this secondary nocturnal being, a question that returned to trouble nineteenth-century neurologists like William James.[24] Medieval witchcraft confessions were

now identified retrospectively as misinterpretations of spontaneous or
induced double consciousness.[25] Under the influence of a number of
eminent French neurologists, notably Jean-Martin Charcot and Pierre
Janet, the hypnotic state was elided with the existing medical category of
hysteria, a term dating from the Hippocratics[26] which by the late nineteenth
century elided a diffuse number of phenomena which had a phasic pattern:
the hysterical patient, usually young and female, returned at intervals,
generally within hours, to her normal state and remained ignorant of the
episode. Symptoms included selective or global amnesia, aphasia,
blindness, anaesthesia, pains, hallucinations or other alterations of the
sensorium, and excited and inappropriate behaviour, together with fits and
paralyses which did not conform with anatomical knowledge but rather
with popular conceptions of what it was to be amnesic, blind or paralysed.
Hysterical loss of sensation in limbs did not lead to the sort of accidents of
neglect such as burns which were found in a disease like syphilis where the
sensory nerves were destroyed. Particularly in the case of men, during a
more extended hysterical fugue they might wander away to turn up months
later with a different name, occupation and personality, seemingly
oblivious to their earlier life. It was noted that hysterical crises and fugues
frequently followed the receipt of bad news or other shocks, and Charcot
distinguished hysterical fits from the apparently similar symptoms of
epilepsy on the basis that, while epilepsy was the direct consequence of
identifiable brain damage, hysterical symptoms seemed to mimic those of
epilepsy. Was the patient responsible then for what were now recognized as
disturbances of 'function' rather than of anatomical 'structure'? In placing
hysteria and somnambulism together with other instances of the 'narrowing of the field of consciousness', Charcot called attention to the *aboulia* –
the apparent loss of will – which characterized all these patterns. Sceptics
maintained that the hysterical patients whose dramatic symptoms he
demonstrated to captivated medical and lay audiences were deliberately
colluding with their doctor, but like Janet he argued that even though these
symptoms might seem to be purposeful (in avoiding responsibility or
forgetting unpleasant experiences or just in gaining the doctor's attention),
the patient could not be held to be fully aware or responsible for her
hysteria. Consciousness[27] was somehow split, or 'dissociated' to use Janet's
term, and the patient seemed blandly indifferent or even unaware of the
impact of her symptoms upon others.

From the 1830s it had been recognized that double consciousness, the
most dramatic form of hysteria, could emerge either spontaneously or in
the course of hypnotic treatment for nervous complaints (and then
sometimes become spontaneous).[28] The patients were characteristically
young women who alternated between two states: the first recalling the
original personality as recognized by her family, often sick, inhibited and

quiet, a prim martyr who might complain of being 'possessed by something'.[29] By contrast her *état second* was flirtatious, untamed and capricious, sometimes self-confessedly 'wicked'. Characteristically there was one-way amnesia, the second personality (as the state was recognized in the more developed and continuing cases – *dédoublement de la personnalité*) being aware of the experiences of the first personality, frequently commenting on it sardonically. A third or subsequent personality might then emerge which had variable knowledge of the earlier personalities. With practice the experienced physician could summon or dismiss these various states through hypnosis or simply by firmly instructing the patient; sometimes personalities volunteered or were given names by which each might be addressed. A classification was established by the French which emphasized separate memory and awareness as the conditions of each self.[30]

The extent to which the physician might recognize and name the emergent personalities as separate individuals inhabiting a single body is well illustrated by Morton Prince's account of Miss Beauchamp, a case in 1890s Boston, which he wrote up as an intriguing and somewhat gothic tale of medical detection. Similar to the other classic cases, the young woman is depicted prior to the onset of her illness as unhappy and nervous, with a tendency to day-dreaming dating back to the imaginary companions of her childhood. As the different personalities emerge in turn during medical consultation, they write letters to each other and to Dr Prince, spy and play tricks (taking a purgative and then departing so that another personality is faced with the consequences), and painstakingly learn a foreign language which another personality already knows. They have different appetites, musical abilities and susceptibility to illness. Yet they seem unified enough to present a single public identity outside the consulting room, to travel and run a household. Prince pursues 'the real Miss Beauchamp', eliciting the help of one personality against another, intriguing, making and breaking pacts with them, yet constantly deceived by the emergence of new personalities and half-personalities or the elision of the existing ones. He attempts to fuse or else 'kill off' some of them; these in turn protest and demand he kills off the others. In their struggles, both personalities and doctor frequently evoke the idiom of demonic possession, Dr Prince threatening to send the lesser personalities 'back where they came from' – to some sort of spaceless limbo (recalling the biblical equivalent in Mark 5.10). His account also recalls a farcical comedy of errors with the personalities either on or off 'the stage'[31] and he begins to wonder if he is perhaps treating a family as he addresses separate letters to each. (Regrettably they steal and read each other's mail.) He encourages one personality to hypnotize another with unforeseen complications. Attempting to reassemble and order the various identities he is constantly confounded by Miss B's aboulia – her loss of will. Prince labels the personalities B1, B2 and so on, and develops increasingly complicated diagrams to illustrate their relative knowledge and control over each other.[32] His gripping reports on the progress of the case in medical conferences and journals become well known, and one of Miss B's personalities herself develops a professional interest in clinical psychology. The personality Prince eventually identifies as the real Miss B reads his final manuscript before publication, requesting him to leave out passages which are offensive; something that sounds like an unpleasant sexual encounter with an older man is glossed over. She marries one of Prince's medical colleagues. Like some other narratives of multiple personality, her published case history is soon made into a successful play. Another patient trains as Prince's research assistant and starts to publish her own clinical papers.[33]

Given recent feminist critiques of psychiatry which emphasize power and resistance to power, one is left not only with a sense of Dr Prince blithely avoiding his patient's conflicting aspirations as he concretizes her potential identities as fascinating serial phenomena, but of Miss B continually outwitting her physician, leading him on, leaving traps, teasing, fighting under the guise of aboulia with the weapons at her disposal – those female characteristics ascribed to her by his medical theories. But that is to impose our common-sense assumptions (and her doctor's) of a unitary self somewhere behind all the personalities. As I shall suggest this might not be altogether legitimate. The medical interpretation of multiple consciousness, as of the hypnotism and spiritism on which it drew, started from the assumption that in the general run of things there is a single bounded and volitional self which shares a biography with the body which gives rise to it, reflecting and directing in turn the experiences of this body, with a characteristic and enduring identity of personal comportments, responses, habits, sentiments, abilities and memories, all of which are experienced and perceived by others, as hanging together and which are potentially accessible to awareness. As Clifford Geertz[34] puts it more strongly in his account of the Western idea of the self, a 'bounded, unique, more or less integrated motivational and cognitive universe, a dynamic centre of awareness, emotion, judgement and action organised into a distinctive whole and set contrastively both against other such wholes and against a social and natural background . . .' But this hanging together becomes unstuck in dreams, or in the usual processes of forgetting and inattention, such that chunks of past experience cannot necessarily be recalled simultaneously; and while such split-off 'complexes' (as Jung was to call them) usually include fairly discrete memories and ideas, under appropriate conditions (brain damage, inherited constitution, emotional trauma, hypnosis) the split-off fragments might be so extensive as to actually constitute a parallel secondary self.[35] Dissociation could be understood along a spectrum ranging from momentary day-dreaming and fantasy to file more extensive and enduring (and pathological) double consciousness. Explanations of extensive dissociation – what Prince termed disintegration, Janet as *désagrégations psychologiques* – fluctuated between the biological and the psychological. The clinical practice which Ellenberger terms the 'first dynamic psychiatry', exemplified by Charcot and Janet, shifted gradually from physical explanations to the mental.[36]

Where does an idea go when one stops thinking it? Where was the memory of the clock striking which only now does one recall having heard earlier? If there was some general agreement on a distinction between those cognitions which constituted immediate awareness and those which were subconscious (to use Janet's term), it was uncertain how much the latter should be considered as distinct (what he called subconscious fixed ideas). And, if they were, whether the subconscious ideas were to be seen as split off from a prior unitary consciousness to which they then became generally inaccessible, or else as clusters of actually existing subpersonalities which always underlay (or perhaps even constituted) the conscious self of everyday life (a process termed by James' subliminal consciousness, McDougall's animism, Prince's neurograms). In either case, their appearance was generally taken as a neurasthenic diminution in 'nervous energy' (Janet's expression again) occasioned by hereditary vulnerability and various traumata, either physical or later by extension psychological: including industrial and railway accidents, unpleasant news, sexual violence and sexual frustration, and conflicting moral demands. Or in the course of hypnotic treatment. Whether this energy itself had an observable physical existence akin to that of magnetic phenomena and of the presumed communication between the newly discovered cells of the brain was arguable: in the 1890s French neurologists were still attempting to transfer hysterical symptoms and even personalities from one patient to another by means of electro-magnets and telepathy, but it became increasingly accepted that the 'magnetism' of the earlier mesmerizers was just an analogy for something rather less concrete.[37]

Advocating a cathartic therapy of purging traumatic memories, Janet suggested that narrowed consciousness, like other hysterical symptoms, had an adaptive function in hiding such memories from awareness; secondary symbolizations could then disguise the primary memories through association or substitution.[38] His brother re-examined Charcot's influential schema of the successive stages of hysteria to argue that they were rather simultaneous personalities serially accessed. Janet was initially a teacher of philosophy who studied medicine to obtain access to these patients who became his central paradigm; as he remarked, the Paris chair in psychology would not have existed without them.[39] Like Ribot, he argued that double consciousness refuted Kant's idea of the unitary self as transcendent, for consciousness was evidently generated in experience; as he put it, the 'members of the old school accuse us of filching their *moi*'.[40] Ellenberger has suggested that Janet's dynamic model of hysteria, which emphasized meaningful experience over bodily constitution, owed much to the Catholic notion of the pathogenic secret in which purgation of guilt for secret crimes, often incest or infanticide, resulted in physical and spiritual healing.[41] The Protestant pastor's 'cure of souls' provided a more secular, at times explicitly psychological alternative, confession now being reframed as a cathartic recall to awareness of the guilty act. Going further, the French neurologists of the Second Republic claimed that they had uncovered the clinical underpinnings of clerical superstition and popular credulity; the guilty secret life of the gambler, criminal and eccentric being recognized as the mischievous 'second self' (alter ego), as Moritz Benedikt called it.

Such a malign shadow or double had been a common preoccupation of Romantic and Symbolist writers (Hoffman, Goethe, Shelley, Hogg, De Musset, Poe, Dostoyevsky, Stevenson, Wilde), now less personified as a daemonic familiar, bisexual changeling or lost sibling than as a deeper and amoral persistence in the mind of an earlier historical and mythopoetic epoch, a schema which was to be elaborated most fully by Jung (whose first publications, like Janet's, had examined mediums as clinical cases). Consideration as natural experiences of phenomena which had been once taken for 'religious' was common given the robust anticlericalism of the French neurologists, but was also proposed by those New England medical psychologists sympathetic to Transcendentalism and even Spiritualism, and who attempted with professional mediums the same hypnotic experiments as with their neurasthenic patients. (In her quest for therapy Dr Prince's Miss Beauchamp had previously consulted a spiritualist.) Many of the Americans, particularly William James, retained an ambiguous attitude to the supernatural, either allowing it entry to the physical through certain extreme bodily states or else advocating a metaphysical dualism by which mind and matter came together and separated under particular conditions.[42] As an organized body of ideas, spiritism was an immediate response to the widely reported experiences of the Fox sisters in 1847, following which popular enthusiasm swept the United States to reach Europe in the following decade.[43] The Society for Psychical Research, formed by British scientists in 1882, was followed by the American Society for Psychical Research and by the French Institut de Métempsycose. Spontaneous communications with the other world became standardized through women mediums who were particularly open to such communications, together with the increasingly routinized phenomena of automatic writing, seances, table rapping, the arrival of ectoplasm and messages from the dead, all of which were demonstrated through spirit photography and other procedures of verification. And the other world itself became less of a celestial destination, more a parallel if cloudy Homeric underworld populated by gloomy and somewhat banal spirit guides. Spiritualism (the overtly religious variant) took itself as establishing a natural religion free from clerical obscurantism and dogmatism; its members were enthusiasts for the idea of biological evolution, for the emancipation of slaves and women, for social welfare and public health:[44] American perfectionists whose ideas and membership overlapped with Christian Scientists (who denied the reality of sickness[45]), and Transcendentalists and Universalists (who denied evil and eternal punishment).[46] Spiritualism has continued to wax and wane, devising systems of spiritual development which have included versions of reincarnation drawn from Asian religions, sometimes ambivalently accommodating them as Christian sects, the contacts on the 'other side' being variously understood as congealed *psychic energy*, or else taking distinct personalities as named *controls*, *guides*, *spirits* or (in the orientalist groups) *masters*.

Psychodynamics and the temporary decline of double consciousness

Between 1900 and 1910 cases of double consciousness suddenly disappeared from the medical literature. French nineteenth-century medicine had attempted to link together what we might distinguish as naturalistic and personalistic explanations, even if individual theorists inclined more to one side or the other; after Charcot's death the two diverged, to come close again only in the computational cognitive science of the 1980s. Charcot's successors at the Salpêtrière, Babinski and Tourette, eased Janet out of the hospital in order to concentrate clinical research on those neurological conditions for which they presumed an underlying physical disease. It was hinted that Charcot's magnificent medical theatre was just a *'charcoterie'*, his working-class patients having been rewarded with permanent lodging in the hospital; they were rumoured to have faked double consciousness, hysteria and hypnotic states, and to have seduced his medical students physically and mentally.[47] Military medicine excepted, hypnosis became a rather doubtful music hall entertainment, marginal to the new American behaviourism which ridiculed 'mentalist' psychology and which, if it approached the self as any object of interest, did so through its motor (neuromuscular) theory of consciousness.

Hysteria and multiple personality were also now less salient in private consulting rooms.[48] Leading in the opposite direction from the behaviourists, Freud's psychoanalysis with its middle-class clientele became the dominant psychodynamic school. Having followed the Parisian and Bostonian move away from hereditary suggestibility to emphasize the meaning for the patient of the precipitating trauma and its resultant symptoms, he then incorporated into his schema crowd psychology, religious practice and artistic innovation, to develop a general model of moral evolution in which our material instincts and appetites, like the *controls* of the spiritualists, sought to translate themselves into higher forms. The central feature of aboulia – the loss of will characteristic of dissociative states – became incorporated into a more dynamic and developmental 'biology-up' unconscious (rather than working down from the unitary consciousness of everyday experience) which explained the popular recognition that people could often act against what seemed to be their overt intentions. Consciousness and intention did not necessarily run together; 'accidents', like the 'forgetting' of traumatic events, were motivated at a deeper level, and moral accountability was thus more complex than in clinical medicine's opposition between motivated agency and unsolicited disease. Those aspects of awareness which were no longer accessible had been actively 'repressed' rather than, as Charcot had put it, just 'congealed'; and repression itself was just one of a number of defences available to the emergent self. Psychoanalysts took Janet's idea of subconscious personality simply as a part of normal functioning, and the self they elaborated was now less coherent and enduring, even less like a soul than the embodied self of everyday assumptions. That this sort of self could then compete for recognition with other entities of the same order, each bearing proper names and associated with the same body, seemed implausible;[49] double consciousness was taken simply as an identification with some unconscious fantasied self,[50] hypnosis as compliance with the quasi-parental demands of doctors or others. Opponents of Freud criticized his subpersonal psychology for apparently reifying its functional mechanisms (ego, super-ego, id) as if these were distinct personalities, but psychoanalytical emphasis on the therapeutic integration of the moral personality in the course of 'analysis', together with a greater interest in the relationship between doctor and patient, seem to have avoided any proliferation of subpersonalities in the course of treatment.[51] Similarly, even if Jung's analytical psychology encouraged the patient to explore unrecognized and devalued aspects of their personality in the form of archetypal images, often represented as the protagonists of myths and fairy tales, it sought to integrate these into a richer, 'individuated' self.[52]

One aspect of Freud's dynamic psychology which was to prove contentious in the resurgence of multiple personality in the 1980s was his rejection of a single traumatic cause for hysteria. Incest and other sexual traumata had often been argued as the immediate precipitant of hysteria when acting on a suitable constitution – emphasized perhaps through the physician's experience of what the psychoanalysts now recognized as the seductiveness of the patient. Employing Charcot's and Janet's cathartic therapy, Freud had come to the conclusion that his hysterical patients had been sexually violated by male relatives early in life but then split off this experience from awareness, only to have it evoked later by some less serious trauma which recalled the original seduction. In 1897 Freud decided this scenario was unlikely and that the original 'trauma' was rather the developing sexual fantasy of the young child which was later actively repressed through social convention.[53] Questions of the feigning or medical suggestion of symptoms were subsumed into the idea of transference and counter-transference (the relationship of patient and therapist to the other through their own unconscious concerns) which ignored the wider political and ideological context; the clinical practice of briskly removing observable symptoms now being replaced by an ever longer therapy focusing on lifetime adaptation, and often carried out by lay analysts. With some exceptions (Switzerland and later the United States), psychodynamic psychotherapy became divorced from medico-legal debates on criminal responsibility and from the clinical dramas of the public hospital. While Freud initially attempted to reconcile the biological to the psychological, psychoanalysis became an increasingly interpretive procedure: the patients bourgeois, the setting private, the relationship contractual.

While the *grande hystérie* of Charcot's clinic now seems uncommon in Europe, casualty doctors in metropolitan hospitals continue to see cases of functional ('hysterical') anaesthesia and paralyses, and to diagnose fugue states, though these are now perhaps less dramatic. The medical consensus in Britain is that somatic preoccupations now provide the appropriate idiom of distress for personal problems which are difficult to acknowledge, but 'hysteria' is still identified in women and in migrants from non-industrialized countries. To take an example from my work at Guy's Hospital: a middle-aged man enters our casualty department obviously agitated and unable to speak. He writes down that he has lost his voice. A surgeon examines him with a laryngoscope and declares he is not physically ill. The duty psychiatrist sees him and decides this is a case of hysterical aphonia, and I admit him to my ward (I retain here the customary possessive terminology). I go and see him sitting up in his bed and tell him I think something is bothering him, so why doesn't he stay in hospital for a few days to sort it out? He nods agreement but won't write his name or address, gesturing that he doesn't know them. He settles into being a compliant patient, easily finding his way about on the ward. After a couple of days his voice returns suddenly but he seems to have no knowledge of his identity or any events prior to his arrival at the hospital, even when I show him what is almost certainly his name on some documents I find in his wallet. Through them I contact his wife: she visits and says Mr Johnson (as I'll call him) had gone off to work as usual on the day of admission but she has not seen him since; she is concerned as he has never been ill before. Her presence clearly annoys him and he tells the nursing staff he wishes to be left alone. A formal psychiatric interview (the 'mental state examination') is difficult because he is now not very cooperative; the diagnosis remains hysterical fugue with amnesia, and at my request the nursing staff offer him reassurance that he will get better when he is able to talk about his worries. Four days pass but nothing changes. He remains irritated with his wife, and now with the staff. A male nurse tells me critically that my patient is a malingerer. I tell Mr Johnson that I am going to hypnotize him; the nurses reinforce this by saying I never fail; he looks nonplussed. I hypnotize him (not very confidently because I did not do it often, and anyway have read Ellenberger and regard the whole thing as a little, well, theatrical). An audience of medical students and my junior colleagues watch fascinated. Not sure whether he *is* hypnotized (or how I could know whether he is), and not wishing to try any tricks of post-hypnotic suggestion in case they fail (and anyway I have an out-patient clinic waiting), I confidently tell him he is now hypnotized. His eyes look suitably glazed and he talks more spontaneously, agrees he has a problem but that it is difficult to talk about. I tell him to wake up, and then continue the next day now using a slow intravenous injection of sodium amytal instead of hypnosis but with my same audience.

Mr Johnson tells his story. He is 54, a West Indian immigrant from Dominica who has worked on the London underground for 20 years. Now a clerk. His life strikes me as rigid, prim and disciplined: a church-going Methodist, not charismatic, never sick, no problems, the wife does her job, a fine woman, has no time for the modern young Blacks now, hates reggae and carnival, thinks Rastas should have their locks cut off, his own children are grown up but rarely in contact, he used to vote Labour not now. Patriotic, rather punitive social values. He once went to evening classes to study but it was evident he would not be promoted. Q: Because you're Black? A: [reluctantly] Yes. Well, on early morning duty in his suburban station, a church acquaintance of his had appeared at the ticket office with a companion. This young man urgently needs to get a monthly season ticket to get to his new job but has no cash. Could London Transport in the person of Mr Johnson loan the money till the following week? My patient replies frigidly that this is not permitted. The friend persists and, frightened lest his supervisor will come over and make a fuss, quite against his better judgement Mr Johnson now makes out a ticket and hurriedly hands it over. The other two depart, and he is suddenly horrified, ashamed, gut-rendingly anxious, nauseated, not believing what he has done – he has stolen from the transport authority! He cannot wait till lunchtime, makes an excuse that he is suddenly feeling unwell to the astonishment of his colleagues, leaves the station to go to the post office, and takes out from his account the appropriate amount of money. On returning to work he guiltily slips it into the till. But now he feels just as bad, waves of anger at his friend alternating with moments of terror. For he had certainly stolen if only for a moment.

That evening he goes to look for the friend to be told he has gone away. Suddenly Mr Johnson knows that he will not be repaid. He feels quite sick, quarrels with his wife, but keeps the affair to himself lest he seem foolish. He goes to bed early yet cannot sleep, ruminating, grinding. The next few days are worse, anger alternating with shame, periods of sweating, retching, pains in his stomach. The day of promised repayment arrives. No young man, no friend. He has been duped. He gets through the day, still half expecting his friend, mistaking people in the distance for him; in the evening he cannot face going to look for him again. Passers-by in the street now seem to know all about it for they look at him in a knowing way: a thief, a gull. The next day on the way to work, his mind goes blank and he finds himself at the hospital. Sweating profusely he asks me if he has had a stroke from the pressure, and will I report him to his station manager? I say of course not. He doesn't look very relieved and, dismissing the medical audience, I talk to him about our natural tendency to dissociate, that the mind protects itself against pain by temporarily splitting bits off, that his problem is not that he is a criminal but rather that he is perhaps too conscientious. He readily agrees to all this and then says he must now go home. I persist, suggesting we need to talk about more general issues, how he copes with life, about his personal goals, about his satisfaction with coming to Britain. He looks suspicious (there has been recent publicity about mental illness being mistakenly diagnosed in the West Indian community). He asks me if I think he's 'mental': I say no, but it might be helpful to talk longer. He insists on leaving, refuses a follow-up appointment but sends the nurses a neat formal letter thanking them for his excellent care.

This episode replays and comments on the issue of double consciousness: the same sort of dissociative fugue as that described in Paris in the 1890s, the same hypnotic treatment and the same doubts about its validity, the half-voiced mockery of colleagues, the ambiguities about personal responsibility, the rather theatrical public treatment now based on the classic accounts. And my explanation to him is one which Janet might have given. What then has changed? I suspect I have less sense of the 'psychological truth' of the illness, that I myself recognize it as a part of wider social institutions including medical power and racism. And I am somehow aware that Mr Johnson and I have worked together on a satisfactory final narrative, one which allows us a reasonable degree of satisfaction with ourselves. (The medical students certainly think it's all terrific.) Indeed we have both played our parts rather well.

From the biology of consciousness to the ethnology of spirit possession: some problems with the standard model

More interested than Freud in the context of illness, Janet had derived hysteria and multiple personality from what he took as primitive modes of consciousness, noted parallels between clinical psychotherapy and popular healing, and traced a development from medieval witchcraft accusations and spirit possession, through magnetism and American spiritism to the neurological clinic.[54] Voluntarily sought possession, as in *shango* and *vodu*, has commonly been regarded by anthropologists as akin to double consciousness; the devotee is entered by a named spirit as she assumes the attributes of this power, a characteristic voice, gestures and personality, employing their particular paraphernalia and insignia, and sometimes speaking different 'languages'. Though such possession normally occurs in a circumscribed context as expressly sought, and to the ethnographic observer retains some motivated quality,[55] the same possessing power, as Alfred Métraux has noted, may 'ride its horse' against volition, in situations of sudden surprise, street accident or even surgical anaesthesia. And it may be exorcised, accommodated or assimilated. On occasion more than one spirit might enter the host to engage in conversation or dispute, yet, divine incarnations aside, spirit and human person are recognized as distinct.

Double consciousness was taken by Janet to be intrapersonal in origin, and thus its Western expression as psychological illness rather than spirit intrusion more truly reflected its origin, as did the new clinical treatment which proposed the integration of what were only subjective phenomena. (For consciousness is now more real to us than the spirits.) Similarly, those anthropological models of spirit mediumship and possession influenced by psychiatry argued that the spirits, representing as they did the personified externalization of standardized psychological conflicts, went along with a generally personalistic reading of the natural world together with animism, sorcery and so forth. The residual Western representatives of this primitive psychology were hysterics and women, regressing back and down (to use the evolutionary topology of the English neurologists which was popularized by Freud) to an earlier level of suggestibility and magical thinking.[56] As we shall see, this evolutionary idiom leaves problematic the recent recurrence of multiple personality in the United States which in many particulars recalls spirit possession as much as it does the hysteria of Janet's observations.

Anthropology's debate on primitive mentality and its interest in the psychological adjustment of the spirit medium need not be detailed here, except to note our shift from an empirical psychology of competences and states given in nature to a sociological reading in which 'consciousness' and 'psychology' themselves represent particular cultural sentiments and memories through local categories of personhood, character, autonomy, moral agency, responsibility and the like; and that these public categories are variably deployed in certain situations, tensions between social sectors becoming salient in the personal experience of socially vulnerable or pivotal individuals – experience then shaped by immediate context and procedures for managing distress whether medical, lay or religious.[57] Students of spirit possession have noted similarities between the contexts of possession ritual, the nineteenth-century American seance and the contemporary clinic: in particular shared idioms of distress which remove moral accountability from the afflicted individual; the manifestation of these idioms through spontaneous or sought (or induced) altered states of consciousness; with a charismatic shaman, medium or doctor directing the proceedings; the altered experience being personified as the entry of a named spirit, control or secondary personality; with a variable surrender of volition and agency to this external power (as the clinician's aboulia); the local response elaborating and validating the altered state, integrating and resolving the presumed psychological split explicitly (in the goals of psychotherapy) or in our analysis (psychological anthropology's explanation of a local healer's efficacy). The theoretical language now adopted is less clinical and of a higher order of generality, allowing incorporation of less obviously medical concerns: affliction or invidia rather than psychological trauma, alternative phases of consciousness rather than hysteria or possession states, indeed creativity rather than pathology.[58]

The 'standard model' of the mechanism of possession trance and multiple personality, however, remains not unlike that elaborated by Ribot and Janet in the 1890s: that these patterns could in theory be specified by psychophysiology alone. Humans have the ability to dissociate their mental processes and do so the whole time – through changing moods, selective attention and putting unpleasant issues out of mind, through fantasy and dreaming – for the potential contents of our awareness are hardly accessible simultaneously.[59] And some experiences are not easily remembered, because they are hardly significant enough to remark for more than a few seconds, because memories of them have not been periodically recalled and thus have faded, or else because they are unpleasant or painful in some way, for forgetting can be active and motivated. And the immediacy of our bodies and surroundings fluctuates, dependent on what we can recognize as intended perception, the quality of our will being variable, dependent on our current interests and customary procedures. You can eat an apple while riding your bicycle but you are not equally 'in' each activity at any

one moment, nor are you generally aware of switching from one to the
other deliberately for your stream of awareness appears a seamless web. To
be 'conscious' is to know you are aware of something, bestowing reality
through perception: an adaptive disposition located in the neo-cortex,
selected in evolution, which enables the human organism to engage flexibly
but attentively with different situations.[60] Your ability to dissociate is
adaptive in switching attention when necessary, in avoiding sensory
overload in severe pain or terrifying and conflictual situations of cognitive
dissonance where all your available responses seem inadequate. Severe
tiredness, fear, pain or startling can result in the experience of numbing
(depersonalization) whose behavioural concomitant ('freezing') might, like
the temporary analgesia of accident or battle, once have had some survival
value.

Dissociation is thus the necessary flip side of consciousness: it allows
detachment of awareness from the immediate passage of events, part of the
evolutionary development of 'self-consciousness' as an internal system of
representation and self-monitoring where the individual's awareness can
then objectivize their own cognitions ('my senses deceive me', 'I was
overcome by emotion'), allowing self-recognition, anticipation, introspec-
tion, creative imagination, recognition of another's motives and possible
identification with them, disbelief, deceit and acting: all requirements for
our complex programmes of intersubjective action.[61] Under certain
conditions such as hypnosis, or standardized types of sensory patterning,
deprivation and overload, through an altered balance between sympathetic
and parasympathetic neural activity, through hyperventilation or the
ingestion of psychoactive substances, dissociation can be facilitated
physiologically to enhance or diminish attention, to day-dream or
meditate, as a sense of shared communality or an out-of-body experience,
as hallucination, anaesthesia, motor passivity or paralysis. Through our
cognitive schema of a bounded self as the usual locus of experience and
volition, whether given in biology or in the responses of others, we may
recognize the distinctive bodily facilitation of these experiences as other to
our volition:[62] like religious conversion or artistic inspiration, they may be
recognized as something alien, reinforcing our notions of external reality,
causality and personal subjectivity through standardized rituals which
enable us to realize our particular schema in immediate situations. In what
may be experienced as 'disturbances' of the everyday self – that is in
situations of extensive dissociation – interrelated memories, sensations and
bodily actions may cease to be recognized as in any way our own, to
become personified as human-like entities, whether these are benign or
malevolent.[63] Out of the alternative possibilities of human awareness a
culture selects its 'ordinary consciousness', its 'characteristic and habitual
patterning of mental functioning that adapts the individual, more or less

consciously, to survive in his culture's consensual reality'.[64]

This rather Kantian model leaves certain problems. In arguing for an increasing historical split (yet one independent of any specific cultural history) between physical states and the cognizing actor, its dualism tends to emphasize the more salient aspects of dissociation, thus facilitating an apparently clear distinction between an autonomous physiological state and the local psychology which it generates and through which it is experienced: as in Durkheim's *effervescences* or Bourguignon's typology of altered states of consciousness.[65] In the generally unremarked fluctuations of our daily awareness it is difficult to make this distinction. Such dualism renders everyday embodied consciousness and moral selfhood relatively unproblematic and fixed, as if given by a constant physiology about which we need say no more.[66] Nor does it allow for our less obviously cognitive but enacted modes of acquiring bodily schemata[67] for a divided self, particularly through the state of pregnancy,[68] but also lactating, menstruating, masturbating and coitus; in dancing, playing, exercising, pratfall, violence, crying, tickling and startling, grooming, gesturing, blushing, swallowing, excreting, soothing pain, sleeping and dreaming.

Affinities between the sub-personal elements of rather different local psychologies have often been remarked. Robin Horton has noted the resemblance of the psychoanalytical schema (ego, id and super-ego processes) to certain West African psychologies (the individual demonstrating agencies deriving from a unique soul, from nature and from lineage).[69] Such elements are not generally experienced or identified as separate centres of awareness, for something like a superordinate 'self'[70] has an enduring existence unified in self-awareness, will, action and memory. By and large, everyday identity does seem fairly unitary, with the development in early life of an internally consistent awareness as the locus of biographical experience, and which is recognized by others as a distinct entity continuing through time which is accountable for its past actions: a single centre of narrative gravity as Daniel Dennett puts it.[71] Both psychoanalytic and West African schemata are accounts which reconcile our understanding that we are unique, self-aware and volitional agents, yet we each share aspects of our identity with animals and with our close fellows. In circumstances where everyday identity does not hang together in the expected way, when our taken-for-granted boundary between action and contingency is radically disrupted by dispute, disaster or sickness, we may emphasize such available distinctions and give the elements a greater degree of personified autonomy such that human-like action between them serves for a more plausible understanding.

Yet our everyday experience as an enduring self is multifaceted. We are not completely here, now, always, in quite the same way. The self 'occupies' a variety of roles, titles, offices and statuses – as woman, adult, member of clan or age set, as latah, patient, parent or master of the fishing spear – without these obscuring some continuing personal identity.[72] We are not distinct individuals in each, and usually these identities do not conflict too much, yet we enact a different comportment and social character (*persona*) in each, context-dependent yet drawn from and representing an enduring individual, even if in certain circumstances we identify ourselves more fully with one or other. The available alternative selves of multiple personalities or possessing spirits may advertise a particular social status, often one to which we do not otherwise have access.[73] For, against the nineteenth-century neurologists, we might now argue that alternative personalities are not simply an existing part of us which is then split off, but rather new social potentials, ambitions, strategems, perversities and imagined identities which we try on to see how they fit, whether aspiring to adopt them permanently, perhaps to become them, or just in game-playing masquerade or private fantasy (for an individual is frequently their own principal audience). And there are all sorts of options and uncertainties along different continua: play-acting, glossolalia and deceit, with personae nominalized not just as ad hoc interpretations of some physiological shift but in social standardization as representing personified values or as historical and cosmological figures. We might recall the medieval morality play where European virtues and vices were each represented on the stage as personified beings – Lust, Charity, Envy and so on – without the play as a whole being intended for a human anatomy rather than as an allegory for humankind.[74]

10. Multiple Personality Returns

Reports of double consciousness in Europe and America declined after 1900. The introduction by the psychoanalyst Charles Rycroft to the 1978 edition of Prince's classic case, for instance, recommended it as the historical document of a psychologically unsophisticated era which had ended with Freud: ritual masquerade had now been replaced by the insights of depth psychotherapy. Sporadic cases of multiple personality occasionally appeared, and the image of the good/bad double was continually replayed through films based on the classic gothic novels and through the cinematic popularization of psychoanalysis itself, where an accessible linear narrative represented personal conflicts as successive and variant personifications or dreams of the same individual.[1]

In the late 1970s, following revelations about the widespread sexual exploitation of female children, cases of multiple personality suddenly began to emerge again in the United States, particularly after the well-publicized account of 'Sybil'.[2] As before, questions of authenticity and medical suggestion were immediately raised. Corbett Thigpen, the psychiatrist who had treated Christine Sizeman – well known through the film based on his 1957 book *The Three Faces of Eve*[3] – argued that spontaneous multiple personality like Eve's was rare. After the film made him famous he was besieged by *multiples*, as individuals with multiple personality disorder (MPD) were now called. Thigpen comments that of the thousands of patients he saw in the following thirty years only one was 'genuine', that is spontaneous and prior to medical intervention.[4] At least one new case emerged immediately after the individual saw the film.[5]

Besides the presumed aetiology of early sexual trauma, multiple personality differed from nineteenth-century double consciousness in the sheer number of personalities, frequently young children, who now appeared. Sybil, the first well-publicized case attributed to repressed memories of sexual abuse, developed 16 personalities. Eve, who had retired from public view presumed cured, returned with 22 personalities, and then recalled having been abused, to chair the recently formed International Society for the Study of Multiple Personality and Dissociation. An increasingly active group of patients, Speaking for Our Selves, publicly attacked sceptical doctors,[6] while those professionals who were sympathetic provided expert legitimation in 1988 with a generally supportive journal called *Dissociation* and devised a number of rating scales to measure dissociation and to determine MPD. Significantly, following the example of Sybil's psychiatrist, therapists now often ascribed to each personality proper names by which they were directly addressed in treatment. The spontaneity of the syndrome has continued to be argued in the medical press, particularly as to whether 'repressed memories' can be truly recalled to awareness decades later.[7] Some doctors maintain that, if properly sought, MPD is found in 10 per cent of psychiatric patients, while popular 'recovery manuals' presume half the female American population have been sexually abused and are thus *latent multiples*.[8] The question of induction through mass publicity or through the particular procedures used (hypnosis, guided imagery, trance work, body massage) is countered with the argument that genuine MPD is the response to a hidden trauma, indeed a type of autohypnotic self-healing in which the pain is so intense that 'the self leaves':[9] the public recognition of 'latent' or 'secret MPD' simply enables multiples to come out and seek the professional support they need or to recognize the condition in themselves – less medical suggestion than appropriate diagnosis.[10] Patients maintain that television reports and films about MPD enable them to give expression to something already there since their childhood rape.

Over a hundred different secondary personalities (now known as *alters*) associated with one physical body have been identified. A single body's alters may have consistent differences in handedness, facial expression, cerebral bloodflow and EEG recordings; up to 60 points difference in IQ scores, with their own characteristic visual abilities, handwriting, vocabulary, speech patterns and immunological responses; they have diverse memories and personal and family histories, and different ages, genders, ethnicity and sexual orientations.[11] They are often suicidal, self-mutilating, self-hating and sometimes violent.[12] As with the early epidemic of double consciousness, the personality immediately presenting to the doctor is troubled but bland, while the secondary personality often admits to being 'playful' or 'wicked'.[13] Compared with its nineteenth-century predecessors, MPD seem less a mimicry of neurological disease; not only do larger numbers of discrete personalities emerge but these seem generally more aware of each, coming and going relatively freely outside clinical sessions, conversing together as they scheme, quarrel, choose appropriate wardrobes, obtain spectacle prescriptions consistent with their various ages, or arrange their own personal television and book contracts; if the multiple is European- rather than American-born, one or other alter may speak only the language of origin.

Medical treatment of the new epidemic initially recalled that of the last century: hypnosis and persuasion to discharge the pathogenic secret and then reintegrate the secondary personalities with the original self, or else exhortations to just 'go back' as Prince had put it. As before, the secondary personalities often objected to being killed off. But now, with the appearance of the multiple activists (and their alters) on television, the support of feminist therapists emphasizing the politics of rape, and through well-publicized court defences that the personality in the dock was not the same one who had committed the crime (for instance the Hillside Strangler) (unsuccessfully, but sometimes only after defence lawyers have persuaded the court that the defendant when giving evidence should be sworn in separately under all their different personalities[14]), the alters have gained a public voice and demand their legal right to an independent life. Frequently young children, these alters are now accommodated rather than integrated or exorcised, for their very existence as secret memories has become a public testimony to the reality of the abuse of young women. Indeed, killing them off is regarded by the multiple movement as murder, as the concealment of one crime by another – 'revictimisation' – as the male physician simply re-enacts the original abuse.[15] The preferred therapeutic option is now to keep all the personalities in play, establishing explicit therapeutic contracts with each to encourage 'mutual awareness and communication' between them in what has increasingly come to resemble family therapy,[16] the goal being termed 'co-consciousness' (although some therapists still postulate an Inner Self Helper as the convener of the group). Hypnotherapists encourage the *survivor* to meet and comfort their abused earlier self, or instruct the alters to 'come out and play' only in dream-time. Drama therapists instruct each individual in their therapy group to take on and role-play one of the alters elicited from one individual, the whole then enacting that body's mental state.

In the 1890s some American doctors sympathetic to Spiritualism had accepted secondary personalities as visiting benign spirits and were less inclined to kill them off.[17] This interpretation too has returned but now in a demonic variant: sexual abuse of working-class children in both Britain and America has been linked (on implausible evidence[18]) with male witchcraft, cannibalism and child sacrifice.[19] Satanic explanations have been encouraged among teachers and social workers by evangelical Christian networks which practise exorcism and generally favour a diabolical interpretation of human malevolence and misfortune.[20] A British psychiatrist with a clinical interest in child sexual abuse has recently stated that 10 per cent of our adult population are practising Satanists.[21] A British textbook for treating survivors of Satanic abuse written by clinicians at London University[22] does not follow American psychiatrists in recognizing alters as alien demons, but suggests rather that the Satanists themselves use hypnotherapy to induce secondary personalities.[23] It proposes that therapists have not taken seriously their patients' accounts of a war-time atrocity in peace-time England. Men and women ... worship Satan as their god in private houses or in churchyards and forests. In so doing they literally turn upside down any moral concept that comes from Christianity. They practise every sexual perversion that exists with animals, children and both sexes. They drink blood and urine and eat faeces and insects. They are involved in pornographic films and drug-dealing as a way of raising money. They are highly organised, successful in their secrecy and have a belief that through their pain and abuse they are getting closer to their god.[24]

The contributors argue that their own therapeutic role must preclude any ascertaining of the 'truth' of memories of Satanic abuse[25] but that those apparently seeking to discredit their work publicly, generally doctors and jurists, are ritual abusers themselves.[26] (MPD therapists frequently present themselves as beleaguered or oppressed pioneers facing 'the pervasive hostile counter-transference' of their colleagues.[27]) The book proposes that survivors should be treated in extended sessions in special sanctuaries to be set up in the near future.[28] A professor of psychology at the University of Utah has argued that the SRA (Satanic Ritual Abuse) conspiracy, involving Satanists, the CIA and Jewish kabbalists, has produced 'cultified multiples' who are currently under surveillance by the Utah Police Department of Public Safety.[29]

American psychiatrists have proposed that the sexual abuse which results in MPD is carried out not only by the child's family, the CIA and by Satanists but by extra-terrestrial *effectors* who abduct, abuse and then return the victim; one Harvard University clinic has now treated more than 70 of these patients or *experiencers*.[30] Nineteenth-century Spiritualists had described visits to alien flying machines, and Schnabel[31] gives a detailed account of the development of the various *experiencer* (or *abductee*) networks involving observers of Unidentified Flying Objects, science fiction writers, psychologists and psychiatrists: coteries who met on the New York cocktail circuit, exchanged clients, franchised new techniques, sponsored conferences and appeared on rival television chat shows. In the late 1940s, with the start of the Cold War, a number of sightings of flying saucers were initially taken seriously by the US Air Force but then discredited by a number of government commissions. (Enthusiasts have continued to argue a collaboration with the aliens by the US government and the United Nations.) Originally green in colour, by the start of the Civil Rights Movement the aliens were observed to have become somewhat darker or at least grey. Accounts of physical abductions of humans first appeared in the early 1950s, initially benevolent in intent but by the 1960s involving 'medical examinations', usually of a gynaecological type with the women's legs spread in stirrups.[32] These accounts progressed in a few years to uncovered memories of rape as the abductees began to discover bruises and other marks on their bodies which to critical observers recalled medieval stigmata. Starting in the 1970s hypnotic therapy was used to 'regress missing time cases' whose memories of the events had been erased by the abductors: by the 1980s more than a thousand women in therapy had successfully recalled being abducted, inseminated and returned to earth, only to be reabducted for the harvesting of their hybrid offspring. (Fewer men were abducted, generally to be sexually aroused and have their semen emitted and piped off.) Extrapolating from a questionnaire study of the public in 1991 suggests that over 15 million Americans have now been abducted.[33] By the late 1980s, the small number of abductee scholars who still favoured benevolent alien intrusion had gravitated to New Age and Near Death Experience (NDE) groups in order to contact these higher powers; those arguing for malevolent agencies aligned themselves with the existing sexual abuse theorists including many in the Christian Right and feminist mental health networks. Under ever 'deeper' hypnosis, some survivors were now able to recall sexual abuse in an earlier life form, as 'Eve' did by 1989.[34] (Multiple personality aside, 28 per cent of American psychotherapists accept that hypnosis facilitates recall of memories from previous lives.[35]) The American psychiatrist John Mack has the belief – might I say faith – that the abduction phenomenon is, at its core, about the preservation of life on Earth at a time when the planet's life is 'profoundly threatened'.[36] Schnabel describes the disputes between the different abductee therapists, their conflicts with rival experts for lucrative television time, film and book contracts, the attempt to monopolize the more important abductees and to discredit those of competing cliques, and the unsuccessful proposal by the psychiatrists involved to exclude amateur therapists from conducting hypnotic regression (backed by their consensus DSM-III diagnosis of Adjustment Disorder with Mixed Emotional Features, i.e. anxiety and depression caused by the alien abduction).[37] Objections that the abductees could be shown by psychological tests to be 'fantasy-prone individuals' (FPIs) were countered with the argument that this personality trait was a response to the abduction. That most abductees reported being removed from and returned to their beds at night has been suggested by sceptics to recall common temporal lobe and hypnogogic phenomena such as sleep paralysis and out-of-body experiences (which may be locally understood as incubi such as Old Hag among Newfoundland fishermen[38]). Indeed, on mapping cerebral localizations of the body's sensory imput, the vagina is represented on the orbital frontal lobes, adjacent to temporal lobe seizures which are not infrequently experienced by women as sexual penetration; while dream-time erection and 'nocturnal emission' are of course common experiences for men.

The multiple selves are variously identified as the possessing aliens themselves, as their hybrid offspring, as the psychological representation or psychic reincarnation of the human perpetrator, as living or deceased family members, as 'transcendent spirit helpers', as new attempts at self-healing, or as the lost person of an abused childhood.[39] Christian psychiatrists and clergy who offer 'deliverance ministry' describe them as invasive incubi, or as congealed ancestral vices and the vengeful spirits of aborted foetuses passing down 'the generation line', an idiom recalling Ribot's rather less dramatic description of the traumatic memory as a 'mental parasite'.[40] These variant identifications are not restricted each to a therapeutic school; university professors of medicine teach their students how to distinguish anthropomorphic alters who are merely split-off psychological functions from those who are to be diagnosed as extra-terrestrials or demonic spirits.[41]

The reality of multiple personality has not gone unquestioned. The spontaneous 'recovery' of memories of sexual abuse in MPD has been challenged in 'the biggest story in psychiatry for a decade'.[42] Therapeutically encouraged legal suits by adults against their parents for having sexually abused them as children and against their earlier doctors for having failed to diagnose their MPD have been met by counter-claims against the individuals' therapists of inducing a 'false memory syndrome' in distressed individuals who are persuaded to recall non-existent sexual abuse (akin to false confessions to the police), encouraged by the expanding 'survivors' movement' with its television volunteering of MPD. Damages against the parent for sexual abuse have been of the order of up to $5 million plus lawyers' and doctors' fees; and the Roman Catholic church in the United States has reportedly paid $500 million secretly to have claims of child molestation against its priests dropped.[43] By 1993 7000 people had joined the anti-MPD False Memory Syndrome Foundation, whose therapists specialize in counter-techniques and who liken the whole issue to the Salem witch trials. Indeed, there have been recent instances in rural American communities of self-accusations of Satanic cannibalism volunteered by newly 'born-again' Christians.[44] The question of legally establishing the reality of abuse is confused by the absence of clear physical signs and the obvious questions as to the suggestibility of child or patient as a potential witness.[45]

The philosopher Ian Hacking proposes that MPD is less a 'condition' than a

> movement ... built roughly as a pyramid. At the top there is a relatively small number of dedicated psychiatrists who diagnose literally hundreds of patients. Then there is a larger number of clinical psychologists who recognize some of their clients as multiples. Next, at least in some

regions, there is a very substantial number of social workers who find the condition in their casework. And finally there are the multiples themselves, some of whom organize themselves into self-help groups, publish newsletters and the like.[46]

As in the 1890s, philosophers of mind have, however, become interested in multiple personality because of the questions it raises about the roots of personal identity in memory and consciousness. And the multiple movement in turn deploys their arguments against an invariate single self. Wilkes is sympathetic to the idea that the neuropsychological correlates suggest that the various identities may be regarded as conventionally discrete. Braude is less concerned with the reality of MPD than using it as a mind experiment in which each personality experiences itself as at the centre of a complete consciousness but through all of which still runs some fundamental Kantian unification. Dennett, like Hacking, emphasizes the narrative assumptions underlying MPD but proposes that its development follows relatively easily on the multiple functions of the mind for there is no unitary centre given in nature, no Cartesian self, material or otherwise, not even a shifting 'searchlight' of awareness, but rather competition between a number of 'multiple drafts': a model supported by recent evidence from neuropsychology such as blindsight guessing or alterations in personal identity after surgical severing of the corpus callosum. Dennett argues there is no single canonical experience or representation of either the external world or our own internal processes at a particular point in space or time: the brain responds to the outside world but the same processes can respond to this response itself – and this is what we reify as consciousness. It is our apparently unitary self that is now taken as problematic, not its dissociation. Why the self is generally experienced as unitary remains biologically mysterious; it just seems an efficient way of proceeding which is developed, perhaps, through social action.[47]

Multiplicity and modernity

Victorian double consciousness and contemporary MPD have sufficient resemblance to each other to justify our comparing them under the common rubric of multiple personality.[48] Continuity between the two epidemics is not only in our analysis, for contemporary multiples and their medical advocates regard both manifestations as the same phenomenon and are familiar with the earlier literature, whose debates they have recommenced, notably on whether a single trauma is necessary and sufficient.[49]

Whether at this point we read multiple personality as an idiom of

distress, as a psychological defence against sexual abuse or as a creative
fantasy, whether we grant it some existence as a distinct psychophysiological entity, socially induced or requiring public acceptance to bring it into
the open, its local context and meanings are significant. Can either wave of
multiplicity be related to a coherent group of professional interests, or to
some more diffuse sensibility of the times, or even to similar changes in
women's social experience? In terms of immediate context, we can
recognize in both epidemics a committed network of male doctors and
psychologists, who accept the phenomenon as a legitimate matter of
clinical importance which requires nosologies and instruments of verification, and whose professional reputation and public career are derived from
it, diagnosing it where others fail, and who are identified publicly with it as
authoritative experts through their newspaper articles, publicized case
histories and, in the second wave, cinema dramatizations and television
shows.[50] And both epidemics furnish evidence for philosophers and
moralists whose conclusions in turn are used to authenticate the
phenomenon.

While he himself was not particularly interested in multiple personality,
Freud's role is significant, for the new wave, both as an observed
phenomenon and in its explanation, returns us to his theoretical position
before he abandoned the seduction hypothesis. Criticism of his apparent
suppression of the evidence for incest has followed the recognition that
sexual rape or seduction of children by adult males in America is far more
common than previously realized; and with this recognition has appeared
an expert therapeutic practice for the 'survivors' which, although partly
influenced by psychoanalytical therapy, has resonances with Janet's earlier
emphasis on the individual's adaptation to a single traumatic event.
Classical psychoanalysis has lost the pre-eminence it held in America from
the 1930s to the 1960s, squeezed out between psychiatry's recent
rapprochement with biomedical experimentalism and the competition
from these more focused, lay therapies with radically shorter and cheaper
training.[51]

Multiple personality disorder is still rarely reported in Britain or
elsewhere in Europe,[52] and the recognition of child sexual abuse has
generally not involved British doctors in demonological quests. 'Our more
bracing attitude is summed up by a consultant psychiatrist who, when
asked what he did about MPD, replied: "We react to any suggestions that
there are two or three more personalities by saying that there are two or
more aspects to one personality and asserting that the individual must take
responsibility for both of these aspects. It works." '[53] Why the British
scepticism? That the sexual violation of children is less common in Britain
seems unlikely.[54] Is it experienced differently in the United States, or are
we to locate MPD in some specific therapeutic intervention? There are far

fewer psychiatrists per population in the United Kingdom (less than 4000 for the whole country[55]), and they have never had the popular and juridical influence of their North American colleagues. They remain within the public hospitals, committed to the treatment of psychosis, and have not been subject to the enthusiastic paradigm shifts of American medicine now engaged with an extensive medical malpractice industry and biomedical ethicists (not to mention the new profession of medical anthropologists). British psychiatrists, like their other medical colleagues, argue a robust dichotomy between 'real' and 'imaginary' symptoms, placing less emphasis on implicit motivations. Their professional interest lies in solving clinical problems briskly rather than maintaining a lucrative clientele of chronic private patients – the preserve of the small number of British psycho-analysts who generally take an 'integrative' view of dissociative symptoms. Dramatic symptoms which engage others are discouraged, doubtless regarded as in rather poor taste, certainly as insincere or exaggerated.

Beyond this perhaps lie wider questions of a society's susceptibility to 'ideas in the air' – as Dostoyevsky put it in the case of Raskolnikov. Why multiplicity? Hacking argues that 'what we do see from time to time in European and American milieux are some very troubled people interacting with their cultural and medical surroundings ... They cast, perhaps, a distorting image of what their communities think it is to be a person'.[56] Kenny characterizes multiple personalities as 'parodies of conventional social roles'.[57] We might invoke broader idioms for contemporary identity and self-transformation, and for the justification of distress and personal failure. It is certainly not difficult to offer homologies between individual and society, such that the experiencing self offers a microcosm of wider issues, the dissociation of the individual standing for the dis-sociation of the collectivity, now less an ordered hierarchy than a contractual network.[58] The nineteenth-century epidemic of double consciousness was regarded by its psychologists and cultural commentators as the mirror of a fragmenting society.[59] It is less easy to show how such correspon-dences plausibly motivate personal experiences. Henri Ellenberger's magisterial study of nineteenth-century psychiatry, on which I have drawn extensively here, has been criticized for taking just such parallels as historically causal.[60] That the self is a mirror of society is itself a local psychology: contemporary Europeans may experience matters that way, or they may not, or more likely they see it that way in certain situations. As Hacking notes, it is a particular local notion of the person that is significant, yet the individual may represent society less as its mirror than as the locus of social fault lines or as the recipient of quite various 'stresses'.[61] Yet expert groups maintain their authority through the importance of their therapeutic intercessions, the illness becoming emblematic of current dilemmas, 'the national disease', 'the sickness of our age', 'our number-one mental health problem': a prototype to which other ills are referred or into which they are subsumed. To be successful, healers need to convince others not only that they cure the individual but that they are, to use La Barre's term, culture healers. The particular ambiguities of psychiatry's concerns with the medical and the moral allow it a privileged place in Western societies in resolving such dilemmas; its conceptions of the mind become popularized as normative models for the mind.[62] Allan Young has argued that the new category of Post-Traumatic Stress Disorder – of which MPD has been seen as a variant[63] – originally developed in American military hospitals as an exculpation for the personal guilt of Vietnam War veterans, transforming them from the aggressors into the victims in their turn,[64] a diagnosis that has now become available for taking on other vexed questions of the attribution of personal or official responsibility in a contractual society.

British class identity still provides some residual location for failure as outside the individual in political contingency, but in the United States, during the late nineteenth century as much as now, personal disappointment requires less some sense of bad luck than of competitive disadvantage or the malevolence of others – and hence recourse to legal redress[65] or else to the sort of 'positive' transformation, eliding religious conversion, self-knowledge and managerial presentation, exemplified by Dale Carnegie and Norman Vincent Peale. The United States has always taken itself as the site for strategic self-fashioning, by which diverse immigrant groups realize themselves as Americans as they move to higher status jobs and improve their education, as they change their residence, neighbourhood, profession, friends, spouses, political affiliation, leisure activities, voluntary associations, and even their name and religion, with associated changes of presentation in mannerism, comportment, language, idiom and dress. With dedication to manuals of kinaesthetics, personal communication and handwriting, earlier selves and practices became incorporated or even forgotten.[66] American identity is achieved in the very process of transformation, in fulfilling some apparently inherent potential, both as the normative expectation of what it is to become genuinely American and as a practical possibility, articulated for men in self-monitoring manuals of salesmanship and entrepreneurial psychology, for women through remodelling their bodies by dieting and plastic surgery: realizing one's personality in the marketing of it, through self-help groups and civil associations which emphasize the achievement of a 'real' or 'positive' identity for minorities and stigmatized groups, currently articulated through a politico-therapeutic language of communication, growth, personal space, realization and authenticity. America is a psychologized society, not just in that psychology is the most popular supplementary subject for its university students, but in that psychology is the national idiom which, reading social power as personal performance, argues for autonomy and self-scrutiny, for consumer choice and therapeutic transformation.

The late nineteenth and earlier twentieth century were characterized by a proliferation of technologies by which a number of objective and replicable characteristics came to constitute the individual – callisthenics, graphology, IQ- and personality-testing, photometrics and somatotyping, the polygraph. Such characteristics could, to an extent, be achieved: to alter your handwriting under professional supervision would change your personality and thus your financial mobility; as expert knowledge these practices were justified by the 'motor theory of consciousness' of William James. Whether they should be regarded as therapeutic or transformative seems arbitrary: the police psychologist's lie detector (galvanometer) emerges as the 'e-meter' of the Church of Scientology, through which repressed traumatic memories, often of past lives, are identified and 'cleared'. What might be regarded elsewhere as an extreme response to current dissatisfaction with personal circumstances – voluntarily disappearing from one's present neighbourhood and family to emerge elsewhere with a new name and personal identity – is now facilitated by a publishing house which has produced over 30 manuals to direct something British psychiatrists would recognize as a hysterical fugue.[67]

I am aware that this is a European's image of the United States, one which since Trollope and de Tocqueville has seen that country as anomic and neotenic, its emphasis on personal self-transformation as the concealment of class conflict, its institutions maintained through periodic moral panics and social dramas, its citizens unable to agree on what constitutes reality without recourse to legal or medical authority.[68] Yet America's 'obsession with self-awareness', what Louis Hartz in *The Liberal Tradition in America* terms the 'peculiar quality of America's hysteria', is well recognized by its own cultural critics.[69] Self-realization through pulling on one's bootstraps has always been central to what it is to be an American – from the frontier regeneration of the Great Awakening and its transformation of self and nature, to Universalism, Transcendentalism, New Thought, Christian Science, pragmatism, 'little man' populism, to Boosterism, Soroptimism and the search for university tenure: a quest for achieved rather than ascribed status, a fundamentally optimistic view that time and space still lie unlimited before one. Relocation, upward social mobility, self-reliance and perfectionism are hardly limited to America;[70] and it is easy to identify in any society a concern with rapid social transformations, the breakdown of family life and traditional interpersonal ties (as did the European pessimism of Herder, Gissing, Pater and Musil) but it has seemed integral to American exceptionalism to regard incompleteness as the appropriate state of affairs. Nor am I necessarily critical of an optimism which reframes mental retardation through 'normalization', which reasserts the moral integrity of stigmatized minorities and the chronically ill in 'the politics of identity', and which can translate misfortune into achievement. Yet we might take an ironically European view and question whether the search for authenticity does not preclude its own goal; that to develop a hundred personalities is perhaps to have none.[71]

In any period of perceived change or creolization, both society and self may be experienced as hollow, fragmented or double, as estranged from a past unity to enter an indeterminate future.[72] If George Gissing bemoaned the end of the nineteenth century as 'decades of sexual anarchy . . . with the laws governing human identity, friendships and sexual behaviour breaking down', now our 'radical democratisation of the personal',[73] our fragmented and commodified assimilation of alternative selves, may be argued to be especially part of a late modern condition where the ascription of risk becomes more significant than the ascription of value.[74] With the decline of Calvinist moral imperatives, American individualism has become, as Jackson Lears puts it, 'weightless and unreal'.[75] Is there anything more specific about contemporary fin-de-siècle America, endlessly self-creating, polyphonic, ludic and multiplex,[76] which suggests closer parallels with late nineteenth-century France? That other daughter of the Enlightenment, which also perceived itself as preoccupied with artifice and representation, which recognized the commodification of sex and marriage, and was confused about civil divorce and public religion, about the sexual exploitation of children and female emancipation – an increasingly contractual and legalistic society characterized by the detachment of the voyeuristic boulevard flâneur posing in the rootless *spleen* of the anonymous crowd; with immersion in new and impersonal *grands magasins*, and increased opportunities for social mobility and travel; enthusiasms for bodily transformation and athletic spectacle; with the intermittent emergence of variant sexualities, and the loss of traditional clerical authority under the governments of the Third Republic: public concerns ambivalently countered by a response which Ellenberger[77] has aptly described as 'Neo-Romantic', irrational, narcissistic, decadent and primitivist, with positivism's project of boundless technical progress and limitless material prosperity now foreclosed, shot through with pessimism and a sense that time was running out with the century, the race exhausted, its vigour dissipated, threatened by its incorporation of aliens, with a quest for secular myths and new heroes, or else for mystical continuities with a natural world that at times seemed exhausted too, with a return to religious orthodoxy or else to domesticated variants of Asian religions.[78] In the United States the resurgence of Protestant fundamentalism in the 1980s required public figures to acknowledge that they had been 'born again' – as having spontaneously achieved a new moral identity.[79] Recalling the fate of double consciousness, this demand for testimonies of spontaneity collapsed in religious scandals and accusations of feigning; we might wonder if the demands for 'born again' experiences should be taken as a response to the perceived fragmentation of personal identity (a spiritual and psychological healing, as argued by its protagonists) or simply a manifestation of it.

It would be easy to delineate parallels between the end of the French nineteenth century and the end of the American twentieth.[80] More specifically we might prefer to note a similar shift in the location of the self, less a dissociation than a deterritorialization of it; the external physical frontiers of a now mechanized nature becoming congested and fore-shortened so that our bodies turn in on themselves, self-sufficient through dietetics and 'body consciousness'. Muscle building as a parody of labour; the perfectable body less the housing of the self than the very self; social controls and standardized rituals becoming internalized as 'self-expression' and 'choice' in transformations attained through potentially unlimited consumption.[81] We have both become lesser than we thought, as simply elements in a natural world which is indifferent to human interests; and greater, in that we recognize that this world is refracted and remade in our cognitions and actions.

Multiple personality was attributed last century to such reshapings of the self in lived time as the photograph, the phonograph, the telephone and the X-ray.[82] Where then did the new telephone conversation take place? We might argue in the emerging world of what we now term 'cyberspace': in the virtual architecture of electronically generated, accessed and sustained memory which we enter through our personal computer or notebook, in interactive television (and more recently virtual reality and other prosthetic embodiments), in electronic mail, the Internet, multidimensional graphical user interfaces and hypertext, in the recorded space of portable stereos, in 'personality profiles' generated by our credit card transactions, in satellite television channels and electronic conferencing, teledildonics ('telephone sex') and cybererotics – an increasingly global modularity which questions individual time, proximity, work, value and ownership, and whose shift from material production to information and representation radically resituates the location of our taken-for-granted physical experience and interactions in a post-industrial and post-corporeal global space, our embodied experience fragmented and commodified.[83] As do the replace-able parts of our biomedical body shop – sperm, egg and embryo banks, fertility drugs and multiple births, cerebral implants of foetal tissue and computer chips, life support machines to harvest organs from the brain-dead, market-ready tissue-typed kidneys, electronic prostheses and gene-splicing. For women these are particularly significant in the 'life versus choice' debate on foetal personhood – the salient schema for two beings housed in one body.[84] And with this has gone a decay of linear or determinist theory, whether as prose, progress or biography, in favour of fragmented, multiple, iterative and creolized imagery, a dissatisfaction with ascribed hierarchies and a preference for market vicissitudes over command economies, a loosely associated milieu of ideas which we might remark in post-colonial aesthetics, social constructivism, evolutionary epistemology, biosociality, non-linear chaos models, fractal mathematics and dissipative systems theory. A similar idiom of multiplicity emerges in 'the new biology' which argues our early ancestors incorporated other bacteria which have become our bodies' organelles and tissues.[85]

In 1986 Bolter proposed that the computer, like the medieval mechanical clock, had become our 'defining technology', an instrumental extension of the body but which was taken as the model for a self in an idiom of inputs and outputs, the body as hardware with consciousness as software. If they have any identifiable locus at all, human minds are now serial virtual machines implemented on parallel hardware, and MPD is just a different program run on this same hardware.[86] But computers are not just a fashionable and accessible metaphor, our latest edition of *l'homme machine*, for the computer network actually embodies rather than merely represents symbolic logic in a virtual space which in each generation seeks to grow ever larger in relation to the physical limitations of its linear circuits and available telephone bandwidth. The computational theories of the 1960s proposed that human mentation, like digital computers, operated by such logic-based manipulations of symbols; practically unsuccessful in such tasks as natural language translation, recent connectionist revisions now evoke the mind as a distributed network of elementary subsystems that work by trial and error rather than from unified design. Cyberpunk novels and ecotechnology, like the not dissimilar 'hard AI' and Artificial Life arguments, offer more than a fantasied model of the self – rather an ad hoc, virtual but potentially immortal multiplex self which has no inevitable locus in the physical body.[87]

> Cyberspace becomes another venue for consciousness itself . . . Animism is not only possible, it is implicit . . . To the body in cyberspace we are the mind. By a strange reversal of our cultural expectations, however, it is the body in cyberspace that is immortal, while the animating soul, housed in a body outside cyberspace, faces mortality.[88]

Customary distinction between nature, agency and technology are elided in robotics, in our recognition of self-organizing inorganic chemical reactions, and in information-based biological procedures such as DNA replication. Proponents of Artificial Life argue that it collapses our categories of matter, life and artefact, the whole universe being a 'cellular automaton'.[89] 'There is no "I" for a person, for a beehive, for a corporation, for an animal, for a nation, for any living thing.'[90]

I do not want to make too much of cyberspace as a fundamental rupture with previous locations of the self. Parallel processing and virtual reality, like the new reproductive technologies, are the latest relocation of our embodied agency in a biosocial history marked by the development of clothes, spear throwers, figurative representation, property, silent reading, autobiography, linear perspective, printing, coordinate geometry, the novel, mechanized transport, military brothels, limited liability, cosmetic surgery and cultural relativism. Each progression may be experienced as a 'dissociation of sensibility'[91] yet taken as the model for ourselves. But if the problem for nineteenth-century philosophers lay in the disintegration of a unitary self given in nature, current interest lies in the opposite – in the surprising synthesis of our sub-personal modules. It is not altered states of consciousness that are now problematic but our illusive experience of unitary consciousness in a data-based collectivization of the human sensorium.

The self as a contesting network of separate modules is found not just in Riemannian space, AIDS and auto-immune disease, in recent cognitive psychology, linguistics and neuro-philosophy,[92] but, significantly for the immediate development of MPD, in the more accessible 'human potential' therapies (derived from the 'ego-centred' psychoanalysis of the United States through the Object Relations School, Primal Therapy and Transactional Analysis): clinical practices and self-help techniques which promote the realization of all our 'selves' aptly recognized under an extraordinary multiplicity of terms[93] – psychological models for the self rather than models of the self. The Ego-State School recognizes a 'federal government over all',[94] while in other American therapies no single state may hold ascendancy (states' rights?). The decisive therapeutic step in concretizing these serial potentials into competing selves 'hiding from each other',[95] and thus into MPD, seems to be in therapist and client personalizing them with a proper name, as in the implausibly named technique of Psychosynthesis.[96] Akin to the earlier guides to self-perfectioning and managerial efficiency, such expert technologies employ a popularized psychoanalytical idiom of unrealized levels of individuation (as in est, Scientology and TM) as potential selves which are to be sequentially realized through a no longer self-sufficient body, in which transformations of identity can have fruitful economic implications;[97] in which our variant identities are neither transitory masks nor imaginary novelties but rather the achievement of something which is authentically there, of which we rest unfulfilled until therapeutically liberated from our repressions, purged of our historical sincerities, lower stages and naive or

hypocritical social obligations. 'Be yourself.' As the philosopher Charles
Taylor puts it, making 'what was hidden manifest for both myself and
others'. One might argue such a practice rather downplays the radical
novelty of any new self while at the same time encouraging us to acquire it –
less the Puritan struggle for arduous refashioning than freedom for
something already there to assume its natural place.[98] Slippery and elusive
though a new persona may be, it works as it is taken by others for an
authentic self.

Multiple personality as experience and practice is not just a reflection of
popular psychology or fiction. As Mark Micale notes of the pervasive idiom
of hysteria in the nineteenth century,

> Once a disease concept enters the domain of public discussion, it
> effectively becomes impossible to chart its lines of cultural origin,
> influence and evolution with any accuracy. Rather, visual, dramatic, and
> medical theories and images become inextricably caught up with one
> another. Eventually, this criss-cross of ideas, information and associa-
> tions forms a single sociocultural milieu from which all authors –
> professional and popular, scientific and literary – may draw.[99]

And patients: if individuals spontaneously develop multiple personality it is
not only as they participate in a pervasive representation of serial
multiplicity through cinema, television, news reports and popular texts.
We know as yet little of the relationship that develops between the multiple
and her therapist except that the therapist vigorously endorses the integrity
of the patient's struggles and her 'unchained memories'.[100] And when the
integrity of the therapist is attacked by sceptics, the patient angrily rallies to
the defence.[101] Ellenberger moves beyond simple ascriptions of 'seduction'
by the hysterical patient (or its recent converse, the 'patriarchy' of the
physician), to propose that such formative theories emerge out of more
widespread cultural preoccupations through the collaboration of a
committed young doctor with an intelligent and engaging patient.
Together they elaborate a mutually agreeable script which both encompasses the woman's distress and the intellectual ambitions of the doctor, a
paradigmatic new illness whose manifestation shapes and confirms the
emerging theory, and which then becomes standardized both as a new
technology and as a legitimate research programme.[102]

The cyborgs of technovisionary bionics and the 'distributed conversation' of the Net,[103] like the sub-personalities of the human potential
therapies and the animism of deep ecology, provide techniques for self-
transformation into alternative identities which are no longer embodied in
the taken-for-granted way.[104] Potential selves are 'accessed' serially
through everyday cultural potentials legitimated and enhanced by

computer games and medical technologies. Undesirable future selves are to be identified through 'risk factors' and then averted through self-monitoring techniques such as stress management.[105] Despite its affinity with the pluripotent roles demanded by post-industrial managerialism, multiple personality is not a phenomenon which somehow emerges as the index of our cultural life but is rather one elaborated in certain expert practices, and now validated in a medico-legal commerce which places the sources of affliction beyond a unitary body which seeks to repossess some 'personal space'. Computer-simulated worlds like Habitat and MUDS structure the 'internal landscape' of the self: psychiatrists are taught to enter cyberspace to advise and direct their patients' alters, escape from dungeons or launch into 'mission[s] to rescue other alters, destroy castle walls, disarm internal computers, rebuild architecture, create safe places ...'.[106] If nineteenth-century double consciousness was recognized as a repression of physical energy,[107] then our current idioms are those of replication and iteration, of intrusive embodiments alien to our still perduring subjectivities.

One of the more unusual modern syndromes including personal identity and body image is *apotemnophilia* – the wish to have one or more body parts (including both legs) surgically removed. We can relate this to *body dysmorphic disorder* – a concern that certain parts of the body, typically ears or noses, are misshapen, also to past descriptions of sexual fascination with mutilation and amputees; but, perhaps more closely, to *transsexualism*, the feeling that one has always felt alien with one's own sex and that one's appropriate gender is the other. As one would-be patient described it,

> The first time I had the feelings of really wanting my leg amputated, that I didn't feel like I wanted this as part of my body, was around seventy-eight or nine, but I can trace that back to when I was four years of age, I saw this man on the street who was an amputee. I knew I just wanted to be like that. It's not part of my body [the leg], the backbone of who I am, it just feels that it ends at my mid-point here on my thigh.[108]

Whether apotemnophilia can indeed be related to a sympathetic medical response and the necessary acceptability of justification for gender reassignment[109] couched in an 'it was always me in the wrong body' idiom, the hospital where a sympathetic surgeon carried out two amputations has now banned further operations of this sort.[110] Both transsexualism and apotemnophilia, like MPD, challenge the way of the self as in the given biological body, a more radical restatement of bodily transformation such as liposuction or cosmetic surgery.

11. Reality, Truth, Power: The Dialogue between Reason and Necessity

What might constitute a 'medical reality' for multiple personality or for the other patterns we have discussed? Presumably that they exist independently of willed intention and that they can be objectively demonstrated as distinct states prior to any local recognition, understanding or therapeutic intervention.[1] As with other contentious Euro-American syndromes (Post-Traumatic Stress Disorder, Pre-Menstrual Tension, Myalgic Encephalomyelitis, Munchausen's Syndrome, Hyperactivity Syndrome, Total Allergy Syndrome), the debate on multiple personality mobilizes supporters and opponents, both medical and lay, who argue for and against its validity; inauthenticity variously being that it is a variant of some already recognized illness such as depression, or else that it is induced by doctor or simulated by patient (this slides into psychodynamic ideas of unconscious motivation), or less commonly that the whole phenomenon is a duplicitous joint fabrication which neither patient nor professional take for actuality.[2] Patient self-help groups on the contrary generally maintain that these illnesses are biologically specified and accuse doctors of implying they are 'only psychological'.[3]

As with ME, PTSD or hysteria,[4] claims to the plausibility of multiple personality can be considered from three positions: biological, phenomenological and dramaturgical.

Biological: there certainly seem to be consistent physiological distinctions associated with the different personalities. But biological variation does not in itself conventionally constitute a disease entity any more than consistent changes in our galvanic skin response (electrical potential) during moments of anger would allow us to characterize this mood as pathological or indeed as any more real than non-angry experience.

Phenomenological: does the reported pattern correspond with its protagonists' experience? There seems little doubt that ME or PTSD are experienced as an illness or that most instances of multiple personality are recognized at the time as genuine and spontaneous new selves, although instances of motivated invention do occur (as after Charcot's death when some of his patients apparently admitted that they had faked the whole thing[5]).

Dramaturgical: if in a particular case we recognize the influence of a theory upon the existence of things which it is held to explain,[6] claims to their independent reality and subjective truth then seem to evaporate, for the individual now has access to the expected scenario through the procedures common to everyday social life – learning, mimesis, strategic role-playing, compliance, deception. Requesting experimental subjects for instance to explicitly 'simulate' hypnosis and MPD leads to the desired phenomena: the extent to which the individuals report the experience to observers controlling the experiment as 'real' depends on the degree of encouragement.[7] Thus Michael Kenny, like Rodney Needham, prefers to talk here of social metaphor.[8] That empirical observations occur within a social context in which they take on more extended meanings and power is not, however, a criterion for denying their claims to provide context-independent truth about the world;[9] and if multiple personality or agoraphobia seem phenomena dependent on the act of informed observation then the private individual is always their own observer, nor can any psychological state be empirically 'real'.[10]

Protagonists and critics of the independent reality of multiple personality of the other patterns tend to agree on an essential dualism: either it just happens to you or else you deliberately do it.[11] Each 'it' is a rather different sort of thing: disease entity versus masquerade. In a number of recent papers I have argued rather for a procedural dualism: we can understand ourselves and the world as a consequence of cause and effect processes, generally independent of, but potentially accessible to, human awareness – the naturalistic mode of thought; yet we can simultaneously understand the same matters personalistically – as the motivated actions of volitional agents employing such characteristically human attributes as intention, representation, narration, self-awareness, inter-subjectivity, identification, deceit and shame. And while Euro-Americans conventionally allocate one or other area of interest to the naturalistic or the personalistic, perhaps objectifying them as separate domains (nature: culture or brain: mind), we can apply either mode of thought to any phenomenon. For the self may be a machine, the natural world may be personified.[12] Psychiatric considerations of such phenomena as self-harm (symptom of depressive illness? intention to die?) or myalgic encephalomyelitis (disease process? malingering?), like medico-legal debates on criminal responsibility (mad? bad?), continually slip between one and the other, for only one mode can be correct at any one time. (The pragmatic legal categories of tort and diminished responsibility generally duck any attempt to examine their mutual relationship, nor can courts easily allocate financial compensation

after accidents according to an index of 'real' versus 'public' disability.)
Neither can be demonstrated as completely true, nor false: we always live
with the two options.[13] As Plato put it in the *Timaeus*, 'The world came
about as a combination of reason and necessity.' But combined how? In
certain areas – anthropology, psychiatry, medical jurisprudence, cognitive
science, ethology and the sociology of knowledge – the practical problems
of reconciling causation and volition become especially salient. As in the
Hegelian or Marxist emergence of mind, in phrenology, phenomenology
and psychoanalysis, in sociobiology and in current neuropsychology and
the philosophy of mind,[14] these generally reduce one position to the other
as prior and essential: whether in ontology, in epistemology or, usually, in
both.

This is not an essay on scientific method and I do not wish to detail
current attempts to resolve the antinomy but rather to take it as an
inescapable ambiguity in our everyday life and thence in expert practice.
Psychoanalysis once attempted to reconcile the opposition through a sub-
personal psychology which showed how the possibility of intention emerges
dynamically from naturalistic sub-personal structures. Its resulting notion
of fantasy (not empirically true, yet not exactly fabricated) elided for
multiple personality the antinomies of physiologically autonomous or
personally contrived.[15] That the professional acceptance of psychoanalysis
now seems inversely related to the recognition of multiple personality
argues against reading the current wave of MPD or PTSD simply as our
postmodern consciousness, for its enthusiasts insist on the objective reality
of both the syndromes as biologically specified and, in the former case, of
its invariant cause, child sexual abuse, a signifier with an all-too-real
signified.[16] And opponents too generally revert to a pre-Freudian
empiricism in denying its existence: no reality to MPD or PTSD because
no causal trauma. This goes along with a shift in the moral economy of our
two modes of thought in the last 20 years in both Britain and the United
States, in an apparently more personalistic and contractual direction –
towards an emphasis on individual responsibility for sickness, unemployment and poverty, and on the rights and responsibilities of the mentally ill,
and on the authenticity of all experiences of subdominant groups;[17] with
diminished space in a contracted natural world transformed by self-
sufficient individuals for underlying 'structures' or 'accidents' – which
remain observable events yet have now become violating traumata
occasioned by the mischief or negligence of others, responsible agents
whom we hold morally and legally accountable for the 'management' of
our risks. Heelas has argued on the basis of locus of control experiments by
psychologists that when there is such a strong emphasis on an autonomous
self, we attribute undesired deviations to some discrete agency external to
this self, whether a personal or technological conspiracy or a cannibalistic

spirit:[18] recalling what Hofstadter has recently called America's 'paranoid political style'.[19] Sexual impulses are particularly likely to be seen as external to the self. Biographies of the Christian Right's apocalyptics indicate that they reattribute everyday agency from their traumatized self to an Antichrist who manifests himself through human malevolence or liberal government policies, final restitution being deferred to the 'end time'.[20]

Access to an experience we might gloss as a severe diminution or even a dissolution of everyday agency has appeared in rather different cultural and political contexts, available to certain individuals through alterations in their brain physiology (naturalistically)[21] and through their enacted situation (personalistically); and this can be occasioned by experienced conflicts and sickness understood through conventional bodily techniques and notions of the self – 'this isn't happening to me, this is happening to someone else'[22] – and by its immediate consequences (recognition by the individual and others, expert encouragement and legitimation).

Despite continued subjective dissociations, the everyday locus of experience and action is a generally unitary and internally consistent individual, bounded, autonomous and fairly undifferentiated, coextensive with a physical body and with that body's history: whether we assume that such unity is given in our body's neural make-up, or else that the idiom of a single rather than a multiplex self has proved rather more successful in our biological and cultural history. Such a unitary individual may recognize himself or herself as losing will, coherence and responsibility, whether in emergencies or at times of radical social change, through diseases of the brain, or in situations standardized as illness, dance, violence and sorcery, or as ecstasy, glossolalia, spirit mediumship, hypnosis, hysteria and multiple personality: occasions when our local representations of a self may provide operational models for multiplicity through mind/body distinctions, psychological faculties or energies, consciousness of physical illness, through humours, emotions, addictions, winds and faces, evolutionary and topographical levels, dream selves, multiple souls, spirit familiars, powers, hidden doubles, guardian angels, many-personed and consubstantial deities, mythical transformations, the identity or otherwise of twins and other products of unnatural fecundity,[23] the differentiation of kin, through onomastics and the avoidance of homonyms, in personifications of the foetus, the dead and the dreamer,[24] through metempsychosis, the sub-personalities of West African psychologies (p. 163) and the human potential movement, and the cyborgs and extraterrestrials of the computer technovisionaries. The loss of volition and control may be recognized as temporary or permanent, as partial or total (the Christian exorcist's distinction between *obsessio* and *possessio*), as a conflict or as a penetration, as loss, rape or theft (*latah, zombi, susto*); or we may recognize our moral agency in the intruding other, simultaneously or serially, whether aware of seeking such an identification or just finding it happen – as 'voluntary' or 'involuntary' possession.[25] (As in those not uncommon situations in which we reflect on some past act and wonder if it really was this same 'I' that performed it.[26]) Context, expectation, access to a particular schema, and the example and response of others organize a variety of standardized narratives, tentative essays, partial stages, elisions and the like, which in turn demonstrate the experiential reality of our local cosmology. Social location facilitates access to particular patterns; thus I would propose that dissociative fugues, like shamanic or cyberspace vision quests, masking and 'central possession cults', are just more available to men, consistent with male access to a more extensive geographical and social space with anticipated movement into a new social persona; in the same societies, 'static' dissociations, involuntary and 'peripheral' possession, latah, hysteria and multiple personality follow from women's restricted mobility or from their experience of pregnancy and something like a sick role.[27]

To take these patterns simply as motivated strategies which the participants themselves prefer to recognize as involuntary[28] assumes that the very articulation of the two modes is voluntary. The recently fashionable personalism of aesthetics, role-play and performance in anthropological theory, however, recapitulates the public assumptions through which eating disorders or MPD now emerge: the particularly Western idea of an achieving self.[29] Reading them, however, in the earlier 'bottom-up' way still favoured by psychologists and physiologists – and participants – leaves us with the contrary problem: that our loss of volition is necessarily non-volitional. The naturalistic idiom is limiting, not just because this is the immediate biomedical context which legitimates these patterns in Western societies but because of the difficulty in making here the customary distinction between aetiology, pathology, symptoms and treatment.[30] (Thus our current emphasis on the contractual rights of the child, proposed as the solution to child sexual abuse, reiterates its perceived causes – the loss of 'natural' paternal responsibility, and the implicit sexualization of an autonomous child with the bodily rights of an adult.)

Let me return to an earlier question. Why women? At a high level of generality, the pattern identified by doctors as the significant pathology may be interpreted as a reconfiguring of the position already ascribed to subdominant individuals;[31] if the female is weaker, sickly and fearful, vulnerable to demons, controlled by others or lacking in moral will, enacting rather than transforming, carrying another being within her, with relatively free access to her body by others, then her 'illness' will become an affirmation of these very characteristics. And MPD is perhaps the extreme variant of those other patterns by which women can negotiate through the characteristics ascribed to them by men; for to be ill is to identify with an image of ourself as being open and vulnerable.[32] In the nineteenth century the neurologist Benedikt wondered if women were more prone to hysteria because they had more to hide;[33] and in the sense that women's 'muted voice', to use the Ardeners' terminology,[34] argues for a double-voiced tradition, simultaneously inside and against the public way of seeing things, double consciousness seems an apt representation (and practical deployment) of their situation. Like the intruding spirit, a disease is something which limits our moral agency; and shared recognition of an external cause, whether spirit or disease, compels others to legitimation and restitution. It is in the inescapable slippage between naturalistic and personalistic that MPD and the other reactions emerge. Sexual abuse, like a disease, is something that seems to happen to us, against volition; the recognition of the violation of female children, the realization that nothing can ever be enough to recompense that child, powerfully compels public acceptance of the reality of the abuse and of its consequences.

Critics of the multiple movement have likened it to the late medieval European witch-hunts, and it will be evident that in this chapter I have recommended analogies between MPD and certain Africanist categorizations of spirit possession and witchcraft: peripheral possession, introspective witchcraft, the direction of accusation, witch-finding, strategic advantage and so on. Without pushing the parallel too far, I find Ioan Lewis' scheme for the relations between possession and witchcraft a potential map.[35] Nineteenth-century double consciousness recalls involuntary trance possession with its emphasis on only partial displacement of the victim's identity, with restitution rather than public redress, while with MPD we approach something recalling witchcraft accusation, greater significance now being attached to a reckoning with a human or human-like perpetrator who is to confess before being (perhaps) absolved. Lewis proposes that both patterns may occur in the same society: trance possession attributed to spirits 'expresses insubordination, but not to the point where it is desired to sever the relationship', whereas witchcraft accusations are frequently associated with themes of incest 'representing as they do a much more direct line of attack, express[ing] hostility between equal rivals, or between superior and subordinate ... and often seek to sunder an unbearably tense relationship'. If witchcraft accusations are indeed frequently directed against coevals in situations of publicly expected amity (but actual animosity, competition and incipient rupturing of domestic obligations or co-residence), then the directions of accusation in MPD – typically daughter to father, or vulnerable young woman to powerful male – suggest increasingly uncertain markings of power and sexuality between childhood and adulthood, female and male.[36] The not uncommon characterization of the jealous refusal of the American mother to protect her abused daughter as a theft of that daughter's identity[37] recalls the 'involuntary' malevolence of the cannibalistic witch mother to her daughter in which she devours the vital essence of her own child.

If illnesses are to be taken as mirrors of their age, then MPD seems to acknowledge the loss of once accepted gender complementarity in a rawer manifestation of male domination, opening up our society's terrible secrets,[38] yet it challenges this through an ambivalent assertion of the rights of the young female to her body. If the spirits of vodu and *sar* present standardized historical memories,[39] and the secondary personalities of the nineteenth-century hysterics were taken by their psychiatrists for factitious neurological signs, for unacceptable sexual desire or for an earlier level of evolutionary development,[40] then the fragmented alters of the current epidemic offer us an unstable multiplicity of now doubtfully welcome children, incorporated aliens, fantasized selves and wounded healers.[41]

Like the other patterns, multiple personality disorder is simultaneously a psychophysiological state, an identity, a medical technology, a disease, a theory of the mind, an allegory of late capitalism and an expressive aesthetic. It is also a political drama. As with certain other illnesses in Western societies, women who demonstrate MPD have now joined together in 'survivors' groups' which play down the idea of 'treatment', sororities through which the symptom is accommodated as a testimony to oppression, but at the cost of continuing propriation.[42] After 1948, opium addiction in China was reframed from an individual psychopathology into a testimony of a colonial domination dating from the Opium Wars, and contemporary feminist therapists have similarly reinscribed a number of women's pathologies as an ambivalent resistance to male power.[43] As in the non-Western analogues (anthropology's cults of affliction) – such as the sar cults of Somalia and Ethiopia or the hernia chiefships of Zaire – sufferers in Alcoholics Anonymous, Agoraphobics Anonymous or Speaking for Our Selves come together to affirm their illness, to strike a contract with it and dedicate themselves to its power, often to gain a sense of heightened control. Not so much a restitution as an accommodation, through which the sodality can then take on less evidently 'therapeutic' roles, in which affected individuals market their experience as emblematic, their suffering as achievement, their recovery as expert knowledge.[44]

The weapons of the weak, to use Victor Turner's well-known expression, not only compel the dominant to restitutive action but may – strategically or otherwise – provide a new identity and material resources for the protagonists, and thence for others. Nineteenth-century women reworked the existing relationship between medical hypnotist and suggestible female, to affirm their weakness as a privileged access to higher knowledge, the medium establishing for herself a professional career which claimed wider solutions to the problems of others,[45] and for the social reformers of the period offering a demystified and natural religion. As contemporary multiples affirm the legitimacy of their several personalities, they too have aligned themselves with contemporary movements for 'the politics of identity' and for women's ownership of their bodies, the stigmata of rape becoming the means of transcending their origin, the ascribed now translated into the achieved, the pathological body becoming a marketable realm of political authenticity.

Notes

Chapter 1

1　Bourdieu 1977: 96.
2　Cited in Fumaroli 1996. Irresolute, humourless, meddling.
3　Cheyne 1734.
4　Brigham 1832.
5　Boudin 1857; Buckle 1856.
6　Stocking 1987.
7　Collingwood 1945; Thomas 1984.
8　M. and J. Bloch 1980.
9　Michaelis 1814.
10　Haraway 1989: 13.
11　Cited by Easlea 1980: 247.
12　John XXI 1550.
13　Stocking 1987: 3.
14　Madden 1857.
15　*Ibid.*; Morel 1860; Bartholomew 1990.
16　Classically argued for psychiatry by Kurt Schneider (1959).
17　E.g. Gaskell 1860.
18　E.g. Beard 1881.
19　Ganser 1897.
20　Birnbaum 1923.
21　For example Birnbaum 1923, Schneider 1959. But on the way apparently reversing Kant's characterization of *form* as subjective ordering, *content* as the physical material: a distinction that goes back to Aristotle's distinction between form and matter in his *Metaphysics*. Without examining the nineteenth-century German philosophical and psychiatric arguments in detail it is not too clear how this happened but, if we assume close links between the two disciplines as Jaspers (1923) assumes, I would suggest something like this: (i) Kant had argued against the British sensationalists in his *Critique of Pure Reason* that perception must involve our subjective ordering of the external natural world to produce the world as our mind can grasp it (that is, as 'phenomenon'). That aspect of our phenomenal world which seemed most evidently subjectively ordered (as opposed to that more evidently produced through immediate sensation of the world but which our minds still ordered) Kant termed 'form'. (ii) German phenomenological studies of psychopathology then became restricted through immediate neuropsychiatric interests to the categorization of the more unusual subjective orderings which were

characteristic of the insane (rather than in the total lived subjectivity of any individual in the world); this 'form' became objectified nosologically as various discrete experiences – the 'phenomena' to be examined in psychiatric inquiry (presumably because hallucinations and delusions had no external reference in the consensual world). (iii) By the late nineteenth century, neuropsychiatry began to divide up between the neurologists who emphasized observable anatomical structure and the psychiatrists who were stuck with insanity where there were no observable one-to-one correspondences between lesion and illness but only altered functioning and experience. (As a residual medical area, psychiatry remains happier talking of 'mental illness' than 'mental disease'.) The more evidently subjective process of generating radically new 'form' (for there was nothing out there which the insane mind ordered except in the case of illusions) became elided with its scientifically more promising (if, for the psychiatrists, only presumed) structuring – altered biology; while that remaining external sensory evidence, which was consensually given and which the mind, insane or otherwise, ordered, became clinically residual as simply shared 'content'. By contrast, the generally more radical French 'science de l'homme', as described by Williams (1994), placed greater emphasis on the environmental and social causation of psychopathology; even if (through Broca's biologization of culture) French psychiatry yielded not dissimilar racist theories by the end of the nineteenth century. It would not be inappropriate to see the French 'tradition as having contributed most evidently to theories of neurosis in the dominant Anglo-American psychiatry of the 1970s–1990s, German medicine as providing the clinical schemata for psychosis. In all three, however, there is repeated oscillation between (and conflation of) what may be distinguished as the naturalistic and the personalistic (Littlewood 1993b).

22 Yap 1974; Lewontin, Rose and Kamin 1984; Good and Good 1981.
23 Littlewood 1994.
24 Jaspers 1923.
25 Weinstein 1962.
26 Littlewood 1993a.
27 Oxley 1849.
28 Kraepelin 1904.
29 Bleuler 1911.
30 Kraepelin 1904. Young (1991, 1993a: 4) has suggested that this model recalls nineteenth-century Positivism in which the chemical determines the biological, the biological the social. The direction of practical diagnosis reverses that of natural causation. While it may appear as excessively concrete – and, when pressed, academic social psychiatrists agree that psychiatric illnesses are not natural entities but rather observed concurrences (e.g. Wing 1978) – something very like this, I would argue, is the clinical psychiatrist's naïve realism (to use our customary term for the epistemology of practising scientists).
31 Birnbaum 1923.
32 Wittgenstein 1958; Geertz 1984.
33 Psychiatric diagnostic categories are ideally monothetic – that is, they have

robust core symptoms which specify that diagnosis and no other. Yet it is perhaps only for schizophrenia that psychiatrists can agree on any defining symptoms which are not found in other illnesses: the 'first-rank' symptoms described by the younger Schneider. Yet these are found in only a half of identified schizophrenic patients in Britain and can be 'overridden' by evidence of organic brain disease (which then becomes the diagnosis). The form/content (pathogenic/pathoplastic) model in comparative psychiatry, like its associated 'category fallacy' in cross-cultural studies (Kleinman 1987) which presumes the European core symptoms everywhere, does seem to produce useful conclusions where there is evidence of invariant biological change which may be said to 'determine' behaviour and experience in a unique way such that they do not seem to occur without it. Examples would be delirium tremens and possibly Gilles de la Tourette's syndrome (although behaviours recalling Tourette's are found with other types of brain lesions and with severe anxiety, and with the experimentally induced hyperstartle response and in such social institutions as latah which encourages hyperstartling). The World Health Organization's International Pilot Study of Schizophrenia (IPSS) produced evidence in the 1970s that a similar core schizophrenic pattern (following Schneider's defining criteria) can be identified in widely differing societies. What it did not show was the extent of the cultural contribution to the illness, supposedly one of the intentions of the study; as Kleinman (1987) has observed, emphasis on the core group, which was shown to have comparable rates across cultures, ignored the cases at the edges where there was a much greater difference in rates such as a three-fold difference between Denmark and India for a 'broad' definition of schizophrenia similar to that actually used in British psychiatric practice. The core symptoms of schizophrenia thus appeared in the IPSS to be a *manifestation* of an underlying disease process; taking a wider category of schizophrenia suggests alternatively that schizophrenic symptoms might also be understood as a *response* to a variety of insults, whether neurological or social. Examining stable societies rather than groups of refugees or communities in the midst of civil upheavals will emphasize intrapersonal biological differences in the aetiology of schizophrenia. (Analogous to the finding that, when studying affluent societies, genetic associations appear more salient in looking at differences in people's height, for we have already minimized one environmental source of variation – nutrition.) Nevertheless, the similarity of core symptoms and rates found in the IPSS argues that we are unlikely to be able to explain all instances of schizophrenia by a more cultural and political understanding as was assumed by anthropologists like Gregory Bateson and by the British anti-psychiatrists of the 1960s. Cultural considerations of the IPSS results have been limited to speculating on the prognosis of an illness whose origin is taken as primarily biological: vague generalizations about industrialization (Cooper and Sartorius 1977), or possible correlations with unemployment in capitalist economies (Warner, R. 1985), or differences in relatives' emotional responses to a person with schizophrenia (Leff *et al.* 1987). While the last named suggests that the response which predicts a poor prognosis in Britain has a similar predictive value when 'translated' to India, this conclusion avoids the problem that one British measure, 'overinvolvement', tended to be generally rated less commonly in the Indian context for all patients (*ibid.*). Nor can we assume that social responses which make for a poor prognosis within a society are those which necessarily differentiate prognosis between societies.

34 Young 1995.
35 The so-called 'neo-Kraepelinian' (Young 1995) diagnostic systems of the 1980s and 1990s such as DSM-III to DSM-IV, which are a reaction against the earlier classification's hypothetic psychodynamics, maintain a hierarchy of diagnostic significance: passivity experiences are still more important in specifying schizophrenia than depressive experiences.
36 Fisher 1985; McCulloch 1994.
37 Rivers 1924.
38 Seligman 1929.
39 Devereux 1956.
40 Kraepelin 1904.
41 *Ibid.*
42 Kiev 1972.
43 O'Brien 1883.
44 Kiev 1972.
45 Littlewood 1993b.
46 Cited by Yap 1967.
47 Young 1995; Jackson 1884.
48 Kraepelin 1904.
49 All used by Kiev 1972.
50 *Ibid.*
51 Carothers 1953.
52 Vint 1932; Carothers 1954.
53 Field 1960.
54 Littlewood 1994.
55 Shweder 1985.
56 Reasons of space preclude consideration of the special case of psychiatric anti-Semitism which has been recently examined by Lifton, Gilman, Degkwitz, Efron, Gay and McGrath.
57 Yap 1967.
58 E.g. Simons and Hughes 1985.
59 By the 1990s, they were acknowledged in the American Psychiatric Association's fourth *Diagnostic and Statistical Manual* (on whose cultural deliberations see Littlewood 1992b).
60 For the changing application of the term see Ritenbaugh 1982a, Littlewood and Lipsedge 1987, Lee 1996, Littlewood 1996a.
61 Neutra *et al.* 1977; Littlewood 1985.
62 Prince 1960.
63 Littlewood and Lipsedge 1987; Lee 1996.
64 Williams 1958.
65 Carothers 1954.
66 Parker 1960.
67 Seligman 1928.

68   *Ibid.*
69   Janet 1925.
70   Devereux 1970.
71   Ackernecht 1943: 31.
72   Devereux 1956: 24.
73   Sargant 1973.
74   Frank 1961; Kiev 1964.
75   E.g. Doi 1971.
76   Sachs 1937; Devereux 1951; to some extent Laubscher 1937.
77   Laubscher 1937.
78   E.g. Roheim 1950; Devereux 1956.
79   E.g. Benedict 1935; Lambo 1955.
80   Such as Ruth Benedict's (1946) study of the Japanese.
81   Following Malinowski 1927.
82   E.g. Jones 1924.
83   Sachs 1937.
84   Notoriously Jung 1930.
85   With rare exceptions: cf. Mannoni 1950; Fanon 1952; Loudon 1959.
86   Kleinman 1988b.
87   Malhotra and Wig 1975.
88   Sargant 1973.
89   Carr 1978.
90   Littlewood 1993a.
91   See Chapter 2 below.
92   E.g. Doi 1971; Kakar 1978.
93   A partial reaction may be found, however, in the anthropological work of Rodney Needham, Scott Atran, Pascal Boyer, Mark Johnson and C. D. Laughlin who have argued against a purely conventional understanding of shared adult cognitions. The extent to which 'culture' and 'nature' may be said to represent not actually existing entities but rather reified modes of thought (Chapter 10 below) is beyond the scope of a brief historical survey; yet we might wonder if the fashionable demedicalization of disease as a biological reality in favour of a cultural understanding is not perhaps the usual (but now postmodern) privileging of Western 'culture' over 'nature'.
94   Kleinman 1988b.
95   Hughes 1985; Hahn 1985.
96   Littlewood 1993a cf. McCulloch 1994.
97   Laubscher 1937; Tooth 1950; Carothers 1953.
98   Lugard 1929; Ernst 1991.
99   The anthropologist Evans-Pritchard, for example, was commissioned to examine the role of prophets in inciting anti-British resistance among the Nuer of the colonial Sudan; in what became a classic text in anthropology we can note that on a couple of occasions he refers to some of them as 'psychotic' (Evans-Pritchard 1940) but this is nowhere developed as any sort of racial or medical theory. While colonialism took for granted a difference between 'higher' and 'lower' levels of civilization, this was not linked to any neurological topology beyond the isolated speculations of Vint, Carothers

and Tooth. By contrast, in the United States, psychiatry was deployed extensively during the nineteenth and twentieth centuries to justify what we may term the internal colonization of Amerindians and African-Americans (Hailer 1970). In the early stages of imperial expansion, domination is explicitly economic or military, and any necessary justification rests simply on evident technical or administrative superiority, sometimes manifest destiny, security of trade or the historical requirements of civilization; only when dominated peoples 'inside the walls ' threaten to achieve some sort of equality do apologies appear couched as a discourse on primitive pathology or biological inferiority (Littlewood and Lipsedge 1982; and see Chapter 2, p. 27). To an extent we may argue that Europe prepared to abandon her settlements well before equality threatened (except for the significant instances of Kenya, Algeria and the French Caribbean: see Vint 1932, Carothers 1954, Fanon 1952), and before colonial administrations had established much beyond a basic mental hospital for the native criminally insane. (Space prevents consideration here of the special case of South Africa.) In North America, arguments in favour of the emancipation of slaves had appeared by the time of Independence only to be countered by medical justifications for continued servitude which invoked such novel diseases as *drapetomania* (the impulse to escape) (Brigham 1832) or even, as argued by Benjamin Rush (1799), that African ancestry was itself an attenuated disease; justifications which became even more necessary for White supremacy after Emancipation. Among Native Americans, for whom collective political action was impossible after they were dispersed on reservations beyond the boundary of a European state, twentieth-century administrators and medical officers developed increasingly psychological – and thence psychopathological – explanations for their high rates of suicide, alcoholism and general failure to participate in national life: the 'internalisation of the frontier' as Andreas Heinz has put it.

100 Tooth 1950; Carothers 1953.
101 Mannoni 1950.
102 McCulloch 1994.
103 Mars 1946; Fanon 1952. Why the English/French difference? Perhaps because French colonialism tended to a model of cultural and biological assimilation, the English arguing more for cultural segregation (Taguieff 1988; Osborne 1994). French psychiatry was (and is) a much more intellectual profession than its pragmatic British counterpart, and medical students from Martinique or Senegal when studying in Paris were more likely to be exposed to political and philosophical debate than they would have been in a London medical school.
104 Rivers 1924; Malinowski 1927.
105 Goody 1995.
106 Lyons 1992; Price 1913; Culpin 1953; Ernst 1991; Barrell 1991; Littlewood 1992c.
107 Neutra *et al.* 1977.
108 Jarves 1872, cited by Mauss 1926; Eastwell 1982.
109 German 1972; but compare the psychiatrist De Jong 1987 who combines the anthropology of local ritual with conventional medical epidemiology.

110 It may be objected reasonably that the very idea of culture-specific pathology is redundant, not just in the normative assumptions which give rise to the idea of 'pathology' for any domain (whether biological, psychological or social), but as a residue of the colonial reading of local practices as medico-legal problems (*amok*) or as superstition (*dhat*), hysteria (spirit possession) or other neuroses (*piblokto*, *latah*) (Littlewood 1984, 1991): patterns which then were rather optimistically fitted into the nosology of European medicine. For 'We predicate of the thing what lies in the method of representation. Impressed by the possibility of a comparison, we think we are perceiving a state of affairs of the highest generality' (Wittgenstein 1958: para. 105). Two related issues remain in dispute: the distinctiveness which by definition any local syndrome must demonstrate relative to the ease with which it can be placed in a more general category; and whether such a category is to be derived from its symptomatology (the current psychiatric preference), from its biological correlates (Simons and Hughes 1985), or else from some more sociological criterion such as local understanding or political context (Chapter 3, this volume); what actually constitutes culture-binding – whether the 'syndrome' is just the local recognition of a global reality (*amok* properly being the psychotic illness schizophrenia), or an inappropriate demonstration of shared sentiments (the *dhat* syndrome as an excessive male concern with South Asian notions of purity and semen loss), or the adult's representation of traumatic childhood experience (psychoanalytical interpretations of the probably factitious Ojibwa *windigo* – Parker 1960), or the manifestation of collective tensions in certain pivotal individuals (Somali *sar*, Lewis 1969) or the conventional resolution of such identified tensions (*ibid.*), or individual self-mastery against particular constraints (Sudanese *zar*, Boddy 1989). The same pattern may be variously identified as norm, illness, aetiology or treatment, as resistance or performance. Restricting ourselves to the local ethnography may allow us to avoid categorization but hardly facilitates cross-cultural conclusions.

Chapter 2

1 For instance Julian Leff (1990a, 1990b) and Raymond Prince (1991).
2 Littlewood 1980; Chrisman and Maretzki 1982; Mercer 1986; Taussig 1987; Kleinman 1988b. Critical medical anthropology (Scheper-Hughes 1990) perhaps excepted: Gaines (1992: Introduction) argues that the Marxist sympathies of critical anthropology give it a 'positivistic' emphasis on a supposedly 'real' (biological) substratum. I have suggested (1992c) rather that the prescriptive quality of critical medical anthropology lies in its homeopathic replication of its antagonist, American medical evangelism.
3 Which was a legitimate subject for medicalization. For example Cooper 1967, Ingelby 1981. Compare Sedgwick 1982 and the essays in Boyers and Orrill 1972, especially Sedgwick's.
4 Szasz 1961; Goffman 1971.
5 Sontag 1979.
6 Podrabinek 1980; Littlewood and Lipsedge 1982; Deleuze and Guattari 1984; Gilman 1985; Muller-Hill 1988; Littlewood 1993a.
7 The work of Peter Sedgwick (1982) perhaps excepted.

8 The term *functional* usually refers in psychiatry to psychoses without gross structural changes, yet whose patterns of abnormality are presumed to have an eventually demonstrable biological origin (Chapter 1). My use of the term in this book is more conventional, referring to the activity of parts of a delineated pattern or process which is recognized as integral to the coherence of some whole (Radcliffe-Brown 1951; Parsons 1952), such that a part *is* its function. Once dominant in the social sciences, functionalism has been criticized for being trivially true (cross-associations between any social phenomena in a given society may be said to contribute to that society's overall coherence) and for its inability to deal with change over time, with external influences or conflict within the system, or with human intentions; and in that not all identified elements of a society manifest simultaneously in each other and that there may be redundant lacunae (or 'survivals' as they were once called) depending on our level of analysis. Analogous problems arise in evolutionary biology with the idea of *adaptation* (Lewontin 1983), a term also used in psychiatry but to refer to patterns which, while they may well be socially functional, are so named because they primarily maintain the coherence and ideal state of the individual. (The social sciences may term this also as 'functional', here coming close to the psychologist's older notion of 'need': Firth 1957). My concern is not with whether a particular model or frame is essentially true but with whether it is the most useful at any point in the development of a discipline to understand the phenomena of interest. Does the methodological individualism of psychiatric theory inhibit our under-standing of the 'individual'? Does the frame we have chosen (whether disease or function) simply generate results which replicate the experimental design? Ultimately the answer to such questions is aesthetic and pragmatic, not methodological nor given by the data.

9 That there are various biological findings associated with schizophrenia (genetic associations, cerebral ventricular size and so on) is immaterial to whether an idiom of pathology need be applied. Although a Whiggish biological psychiatry would argue that any disease entity obtains its social coherence through recognition of its biological regularities, and that until a biological aetiology is clearly established a disease is often seen in moral terms – as has happened with thyroid disorder, leprosy, syphilis and tuberculosis to take the usually cited instances (Wing 1978; Sontag 1979). Certainly, once a biological causality is established, then any consequent treatment replaces direct moral interpretations by questions of hygiene or access to treatment, and one might presume this is happening with AIDS.

10 Such as Adolf Meyer's early twentieth-century psychobiological schema which is little more than an empirical system of collecting and ordering psychiatric data, and which still provides the rationale behind psychiatry's 'mental state examination'.

11 Métraux (1959) describes spirit possession in Haiti after traffic accidents. Already in 1972 Bastide noted a move away from psychiatric consideration of Afro-American possession states as illnesses to regarding them as therapeutic responses to misfortune including serious psychotic illness.

12 Teoh 1972; Murphy 1973.

13 Murphy 1973; Westermeyer 1973; Carr 1978; Lee 1981. (And similarly perhaps a greater number of Amerindian shamans are now seen as psychotic: Murphy 1973). Tan and Carr (1977) warn that amok in Malaysia is now less a distinct behavioural sequence than a quasi-legal decision for all cases of bizarre violence made particularly by Malay officials. Similarly, Diethelm (1971) describes how *tarantism, fascination* (evil eye) and *lycanthropy* passed from being normative social beliefs in Europe to become first experienced pathologies and then folkloric curiosities.

14 Loudon (1959) criticizes Gluckman's (1954) anthropology of *nomkubulwana* for not deciding whether participants were 'aware' of the symbolism he himself identified: Loudon argues that only if something like his sociological interpretation is articulated by the actors themselves is it valid and thence presumably 'therapeutic'.

15 Littlewood and Lipsedge 1982. Just as Aristotle wriggled out of confronting the injustice of slavery by saying that slaves lack the power of moral reasoning (and are thus things) and as nineteenth-century medical positivism transformed radical politics, prostitution and vagrancy into biological diseases (Gilman 1985; Littlewood 1993a).

16 In the United States (Teish 1985; Adler 1986), North-West Pacific Coast (Jilek 1982) and Hawaii (Shook 1985).

17 Sidel 1973. If the individual addict was exculpated, those who continued to trade in opium were, however, liable to capital punishment.

18 Kleinman 1986.

19 Good and Good 1988. A variant: the massacres in Matabeland by troops of the newly independent Zimbabwean government left a sense of personal pollution in the survivors which had to be eradicated by 'healing' by traditional diviners as well as in the development of new cults (Werbner 1991). 'Healing' itself has a moral connotation in Western monotheisms – frequently identified with conversion and repentance (Littlewood and Dein 1994).

20 Ngui 1969. Shirley Ardener (1975) shows how Nigerian women's immediate response to an insult to their gender by their men – genital display and verbal abuse – was successfully redeployed against the British imperial administration in the Women's War of 1929. Compare the 'reverse' deployment by Indonesian women of *latah* against their own menfolk.

21 Rip 1973; Scheper-Hughes 1979; Swartz 1989; Sachdev 1990; Littlewood 1993a.

22 Deleuze and Guattari 1984; Littlewood 1993a.

23 Fisher 1985; Scheper-Hughes 1979; Littlewood and Lipsedge 1982; Littlewood 1992a; Fanon 1965. Ironically pathology has itself become 'pathologised': the Greek παθos may be glossed as emotion or feeling, often but not always in a context of distress. In the seventeenth century *pathognomic* in English still had this general connotation (as *pathetic* and *empathetic* still do) but *pathological* now referred to (physical) disease. Only in the early nineteenth century did the word *pathology* become one sometimes applied to mental illness (Jeremy Bentham, *cit.* OED).

24 Classically Wootton 1959; and for South Africa, Rip 1973. And ethologists: Konrad Lorenz (1970, *Nobel Symposium 14*, pp. 409, 406) described student

rebellion as 'the hypothalamus [in the "lower" point of the brain] at the helm
... it must be emphasised that this failure to identify with the social norms of
the parental culture is the direct cause of truly pathological phenomena'.

25 Wootton 1959:14.

26 Sontag 1979. 'Social divisions' can be overcome journalistically and politically
speaking by 'healing' or if occasion should warrant by 'radical surgery'.

27 Such as John Wing (1978).

28 Schneider 1959; Wing 1978: 22. And thus we can talk of the 'abuse of
psychiatry'. The sociological critiques in the 1980s led psychiatry to burrow
even further into neurophysiology (as if in a different – but the same –
direction as the absconding deity of the early Scientific Revolution pursued by
physics).

29 Quoted in Rosen 1968.

30 Chapter 1: note 33.

31 Or even as that with which doctors are concerned. See Long 1965, Kendell
1975, Boorse 1975, Sedgwick 1982, Good and Good 1992 for partial reviews.

32 Schizophrenia is still variously but convincingly described as a discrete
biochemical disease with specific genetic causation, as the by-product of the
evolutionary selection of creativity, as the universally recognized category of
madness, as cerebral adaptation to brain damage, as faulty neurocognitive
processing, as the response to faulty parenting or family communication, as
the consequence of birth trauma, maternal influenza, rapid social change,
capitalism, unemployment or racism, and as the social marginalization of
deviance.

33 The emphasis on pain or suffering as the central concern for psychiatry
(showed by both the older comparative psychiatrists (Leff 1990a) and the
'new cross-cultural psychiatrists' (Kleinman 1988a)) assumes the subjective
experience can be allocated to a positive or negative hedonic tone (to use the
psychiatrists' term); yet in Crete, for example, *raimos* connotes intense grief
but also the satisfaction of an overwhelming preoccupation, and *lakhtose* is
both acute anxiety when anticipating an accident but also sexual longing.

34 As Leff (1990a, 1990b) has argued against an earlier presentation of these
arguments. Doubtless a postmodernist would welcome this frank acknowledgement that it is social meaning and action not the natural world that
characterizes psychiatry's subject. And that ultimately it is concerned with
biology because it is concerned with personal experience.

35 At one level we are ourselves historically constituted by 'disease', not only in
that we share certain nucleotide sequences with bacteria, but because
contemporary humans are determined through millennia of epidemics in
which each generation of survivors constitute our ancestors. (Survival is in part
a function of antigenic complementarity, while the correlates of one identified
pathology may of course be the decreased likelihood of another.)

36 Young 1980a, 1980b; Littlewood 1993c; Chapter 3 this volume.

37 E.g. Gaines 1982b.

38 Leff 1990a.

39 Dyschromic spirochaetosis has been one of the standard instances advanced in
favour of cognitive relativism (like the supposedly extensive Inuit lexicon for

'snow'). That a biological reality recognized by Westerners as a disfiguring skin disease is actually taken by an Amazonian society as 'normal' and a prerequisite for marriage has been recently questioned (Gilbert Lewis: personal communication).

40 A poignant instance is Mark Vonnegut's memoir (1976) in which he describes how the hippie commune in which he lived, after debating for some time how to cope with his schizophrenia, eventually took him to the local psychiatric hospital for electroconvulsive therapy.

41 Littlewood 1993b, 1993c.

42 Particularly subdominant groups who perceive themselves through the eyes of the dominant: Morris 1985, Scheper-Hughes 1979, Fisher 1985, Robins 1986, Littlewood 1993b.

43 Lane 1988; Sachs 1989.

44 De Salvo 1989; Caramagno 1992.

45 Ingold 1989. Or in family therapy; my difference with the latter is that it still employs the terms like 'dysfunctional' or 'embedded' in normative senses even when it claims to deal only with illnesses as these are recognized and put forward by the families seeking therapy.

Chapter 3

1 Notably Chesler 1974; Allen 1984.

2 Essentially Usher's (1991) position.

3 Essentially Showalter's (1987a) position. To be fair, both Showalter and Usher take up both positions but the former examines more closely the relationship between diagnosis and historical context. Position A (vulnerability and differential stress) is also that of most medical commentators, B of most feminist sociologists who invoke idioms of 'social construction'.

4 Littlewood and Lipsedge 1982.

5 Nineteenth-century hysteria is perhaps an exception: see Showalter's (1993) critique of recent Lacanian proposals that the Victorian hysteric demonstrated a bodily proto-resistance – self-aware or more usually implicit – to patriarchal logocentrism.

6 As Usher 1991: 10.

7 Baier 1994.

8 Jack 1992; Van der Waals *et al.* 1993.

9 Cooperstock and Sims 1971; Dunbar, Perera and Jenner 1989.

10 Gabe and Williams 1986.

11 Parry *et al.* 1973; Lock 1993: 297.

12 Cooperstock 1971.

13 Stimson 1975.

14 Seidenberg 1974.

15 Prather and Fidell 1975.

16 Paragraph references: Hodes 1990; O'Brien 1986; Kreitman and Schreiber 1979; Jack 1992; Morgan *et al.* 1975; Hawton *et al.* 1982.

17 Paragraph references: Bancroft *et al.* 1979; cf. O'Brien 1986; Kreitman *et al.* 1970; Chiles *et al.* 1985; Hawton *et al.* 1982.

18 Jack and Williams 1994.

19 Ramon *et al.* 1975.
20 Hawton *et al.* 1981.
21 *British Medical Journal* 1971; Shauer 1975.
22 Lewis 1971.
23 Turner 1969, following T. S. Eliot (*The Family Reunion*) and before him Oscar Wilde.
24 Newman 1964; Salisbury 1966, 1967; Koch 1968; Langness 1968; Clarke 1973; Reay 1977.
25 Newman 1964.
26 Clarke 1973: 209.
27 Newman 1964: 3.
28 Eliade 1964.
29 Jones 1971.
30 Firth 1961.
31 *Ibid.* 12.
32 Harris 1957.
33 *Ibid.* 1054, 1060.
34 Lewis 1966, 1971.
35 Lewis 1971: 75, 76.
36 Turner 1969.
37 Harris 1957: 1064.
38 Richards 1982: 169.
39 Harris 1957: 1060.
40 Firth 1961: 15.
41 Ortner 1974; although many 'second-wave' feminists – Cixous, Chodorow, Daly, Dworkin, Irigary and Rich (cf. Kristeva), like earlier psychiatrists, have re-essentialized all women as biologically 'closer to nature': nurturant and emotionally authentic, not driven by the male quest for social power over their fellows (Littlewood 1993b).
42 Hage and Harary 1983.
43 Van Gennep 1960; Peters and Price-Williams 1983; Wilson 1967; Turner 1969.
44 Harris 1957: 1061.
45 Leach 1961: 135–6.
46 Langness 1968: 2762
47 Newman 1964.
48 Scheff 1979.
49 Corin and Bibeau 1980. Note the 'occasionally'.
50 Ogrizek 1982; Boddy 1989.
51 Janzen 1978.
52 Corin 1978; Spring 1978; Janzen 1979; Lee 1981.
53 Leach 1961.
54 Lee 1981.
55 Young 1976.
56 Good and Good 1981.
57 Ginsberg 1971.
58 *Ibid.*, cf. James and Hawton 1985.

59   Classically described by Parsons (1951) as the *sick role*.
60   Young 1976.
61   Ortner 1974.
62   La Fontaine 1981: 347.
63   Lock 1993.
64   Broverman *et al.* 1970.
65   Phillips and Segal 1969; Gove and Tudor 1973; Horwitz 1977.
66   Jordanova 1980.
67   James 1963.
68   'Or, a Staff of Aesculapius Gules within a bordure Sable charged with four Butterflies of the Field ... And the Supporters are on either side a serpent or Langued Gules.'
69   Ingelby 1982. Notably Chesler 1974; Jordanova 1981; Showalter 1987a; Usher 1991.
70   Jordanova 1980.
71   Turner 1984.
72   Hage and Harary 1983: 116.
73   Whether 'the charisma of dominance comes from a particular power – that of ultimately defining the world in which non-dominants live – to reveal it will require more than the examination of crude, arbitrary cruelties or exploitations' (Ardener 1989: 186).
74   Smith-Rosenberg 1972.
75   Freud 1946.
76   Gilman 1892, cited by Usher 1991.
77   Turner 1984.
78   Smith-Rosenberg 1972.
79   Ellenberger 1970.
80   Eisenberg 1977.
81   Chapter 4.
82   Indeed Bryan Turner (1984) has proposed the term 'sacred disease' for those Western patterns of psychological illness which are represented by male control over women and thus representing the essence of social power within the community. (*The Times* 1990; compare suffragettes on hunger strike refusing food.)
83   James and Hawton 1985. We do not know whether female doctors are more likely to sympathize with the overdosing patient than are male doctors. From evidence with other medical conditions (Weissman and Teitelbaum 1985), we might predict they would show more 'understanding'.
84   As Bateson put it, comparing a map to its 'territory' (reality).
85   Geyer and Van der Zouwen 1986.
86   Sakinofsky *et al.* 1990.
87   As argued by Lee and Kleinman (2000) in their account of contemporary Chinese suicide.
88   The rate for death by suicide is 100 times more common in those who have deliberately self-harmed than in the general population (Crawford and Wessely 1998).

Chapter 4

1   Robins *et al.* 1984.
2   Marks 1970.
3   Bell and Newby 1976.
4   De Swaan 1981.
5   Symonds 1971; Al-Issa 1980; Hallam 1984.
6   Goldstein 1973.
7   Goldstein and Chambless 1978.
8   Goldstein 1970.
9   Wolpe 1970; Fodor, I. 1976.
10 Symonds 1971.
11 Hudson 1974.
12 Andrews 1966.
13 Buglass *et al.* 1977.
14 Parsons and Fox 1952; Lazarus 1972.
15 Fry 1962.
16 MacFarlane *et al.* 1954.
17 Ardener 1989.
18 National Organisation for Women 1974.
19 Durkheim 1951.
20 Tilt 1862.
21 McKinlay and Jeffreys 1974; Lock 1993.
22 Townsend and Carbone 1980; Flint 1975; Lock 1993.
23 Maranhao 1986.
24 We have physicians, they have healers. Contrast the titles of two recent influential texts of medical anthropology, Kleinman's pan-cultural *Patients and Healers in the Context of Culture*, and Hahn and Gaines' *Physicians of Western Medicine*.25
     Entralgo 1969. Maranhao (1986) himself relates the therapeutic discourse back to Socratic method. In psychoanalysis this discourse, purged of any technological interruptions, stands as the very process of healing.
26 Littlewood 1984 (following Lévi-Strauss and Needham).
27 Turner 1984; Donzelot 1977.
28 Hillbrand and Pope 1983.
29 Stephen 1987.
30 How 'radical' Mrs Savage was at the time of her suspension remains a matter of debate and some have suggested that her rate of surgical intervention in childbirth was not significantly different from that of male colleagues, and that support for her became increasingly less personal as she evolved into a symbol of opposition to masculine gynaecology.
31 Goody 1982.
32 Gaze 1987.
33 *Ibid.*
34 This is decreasing with the slow untying of biological sex from social roles (Littlewood 1984), although the heterosexual male nurse has to continually justify his sexual interests without compromising his 'feminine' task.
35 *Nursing Times* 1987a. It is illustrated with a handsome muscle-bound male

nurse wielding a threatening syringe, bare-chested beneath his uniform. The male nurse, traditionally at the bottom of the nursing status scale (custodial care), was working-class, while the nineteenth-century nurse was middle-class and thus 'charitable' (at least as an ideal). To an extent this compensated for the men at the bottom of the hierarchy. By contrast women doctors come from a higher class status than most nurses, the London teaching hospital nurses perhaps excepted.

36   Patient: 'Nurse, kiss me goodnight!'
     Nurse: 'Certainly not!'
     Patient: 'Go on, nurse, please, a goodnight kiss!'
     Nurse: 'I'm sorry, no, I shouldn't even be in bed with you.'
     While Kalisch *et al.* (1983) suggest this sexualization of the nurse is a recent phenomenon, a response to the women's movement, nineteenth-century evidence suggests otherwise (Maggs 1983). To argue, as many apologists do, that a non-consummated sexual flirtation with a nurse may be a way for male patients to reduce their distress in the face of life-threatening illness may be true, but this does not explain the social conception of the 'frilly' nurse. In the hospital where I studied it was the orthopaedic ward (where there was little anxiety about serious illness among the men confined to bed) which was characterized by the quantity of sexual badinage. Flirtation as a response to loss of power, yes, but not primarily as a sublimation of terror.

37   Gaze 1987: 27.
     [witness:] 'I don't know what you mean by kinky. I've had a few who liked me to dress up in a maid's uniform or a nurse's uniform . . .'
     Mr Justice Caulfield: 'What? Somebody coughed. I thought she said a matron's uniform.'
     Mr Michael Hill QC, counsel for *The Star*: 'I think she said a French maid's uniform.'
     Mr Justice Caulfield: 'I was a bit surprised at a matron's uniform.' (*The Times* 1987)
     The sexual attributes of the nurse demonstrated in this interchange were the subject of caustic comment in the *Nursing Times* (1987b): 'Clearly Mr. Justice Caulfield sees nothing "kinky" about a prostitute dressing up as a nurse but draws the line at one dressing up as a matron.'

38   Hutt 1985.
39   Simnet 1986.
40   Cassell 1987.
41   Similarly, the attempt to ground an alternative to the physician's diagnosis in such categorizations as 'the nursing process'. Recent attempts to provide entry into the profession through a preliminary period of university study are bedevilled by what, apart from biomedical sciences, this might include. Can the professionalization of the nurse be achieved without loss of the 'nurturant' role? What academic discipline could be central? A promising candidate has been social anthropology which might be felt to offer a rigorous approach to 'healing' and 'care', one grounded in 'holistic' assumptions of 'wellbeing' with a notion of 'positive health' beyond that of the absence of disease. Chrisman (1982) emphasizes that the notion of 'care' is fruitfully open to articulate lay

notions of sickness and patterns of health-seeking behaviours.

42 Armstrong 1987.

43 Henderson 1978.

44 For instance, the interviews in *The Midwives' Dilemma, Sunday Times* magazine, 23 August 1987, in which the radical midwife and the unique male midwife share a similar political perspective.

45 Cassell 1986.

46 And earlier. For a brief review of fictional representations see Maggs (1983, 172–95): 'The nurse as sexual vampire' exploited the patient in the pre-Nightingale period and then turned her attentions to the young doctor to divert him from his work for 'sex and professional incompetence are not too far apart' (p. 178). But see text below.

47 Cassell 1987.

48 Although the GMC has recently become more lenient in cases of 'love affairs' between general practitioners and their patients. In the past, it was a 'striking-off offence' incompatible with the practice of medicine. As in other areas of Western life, there has been some loosening of physical sex from gender-specific social roles.

49 For instance, *Danish Dentist on the Job*.

50 E.g. Carpenter 1978; Maggs 1983. Following the now extensive literature on the history of hysteria in the nineteenth century, I have argued elsewhere that Freud's theory was a psychological presentation of what was really a sociological relationship of power. The popular perception of resistance to psychoanalysis as due to its sexualization of the doctor–patient couple (e.g. John Huston's 1962 film *Freud*) is itself a 'resistance' to the tacit recognition of the power embedded in that relationship.

51 *Ibid.*

52 A survey of junior hospital doctors showed that a fifth had recourse to drinking bouts or drugs (Firth-Cozens 1987).

53 Parodied by medical students as:
    Q: How many legs has a cow?
    A1: Three (diagnosis – Ganser's syndrome)
    A2: I'm a cow (depression)
    A3: You're a cow (paranoia)
    A4: Four milk bottles (schizophrenia)

54 The British physician appears to lack the rich lexicon available for such patients in America – 'albatross', 'goner', 'turkey', 'crock' and 'troll' (Stein 1986). Helman (1985) introduced the useful notion of *pseudo-disease* to characterize patterns of sickness resembling recognized syndromes but which are not characterized by a discrete and invariate pattern of pathophysiological evidence (clinical signs, laboratory investigations). As he shows, pseudo-disease is a function of culture, personality, current life events and lay explanatory models, with the whole pattern being then developed through biomedical context. 'Factitious illnesses' is not quite the same for it includes 'real' pathophysiologies ('diseases') which have been induced by the patient, to an extent shading into 'deliberate self-harm' – mutilations and overdoses. Helman's pseudo-diseases include the iatrogenic development of syndromes

through the medical context: a category which most doctors ignore.
55 *Hospital Doctor*, 7 November 1991: 48.
56 Aber and Higgins 1982.
57 An individual illness is multi-referential, polysemous. I am offering here a simplified account, without details of the psychodynamics of the sessions or of the personal significance of the particular practice she adopted. An external description of this sort does not, of course, do justice to her own feelings and experiences in the face of suffering and death (Davidson and Jackson 1985). 'To determine the extent to which the reactions are conscious: pragmatic attempts at adjustment are difficult: whilst to the theorist there is an element of parody in all of them, the irony is only rarely perceived by principal and audience. Participants certainly experience despair and self-hatred' (Littlewood and Lipsedge 1987). Nor should this account be taken as an instance of the superior benefits of psychiatry compared with general medicine: to an extent I was part of the same institutional context, articulating the same set of symbolic power values. The justification of an anthropologically informed psychiatry is only that of empowering the individual through constructing with them some more sociologically grounded interpretations of the origins and meanings of their illness and coping strategies. It might be reasonably objected that my use of the term 'ritual' is rather loose, indeed pejorative in the popular sense. Nevertheless, I would maintain that we are dealing here with a situation in which 'inequalities in status are stressed, dramatically displaced and underwritten by graded mystical powers' (Herdt 1982) if *disease* functions as an ultrahuman 'mystical' sanction (Chapter 3). Rituals subsume individuals under specific roles which embody their ideological status, and within which there is room for individual interpretations and personal meanings.
58 Curiously recalling the medieval mystic Benedetta Carlini who surreptitiously took blood from herself to smear on her hands, to be recognized as the stigmata of Christ's passion (Brown 1986).
59 Sneddon 1983.
60 Also known as Doctor Shopping or Maternal Hospital Addiction (Meadows 1984). (It is sometimes called Polle Syndrome, after the daughter apparently born to the real Baron Von Munchausen (fictionalized in Raspe's tales) when aged 74 and his 17-year-old wife Bernhardine Von Brumi: her existence has been doubted.) Meadows, who first described it in 1977, has recently pointed out that the publicity itself has led to a number of cases of 'factitious M.S.P.' in which he was telephoned by parents who claimed (falsely) to have it.
61 Meadows 1984.
62 *Ibid.*
63 See note 20, Chapter 10.
64 *The Times*, 15 May 1993.
65 Showalter 1998.
66 *Ibid.*
67 Kilshaw 2000.
68 Norman 1993.
69 Kilshaw 2000.
70 McEvedy and Beard 1970.

71 *British Medical Journal* 1970. I have not separately referenced the quotes. The debate has not ended – a more recent book (Ramsay 1986) restates the viral hypothesis but agrees there may have been some 'hysterical overlay'.

72 An ironic comment, given that the diagnosis advanced by Ramsay of post-viral fatigue is the one described in the *Sunday Express* (Markham-Smith 1987) in its article 'Career women struck down by Yuppie plague'. Irving Salt, the professor of medicine interviewed by the paper, pointed out that it only affected professional women in their 'desire to drive to succeed in their professional careers ... This weakens their immune systems.' The social history of 'post-viral fatigue' remains to be written.

73 Ramsay 1986.

74 Ellenberger 1970; Chodoff and Lyons 1955.

75 Bartholomew 1990; Wessely (1987) provides a useful review.

76 Chodoff and Lyons 1955; Chapter 9.

77 A more appropriate term for this type of mass hysteria is Kleinman's 'acute somatization': social context or stress cause autonomic over-arousal leading to physiological symptoms – sweating, trembling, etc. – which, aided by context (including medical interventions) are systematically focused on and amplified by the individual who minimizes and thereby damps down their affective and cognitive concomitants (Kleinman 1986: 61).

78 *The Times*, 20 December 1990.

79 *Sunday Express*, 22 March 1987: 'Career women struck down by Yuppie plague'.

80 National Task Force 1994; Ciba Symposium 1993.

81 National Task Force 1994: 113.

82 *The Times*, 8 May 1993; *The Times* 5, 6 April 1982; *The Times* 23 March 1990.

83 *Straits Times*, 13 November 1983.

84 Philen *et al.* 1989. Similar concerns in the 1970s in the United States after an epidemic of 'Lyme Disease', in which an environmental cause (ticks) was implicated, led to public calls to defoliate American suburbs and provision of presymptomatic antibiotic prophylaxis (Aronowitz 1998).

85 Gruenberg 1957.

86 Rosen 1968: 204–8.

87 Showalter 1998.

88 A situation recalling that of contemporary Chinese. During and after the Cultural Revolution, when depression and psychological distress were regarded as feudal relics, they have had recourse to the highly somatic idiom of 'neurasthenia' to express and communicate distress (Kleinman 1986).

89 Now actually codified in new government guidelines for assessing 'quality control' in the economies of hospital service provision. One might speculate that the pattern was pioneered by Florence Nightingale herself: 'If, in her condition of bodily collapse, she were to accomplish what she was determined that she could accomplish, the attentions and the services of others would be absolutely indispensable' (Strachey 1918: 152). As Arthur Kleinman has put it, Nightingale's illness 'gave her the sentimental authority of wheelchair and sickbed whilst she negotiated reform' (1986: 150).

90 Allison and Roberts 1998.

 91 Richards 1982: 164–5.
 92 Crapanzano 1973.
 93 Littlewood 1984.
 94 Apter 1982.
 95 Chesler 1974.
 96 Devereux 1970.
 97 Symonds 1971.
 98 Firth 1961: 15.
 99 Lewis 1971; Janzen 1979.
100 Turner 1969.

Chapter 5

 1 Good and Good 1992: 257.
 2 The physician George Beard (1881, page vi, Beard's emphasis). Beard argued such mental debility was the consequence of contemporary urban life; contrariwise, the French psychologist Théodule Ribot argued rather that his universal Law of Least Effort explained how modernity followed from the psychology of technological efficiency and tolerance.
 3 Lock 1992; Showalter 1993.
 4 Kenny 1986: 180. Neither are medical historians immune as Micale (1995) notes.
 5 H. Geertz 1968: as a symbolic resistance to hierarchy by marginal individuals, particularly those who were the servants of Europeans.
 6 Simons 1980.
 7 Kenny 1983. Winzeler (1995) provides a recent review of the latah debate, noting how the pattern was subsumed into the nineteenth-century category of hysteria as an instance of narrowed consciousness and failure of will.
 8 (As Umberto Eco has recently termed exegetical overkill.) Simons 1983b,c.
 9 Littlewood 1993b. As Kenny (1983) puts it, 'Perhaps there is no problem here at all, and latah in its cross-cultural distribution no more of a paradox than is the fact that all people have hands, but only some cultures have exploited the fact in requiring them to be shaken in formal greeting. If that is the case, then the latah performance is taken out of the province of biomedical reductionism and is seen in what I take to be its true light – as theatre.' In the case of, say, eating disorders or multiple personality, are there 'fracture lines' given in advance by physiology, or are we talking, as Kenny (1986) does, of intentional 'parodies' of everyday social roles? Can we distinguish the two?
10 Paragraph references: Littlewood 1991; Simons and Hughes 1985.
11 As Lloyd (1990) argues more generally in relation to the idea of mentalities. The psychiatric and anthropological debate has its counterpart in recent critiques of Foucauldian discourse analysis in other human sciences: is a dominant discourse necessarily independent of individual agency, continually engendered in linguistic practices as an inescapable mode of thinking and talking?
12 To something closer to Durkheim's (1901) social currents, or to Moscovici's (1976) social representations, Foucault's (1973) micropractices, Sperber's (1985) epidemiological representations, or even Dawkin's (1982) memes.

13   Lock 1992.
14   *Asahi Evening News*, 1984, cited by Lock 1992: 99.
15   Cited by Lock 1992: 105.
16   Following Mary Douglas' Durkheimian argument that the body often reflects the wider society in its boundaries, entrances and exits, we can argue the family as another common image of the collectivity. It is not just that the integrity of the family is invoked as the place where a society's own integrity is engendered and maintained, but that the health of the unit stands for the health of the whole. We might wonder if the integrity of the nuclear family is an especially apt representation of the modern nation state.
17   Prince 1983, 1985.
18   E.g. Russell 1990.
19   There are continuing debates as to how 'autonomous' the illness becomes from initial social constraints and personal volition (as a consequence of starvation and damage to the hypothalamus).
20   Bemporad *et al.* 1988; Brumberg 1988; Di Nicola 1990; Russell 1990; Garner *et al.* 1990; Ritenbaugh and Shisslak 1994. The medical debates as to whether anorexia and bulimia should be properly understood as two separate illness, or as one, is irrelevant to my argument.
21   Paragraph references: Caskey 1986; Garner and Garfinkel 1980, 1990; Ritenbaugh 1982a; Feldman *et al.* 1988; Salmons *et al.* 1988; Patton *et al.* 1990; Wardle and Marshland 1990.
22   Ritenbaugh 1982b; through television and radio programmes, newspaper and magazine articles, advertisements, slimming contests and less directly through norms of beauty in fashion articles and a general preference for slimmer girls in illustrations and interviews.
23   Nylander 1971. Grimm (1997) argues that Christianity's emphasis on renunciation of the external world laid the grounds for the thin body as the ideal.
24   Stuart and Jacobson 1979.
25   Garner and Garfinkel 1980. Other estimates of its frequency in particular groups of dancers have been much higher. (The acceptable public term for a prostitute – the woman who most obviously separates accessible – but passive – sexuality from active childbearing – is *model*.)
26   Ritenbaugh 1982a.
27   Brumberg 1988.
28   Elder 1969; *Daily Telegraph* 1984.
29   Millman 1980; Maddox *et al.* 1968. Because members of immigrant minorities or established minorities are less likely to recognize that slimness equals success or because they see this route to achievement as blocked because of racism and thus do not commit their bodies to the market.
30   *Daily Mail.* (Around 1986, I have mislaid the exact reference.) She had other characteristics of the Butterfly (Chapter 3, this volume) – having been a sort of nurse, and according to her biographer being driven to attempt suicide by the demands of her husband's family.
31   Shorter 1983.
32   Garner and Garfinkel 1980.
33   Millman 1980; Cranshaw 1983. There are periodic attempts, generally

unsuccessful, to sexualize the pregnant woman as in the *Vogue* cover photograph in 1992 of a model familiar to the usual readers but now naked and in the last trimester of pregnancy.

34   Polhemus 1978; Furnham and Alibhai 1983; Brown and Konner 1981; Lee *et al.* 1992; Klein 1997.

35   MacCrae 1975.

36   Polhemus 1978; Caskey 1986. And of prestige and differential power; being able to stop eating because one does not wish any more, rather than because the food has run out, is historically and cross-culturally an unusual choice.

37   Prince 1985. Yet industrializing countries such as Argentina, where eating disorders are known as 'fashion girl syndrome', may have particularly high levels – reported as 10 per cent of the adolescent female population (Faiola 1997). For reviews, see Di Nicola 1990, Dolan 1991, Dolan and Ford 1991, Davis and Yager 1992, Ritenbaugh and Shisslak 1994. 'Frequency' may be a function of the availability of hospital admission and clinical interests; and the cross-cultural validity of some of the measures used has been questioned: King and Bhugra 1989, Banks 1992, Ritenbaugh and Shisslak 1994.

38   Bell 1985; Bynum 1987.

39   Brumberg 1988; Bynum 1988.

40   *Working Woman*, London, December 1984. The magazine has since folded.

41   Crisp 1980; Chernin 1985.

42   Boskind-Lodahl 1976.

43   There are some suggestions that anorexic girls are more likely to have been subject to paternal incest. Warner (1983: Chapter 7) suggests that 'androgyneity' may serve as an avoidance of incest with the father (as well as offering a challenge to men).

44   Minuchin *et al.* 1975.

45   Crisp 1980.

46   Ritenbaugh 1982a. Albeit in the restricted sense of a locally recognized category (p. 413).

47   Ritenbaugh 1982b.

48   Millman 1980.

49   Orbach 1978, 1986 but see Mabel-Lois' (1974) engaging paper 'Fat dykes don't make it', *Lesbian Tide*, October, 11–12.

50   Millman 1980.

51   *Ibid.*

52   At both extremes of weight, endocrine changes result in a cessation of menstrual periods and the development of facial hair, recalling St Uncumber, the Christian heroine who to avoid an unwelcome marriage grew a beard (Warner, M. 1985).

53   Millman 1980. And for Black women in the West, hair-straightening tongs and various caustic lotions to lighten the skin; and in non-industrial societies at various times clitoridectomy, foot-binding, ear and neck lengthening, scarification and forced feeding – the list is endless.

54   If nineteenth-century hysteria was concerned with the straightforward suppression of female desire, then anorexia nervosa is concerned with its 'manufacture, extension and detail' (Turner 1984).

55 Berger 1971: 47.
56 Rampling 1985; Gremillion 1992.
57 And indeed lay understanding (Furnham and Hume-Wright 1992).
58 Swartz 1987.
59 Gremillion 1992.
60 Banks 1992.
61 As argued, for instance, by Caskey 1986.
62 *Ibid.*; Gremillion 1992.
63 And thus with Lévi-Strauss' 'complex' forms of marriage where kinship terminology centres on an individual's personal position.
64 An equation of geographical state with language and ethnic identity or 'industrialisation' or Westernization (Deutsch 1991).
65 Hall and Jarvie 1992. Our very distinction between these three domains is an attribute of modernity.
66 A shift from what Gaines (1982b) (following Crapanzano) calls indexical personhood (individual choices are a measure of others' interests) to referential personhood (in which the individual takes himself or herself as the measure).
67 Hall and Jarvie 1992, cf. Parkin 1993. And the determining institution in modernization has variously been taken as urbanization, industrialization or 'cultural'.
68 And statuses. Japan and the Western Pacific Rim arguably an exception; perhaps also Islamic countries as a whole, although here this may be said to go against the preconditions for industrialization – Kennedy 1993, cf. Gellner 1992.
69 This cannot, of course, ensure an exact equivalence of meaning and action in each, for the individual in transition is in some sense not fully 'in' either, and perhaps ascribes new and third meanings; but we can at least come somewhat closer to examining how pattern and context hang together.
70 Not that the measure of excessive fatness is calibrated differently; the debate is not simply circular (every society has its ideal weight) for we can distinguish average from ideal in different groups.
71 Maddox *et al.* 1968; Huenemann *et al.* 1966; Gray *et al.* 1987.
72 Morris and Windsor 1985; Pumariega 1986; Furnham and Alibhai 1983. Davis and Yager (1992) provide a useful review, but too late for some of the more recent British material gathered since the mid-1980s.
73 Using factor analysis of data obtained from interviewing possible 'cases' in Lahore (Mumford *et al.* 1992) and Cairo (Nasser 1993). Cf. other studies in Mirpur (Choudry and Mumford 1992) and North India (King and Bhugra 1989). It does not necessarily follow from the elicitation of similar factors that we are dealing with a single 'disease'.
74 Lee *et al.* 1992. Ritenbaugh and Shisslak 1994 argue that 'fear of fatness' – necessary for an American (DSM-III-R) diagnosis of anorexia, and as a 'persistent overconcern' for bulimia – be dropped from the revised diagnostic manual (DSM-IV).
75 Di Nicola 1990.
76 Mumford *et al.* 1992. They leave open the question of whether a concern with

dieting in Lahore, their area of study, has developed independently of the West; perhaps significantly, the average body mass index of their urban subjects was similar to that of Pakistanis in Britain.

77 Nasser (1986) using the Eating Attitudes Test; Dolan *et al.* 1990; Mumford and Whitehouse 1988.

78 The EAT and the Body Shape Questionnaire, Mumford *et al.* 1991; cf. Arya 1992. Other psychiatric studies have argued that 'culture-change' causes psychiatric illness in Asian Britons. Although immigrants from the Indian subcontinent have been said to have fewer neurotic symptoms than the native English, it is unmarried and upwardly mobile Indian women who are 'less well adjusted' (see Littlewood and Lipsedge 1982 for a review); being successful and hence autonomous in something approximating to a male Western norm may have led to considerable identity conflict for these women. Merrill and Owens (1988) have found that drug overdoses are more frequent among women of Asian ethnicity in Britain than among Whites (but less common for Asian men compared with White men) and identify 'culture conflict' six times more commonly in these women than in the men. Raleigh and Balarajan (1992) argue similarly for the increased suicide rates in Asian migrants to Britain. Just as feminist critiques of psychiatry have emphasized that eating disorders are less of a symptom than a struggle, so critiques of cultural psychiatry in Britain have argued against a simple pathologization of migrant family experience as the consequence of 'culture conflict' (Littlewood 1992d). Criticizing the assumption of assimilation that lies behind the 'traditional' versus 'Western' dichotomy, Hutnik (1991) argues that Asian Britons may actively recreate a variety of rather different ethnic identities, and indeed an individual may flexibly use one or the other in different situations; a public acceptance of 'British identity' may be quite compatible with an enhanced 'Asian identity' in another context.

79 To quote Di Nicola 1990.

80 It may be relevant that eating disorders are less common among the children of African-Caribbean migrants to Britain than among Whites (Dolan *et al.* 1990): a predominantly working-class group who came from almost equally poor societies as the South Asians – but which were arguably 'modern' in the absence of fixed hierarchies or of prescriptive and economically determined patterns of marriage, and in their own valuing of relative gender equality and personal autonomy (Littlewood 1993b). At the same time, we might argue they seem less likely to be expected by their families to attain a new professional status (which for them would already have fewer implications for women's autonomy relative to men (Hutnik 1991)).

81 Hutnik 1991.

82 Merrill and Owens 1988. One cannot assume that because the family provides the everyday locus for ambiguities over autonomy it should be regarded as primarily responsible; the ambiguities may be less 'cultural' than 'social', less about challenging family norms than about economic experiences and actions outside the family, including racism and restricted opportunity.

83 Schmidt and Bakshi (unpublished data). Students in urban Jaipur (predominantly Hindu), and British students of South Asian origin or ethnicity,

and White British students, were asked general questions and given: the Bulimic Investigatory Test, which looks at bulimic conceptions and actions, using a conventional cut-off point to distinguish between possible clinical 'cases' and 'non-cases', together with information about height and weight, attitude to weight and body shape, any menstrual problems, and attendance at slimming clubs; an 'acculturation questionnaire' devised for Hispanic migrants to the United States which asks about the family choice between 'traditional' and 'modern' activities and behaviour, including questions about the type of food eaten at home, language spoken, and dress; a questionnaire assessing 'traditional' versus 'non-traditional' concepts of family relationships, marriage system and the emancipation of women (adapted from an 'intergenerational conflict questionnaire' originally devised for a Kuwaiti population).

84 Goody (1982, 1990) argues that, compared with Africa or elsewhere, a common Eurasian system of settled agrarian communities developed historically 'with use of the plough or irrigation. It remains characterized by a relatively high population density, social stratification with each sector having distinctive relations to agricultural and other production, with bilateral kinship and thus conjugal joint families rather than corporate lineage groups, *with* marriage outside these families but within the wider stratified sector (certainly for North Indian Hindus), and with transfer of wealth at marriage to the groom's family from the bride's (dowry). Mandelbaum (1988) argues for close similarities between Hindu and Muslim female norms and values in northern South Asia, in which the purity of women guarantees male (and family) honour.

85 And any experienced change is mitigated through students already tending to have more 'modern' parents. The experiences of 'modernisation' may be quite different from rural non-elite groups where value changes may be experienced as something quite external to the bounded family unit rather than as conflicting personal choices within it.

86 Indeed the very openness to recognize differences of norms between self and parent is itself arguably 'modern', but the majority of the modernization questions were relatively descriptive rather than evaluative, and parent–child differences were described particularly against a possible consensus norm.

87 To adequately demonstrate this requires a greater variety of samples. In Lahore, a Pakistan city with an established 'dieting culture', a concern with the body shape does seem to correlate with 'pathological attitudes' to eating (Mumford *et al.* 1992).

88 While Asian British men and women were similar to the Whites in terms of weight and shape dissatisfaction, this went with higher prevalence of symptoms. Mumford *et al.* (1991) and Dolan *et al.* (1990) found more abnormal attitudes to eating among Asian girls in Britain than among Whites but no greater concern with body shape. Hutnik (1991) argues that Asian Britons seem less likely than White Britons to define themselves through their body.

89 As Hutnik suggests that individuals in migrant groups may actually adopt a more 'modern', universalizing perspective than that found among the majority (European) group.

 90 Schmidt *et al.* 1993.
 91 Bynum 1988. A psychoanalytic study of migration emphasizes the importance of food during the early stages of adjustment which sometimes takes on aspects of 'compulsive eating, in a frantic search to recover the lost objects' (Grinberg and Grinberg 1984), and Bulik (1987) speculates that attempts to adapt to the new society may lead to eating disorders in a rapid identification with the more immediately accessible aspects of that culture such as female slimness. The middle-class Asian Britons in the Schmidt–Bakshi study were not, however, recent immigrants; indeed, they seemed similar to their White British peers in terms of their personal norms. However, precisely this degree of sought personal autonomy might have led to enhanced constraints within their family of origin, especially for those Asian Britons who considered themselves more 'Westernised' than their families but who were still living at home. Hutnik (1991) found that 'low self-acceptance' – commonly described by doctors among patients with eating disorders – may, among Asian British girls, be associated with conformity to parental wishes; and among young Americans bulimic symptomatology goes along with a perceived lack of family cohesion (Coburn and Ganong 1989).
 92 A study of schoolgirls in northern India found that nearly a third scored above the cut-off point on the Eating Attitudes Test (King and Bhugra 1989).
 93 Mandelbaum 1988; Goody 1990.
 94 Lee *et al.* 1992; Kakar 1988.
 95 Goody 1982.
 96 Bharati 1985.
 97 Masson 1970; Guzder and Krishna 1991.
 98 Kakar 1978: 4.
 99 Guzder and Krishna 1991: 260.
100 Grottanelli 1982.
101 Hershman 1977; Mandelbaum 1988.
102 Guzder and Krishna 1991.
103 Mandelbaum 1988; Goody 1990.
104 Kakar 1978, 1988; Roland 1988.
105 Bharati 1985.
106 Shah 1960.
107 Murphy 1982; Guzder and Krishna 1991; Merrill and Owens 1988; Raleigh and Balarajan 1992.

Chapter 6
 1 The relatives of depressed women have a disproportionate tendency to anti-social behaviour (Winokur 1973) arguing that it may be an 'analogue' of depression (although, of course, also a possible cause, unlikely as that may seem).
 2 Simons and Hughes 1985.
 3 Winzeler 1990; Grottanelli 1985.
 4 Leslie 1991; Harlan 1992. And similarly Ibo male suicide and Japanese *shinju* (Pinquet 1993).
 5 Bourdieu 1977.

6   Edwards 2000.
7   D'Orban 1976; Palmer and Noble 1984.
8   Teoh 1972.
9   Ashton and Donnan 1981; Gould and Shaffer 1986; Schmidtke and Hafner 1988.
10 Cf. Sperber 1985.
11 Simons and Hughes 1985; Westermeyer 1973.
12 Girard 1977, 1978; Taussig 1993; Melberg 1995.
13 Chapter 4; Winzeler 1990; Platt 1987.
14 See Chapter 10.
15 For example: D'Orban 1976; Palmer and Noble 1984; Kennedy and Dyer 1992; Scott 1978; Anon. 1993.
16 Lewis 1969; Mulvey 1987; Turner 1969.
17 Alexander 1979.
18 Kupperman and Trent 1979; Nandy 1995; Netanyahu 1995.
19 Anon. 1993.
20 Kupperman and Trent 1979; Netanyahu 1995.
21 Guelke 1995; cf. MacPherson 1988.
22 Girard 1977; Cohn 1993.
23 Nandy 1995: 26.
24 Kobetz 1975. While the usual police term, 'domestic siege', is not a criminal offence as such, and estimates of frequency have to be drawn from recognized offences recorded by the police, *kidnapping* in England and Wales increased from 102 cases in 1982 to 1059 in 1993, *abduction* from 86 to 356 over the same period (personal communication, Home Office Research and Statistics Department). Where more than one offence takes place at the same time, however, only the most serious is counted in summary statistics: thus kidnapping ending in homicide is recorded as homicide not kidnapping. Abduction is generally classified as a sexual offence and would not generally fit our model of domestic sieges. If hostage-taking during domestic sieges may include a number of offences, then the figure for 1992 court proceedings for kidnapping was 568 (145 found guilty), for hijacking 6 (2), and for false imprisonment 276 (117); the relatively low proportion of findings of guilt probably reflecting reduced and dropped charges as much as aquittals (*ibid.*). I was not able to obtain figures on 'hoax' sieges but was told by police that these are now increasingly common.
25 Compare (i) equivalents in eighteenth-century London (Stevenson 1979); (ii) representations of amok in Javanese theatre which may pass out into reciprocal violence among the spectators like grenade amok at the Laos *boun* festival (Geertz 1966); (iii) or the variably stylized violence of street carnivals and football crowds: 'A spatial structure of inversions is crucial to the symbolic language of Carnival, but there is also another, alternative, structure that exists in time, in the process of ritualised change from one state to another, from everyday norm to the licence of disorder and *back again*. This tripartite structure allows cultural forms and rituals to be used to express disruptive desire, both the desire repressed by a Symbolic Order and the Law as such, and the desire of the oppressed for change. In this sense it is integrative and

arguably conservative providing, in the last resort, a social safety valve for the forces of disorder. Disruption is followed by restoration of the status quo, in a manner that is reminiscent of narrative patterns . . .' (Mulvey 1987, emphasis in the original). On occasion the social tensions represented in carnival masquerade may manifest as continuing violence or be translated into political process. Our customary Western distinction between 'ritual' and 'reality' is by no means obvious.

26   Thus two separate domestic sieges were dramatized on television on the same evening (14/9/95): ITV *The Bill*, BBC1 *The Backup*.

27   Palmer and Noble 1984.

28   Devereux 1970; Scott 1990.

29   Section 1 of the 1989 Childrens Act (on the law relating to a child on the breakdown of the parents' marriage) emphasizes that decisions must be based on 'any harm he has suffered or is at risk of suffering', including physical or psychological injury caused by either parent.

30   Thus Kennedy and Dyer (1992) describe three parental hostage-takers who appeared to have been recognized as having psychiatric illness or alcohol intoxication.

31   Gardner 1989.

32   In an extensively reported incident in 1986, a solicitor, who was being sought by the police in connection with the murder of his wife while he had been having an affair with a French woman, escaped to France where, pursued, he clung to a gargoyle on Amiens Cathedral to the interest of the crowd which gathered in the square below; he harangued the spectators, who eventually became bored and vociferously invited him to jump.

33   Van Gennep 1960.

34   Simons and Hughes 1985.

35   Parkin 1992; Van Gennep 1960.

36   Keillor 1993.

37   Cited by McKee 1992.

38   *Ibid.*

39   Hardy 1997; Kamphris and Emmelkamp 2000.

40   Hardy 1997.

41   Mair 1995: 11.

42   Hardy 1997.

43   *Ibid.*

44   Girard 1977.

45   Classically, Hubert and Mauss 1898.

46   Girard 1977.

47   Seaford 1995.

48   See note 25.

49   Grottanelli 1985.

Chapter 7

1   Has 1990; Reyna and Downs 1994; Nordstrom and Robben 1995; Richards 1996.

2   African Rights 1995.

3   Winkler 1991; Brownmiller 1975; Nordstrom and Robben 1995: Intro.

4   Ilen and Gardwin-Gill 1994; World Vision 1996.

5   As did Malinowski 1941.

6   E.g. Amnesty International 1993a; Asia Watch 1993; Human Rights Watch/Africa 1990.

7   Human Rights Watch/Africa 1990.

8   Laber 1993. Whilst military rape and sexual mutilation have been reported by armed Croats, Bosnians and Serbians, it is the last-named who are particularly under international scrutiny. The ratio of the number of rapes to resulting pregnancies is generally taken to be around one hundred to one (Human Rights Watch/Africa 1990).

9   Olujic (1995) notes that this has often had serious consequences for the women themselves, media exposure being followed by family and community ostracism. The newly independent Bangladesh government's attempt to promote raped women as national heroines and to offer dowries for them was a similar failure.

10   October 1995.

11   Human Rights Watch/Africa 1990.

12   Asia Watch 1993.

13   Amnesty International 1993c: 6.

14   *Ibid.*

15   Amnesty International 1993a.

16   Das 1996.

17   African Watch 1993; African Rights 1993.

18   Amnesty International 1993b, 1996; Immigration and Refugee Board (in Canada) 1993.

19   Bradbury 1992.

20   Howard *et al.* 1995.

21   Laws are silent in war. Or, as Livy put it more cogently, '*vae victis*' (woe to the defeated).

22   E.g. Walter 1950; D. Young 1993.

23   *Independent* 1996.

24   *The Times* 1996c.

25   A common modern image of the peasant (or proletarian: cf. Zola's *Germinal*, Malinowski 1941, Grottanelli 1985). 'Head hunting' was however institutionalized among nineteenth-century Balkan soldiers (Boehm 1983).

26   Sahlins 1983: 88.

27   Ehrenseich 1997.

28   McManners 1994: 114; Adams 1993.

29   Cf. Kanitkar 1994.

30   Compare Melanesia (Herdt 1984).

31   See Polhemus 1978.

32   Rooth 1971, 1974.

33   Berger 1971: 47.

34   Rooth 1971.

35   *Ibid.*

36   E.g. Reich 1975.
37   Holmes 1994.
38   Brownmiller 1975: 105.
39   Lifton 1986.
40   The same period when European societies began to abandon physical pain as a judicial punishment.
41   Bailey 1972; Howard *et al.* 1995.
42   McManners 1994.
43   The notion of war as a delimited game goes back to classical Greece (Hanson 1989), but nineteenth-century Europe's national wars were characterized, as if they were a military tattoo, by interested spectators carrying maps, telescopes and picnic baskets, whose only danger was off-target artillery or an unwise inclination to join in (*Vanity Fair*, *War and Peace*, *Le Débâcle*). Recently reading again Zola's novel about the Battle of Sedan in the Franco–Prussian War, where armed civilians and snipers were certainly an issue, as the author's generally accurate account notes, it appears there was only one case of reported rape during the prolonged German siege and occupation of the city; unlike the Commune that followed, which allowed extensive French-on-French sexual violence.
44   The use of military idioms begs a number of questions but we need some agreed denotations.
45   Which gave international currency to the term *guerrilla* (little war).
46   Compare the American Civil War where the Confederates initially shot those captured Union troops who were Black.
47   Inevitably one wonders about the ethnic origin of their rapists whom the Americans chose to execute.
48   E.g. Brownmiller 1975; Guinan 1993; Human Rights Watch/Africa 1990; cf. 'opportunistic rape' – World Vision 1996.
49   As Jacobo Timerman (1985) has argued.
50   And these are perhaps not easily distinguished. Allan Young (personal communication) has told me of the large number of Americans in Veterans Administration's hospitals diagnosed with post-traumatic stress disorder who still carry photographs from Vietnam of body parts of enemy combatants and civilians dismembered and arranged in piles; some soldiers on active service sent such pictures back to their families.
51   Cf. Barth 1969: 33.
52   Cf. Malinowski 1941.
53   Allodi 1988; Amnesty International Medical Commission 1989.
54   Adams 1993; McManners 1994.
55   Girard 1977.
56   Robben 1995: 92.
57   Cf. Gregory Bateson's schismogenesis or the ethologists' ritual agonistic behaviour. Why, anyway, are wars (like sex) fought between *two* sides? In practice, of course, they are not, and the boundaries sought cut through active neutrals, doubtful allies, unstable coalitions, issues of morale, treason and incompetence.
58   Kerrigan 1996.

59 Kagan 1996; cf. Otterbein 1994.
60 Cited in Kerrigan 1996.
61 Keegan 1995. But maybe not chemical warfare which requires more expensive delivery systems and manufacture effectively limited to national institutions; if military rape is to be considered as a pragmatic strategy, it must be included within a number of other possibilities available to a particular social formation of combatants. Rules depend on affordable hardware and ideological interests, including the allocation of accountability to civilians (Guelke 1995).
62 Kerrigan 1996.
63 Campbell and Gibbs 1986.
64 For soldiers are trained to do things by rote: five minutes of sexual intercourse were allowed for each private soldier in the French regimental *bordels militaires de campagne.*
65 British military historians (Holmes 1994; McManners 1994) have argued that American atrocities in Vietnam were encouraged by the preliminary military–psychological training which employed images of 'female orientals' as subhuman. Compare the almost legitimated murder of prostituting women or Brazilian street children, both with a public 'spoiled identity'.
66 African Rights 1995.
67 Chagnon 1990.
68 Human Rights Watch 1995.
69 On fictive or reconstituted households in wartime: American soldiers on leave in Vietnam hired local prostituting women with whom they lived for their period of leave in 'counterfeit domesticity' (Holmes 1994: 99). In Somalia, girls were married off early for their own security, or to establish alliances with local militia to safeguard their families; in Uganda, the Lord's Resistance Army allowed its officers four 'wives' (captured girls), some were traded for rifles in the Sudan (World Vision 1996).
70 African Rights 1995; Human Rights Watch/Africa 1990.
71 Brownmiller 1975.
72 Holmes 1994; McManners 1994.
73 McManners 1994: 115.
74 Brownmiller 1975.
75 Personal communication: gelada baboons.
76 McManners 1994.
77 Amnesty International 1993a.
78 As with recent accounts of child sexual abuse, we can only with difficulty distinguish atrocity stories (with their own purpose of promoting retribution) from actual events which we ignore under the pretext of lack of verification.
79 *The Times* 1995.
80 A number of people have pointed out to me that there are very different and non-Islamic precedents for the pre-execution rape of young women; nominally at least this goes with a disinclination to execute 'children'. Islam has always argued restraints in war, and the established feuding of patrilineal groups in Afganistan and Morocco rarely involved rape in a standardized cessation of hostilities: 'Do not let the blood of women or children or old men sully your victory' (Abu Bakr).

81 What Erik Erikson called 'pseudospeciation'; compare the equivalent issue in slavery (Spiegel 1996).
82 In *The Seven Pillars of Wisdom*.
83 Holmes 1994.
84 Young 1995. Including Robert Lifton, who elsewhere (1986) has argued powerfully for the personal accountability of Nazi medical torturers.
85 Ironically, PTSD has now become the major medical justification in Europe for granting asylum to civilian refugees from war zones.
86 Human Rights Watch/Africa 1990.
87 October 1995.
88 Holmes 1994: 390. (Brownmiller (1975) doubts Ehrenburg's authorship of this military pamphlet; but compare Rubenstein 1996.) A similar rationale for inter-group rape as the victim's resolution of racism is found in Eldridge Cleaver's *Soul on Ice*.
89 Smuts 1992.
90 Reich 1975; Fromm 1977.
91 Jukes 1993.
92 Only rarely is the woman allowed to wash herself in between rapes, and while in Rwanda HIV infection was a serious concern for the abused women, it seldom seems to have put off the rapists (African Rights 1995: Chapter 10).
93 Rwanda militias (*interahamwe* – 'those who kill together') seem to have encouraged all Hutu men, including non-militia, to participate collectively in sexual violence, more to affirm their immediate loyalty than to (as the authors of the report argue) spread later responsibility (African Rights 1995). The extent to which the rapes were centrally directed by Hutu public officials is still debated (*vide New York Review of Books*, 19 September 1996: 79–80).
94 Otterbein 1994. Obvious counter-examples include Muslim and Eastern European feuds where rape is unusual.
95 Walter (1950) provides an early instance, D. Young (1993) a 'symbolic' account, Eibl-Eibelsfeldt (1979), Shaw and Wong (1989), O'Connell (1995) and Wrangham and Peterson (1998) more in line with current ethology. The image of a new growth emerging from immolation was not uncommon during the Great War, and for Romantic irrationalism, 'The whole earth, continually steeped in blood, is nothing but an immense altar on which every living thing is sacrificed without end, without restraints, without respite' (De Maistre, cited in Holmes 1994).
96 An obvious objection is that while the rape and the killing of women are often associated, no invariate psychophysiological mechanism has been identified, but contemporary ethologists are less concerned with hard-wired biological inevitability than with contingent and statistical reproductive outcomes. Something analogous to rape and simulated rape of defeated males and females occurs among chimpanzees, the one species of non-human primates who on occasion engage in behaviour that recalls 'war' and 'bride capture' (Goodall 1986).
97 Brownmiller 1975.
98 *The Times* 1996d.
99 Walter 1950.

100 Human Rights Watch/Africa 1990.
101 African Rights 1995: Ch. 12.
102 Laber 1993.
103 *Ibid.*
104 *Independent* 1996.
105 *The Times* 1994.
106 E.g. Nordstrom and Robben 1995: Intro; cf. Keen 1996.
107 Hobsbawm 1994.
108 Bartov 1996.
109 Keegan 1995.

Chapter 8

1 Sawbridge 1988.
2 Strickland 1993.
3 Some post-adoption counsellors report it is fairly uncommon, others that it was virtually universal when clients were asked sensitively. I would estimate from their reports that over 50 per cent of current clients seen in London have experienced strong sexual feelings in reunions. The term 'genetic sexual attraction' was coined by Barbara Gonyo (1987), who has described it in various post-adoption newsletters, and is preferred by counsellors to the emotive term 'incest'.
4 Legal, popular and academic definitions of incest vary considerably (La Fontaine 1988). As anthropologists have often noted, categories for prohibited marriage and for prohibited sex do not necessarily correspond (Fox 1980; Arens 1986; Leach 1991). In Scotland, bans on sexual relations do correspond with those on prohibited marriage, while in England sex may be legal in relationships where marriage is not – with parents' siblings and certain step-relatives. In France intrafamilial sexual relations are not in themselves illegal. The English legal category of *incest* refers to vaginal intercourse and thus to only a proportion of intrafamilial sexual acts: it applies to less than a quarter of adult sexual abusers of children (La Fontaine 1990). 'Incest' is not altogether a helpful term and it has been criticized for essentializing social relationships: societies may not have a single term for sexual acts with all unmarriageable kin or affines, particularly when marriage is prescribed between certain categories of kin, when the group of non-eligible marital partners may be identified by a single category as, for example, 'sisters'. In this paper 'incest' is retained to refer to sexual sentiments and physical relations between first-degree biological kin.
5 Reynolds 1991; Lumsden and Wilson 1983.
6 Lévi-Strauss 1949; Fortes 1983.
7 La Fontaine 1988; Leach 1991.
8 La Fontaine 1990.
9 Masson 1984.
10 Twitchell 1987; Shaw 1992.
11 Russell 1984.
12 La Fontaine 1990.
13 Durkheim 1898; Malinowski 1927.

14 Lévi-Strauss 1949.
15 Parsons 1954.
16 Lumsden and Wilson 1983.
17 Reynolds 1980.
18 Shepher 1983.
19 Blovin and Blovin 1988.
20 Fox 1980.
21 *Ibid.*
22 Shaw 1992.
23 Sahlins 1976; cf. Fox 1980; Lumsden and Wilson 1983.
24 Twitchell 1987; La Fontaine 1990.
25 Mayr 1988.
26 E.g. by Jane Austen (1814: 3–4).
27 Westermarck 1894: 80.
28 Shepher 1983.
29 Wolf 1970, 1994.
30 Malinowski 1927; Fortes 1983.
31 Freud 1913.
32 Ingold 1986; Littlewood 1993b.
33 Erickson 1993; cf. Littlewood 1993b.
34 Vidal 1985; cf. Shepher 1983.
35 Mayr 1988; Reynolds 1991.
36 Shepher 1983; Blovin and Blovin 1988; Yamazaki *et al.* 1988.
37 Hayashi and Kimura 1978; Roscoe 1994.
38 Fox 1980.
39 Gavish *et al.* 1984.
40 Shore 1993.
41 Fox 1980.
42 *Ibid.*
43 Chagnon 1990.
44 Fox 1980; Arens 1986.
45 La Fontaine 1990; Erickson 1993.
46 Giddens 1992.
47 Strathern 1992; Littlewood 1993a.
48 Strickland 1993.
49 Quoted in *ibid.*
50 Sorosky *et al.* 1975.
51 Triseolitis 1973.
52 Erickson 1989.
53 *Eros*, from *agape*, to use the classical Greek differentiation (cf. Sternberg and Barnes 1988). On the cultural deployment of biological attachment, Shore (1993) notes that in Samoa, where distant kin may be classificatory 'siblings', accusations of incest cloud virtually any erotic attachment.
54 Sternberg and Barnes 1988; Erickson 1993.
55 Twitchell 1987.
56 Sternberg and Barnes 1988. Dating agencies use detailed lists of personal characteristics, including personality and physical appearance, to 'match' (in

both senses) their clients: they assume a correspondence facilitates successful introductions. Such *sympathy*, seeing oneself mirrored in the other (Van Sant 1993), was commonly recognized in Renaissance and Romantic literature as the prelude to incest (Twitchell 1987).

57   Bowlby 1982.

58   Cf. Erickson 1989. It is significant that some of our informants described their adoptive families as 'cold', perhaps suggesting little affective bonding. Early attachment behaviour (proximity-seeking behaviour) is usually distinguished from the attachment bond (the type of relationship) which, after the first year, involves representational models of the self and others (Bowlby 1982; Vidal 1985). Ainsworth's (1977) modification of Bowlby's original theory proposes three types of bond: *secure*, in which the infant seeks proximity and is comforted on reunion; *insecure avoidant*, in which proximity is avoided; and *insecure ambivalent*, characterized by distress and uncertainty. As Cicchetti *et al.* (1990) argue, it is difficult to identify these in an older child or adult. In the post-adoption reunion, child attachment behaviours are recalled by the recognition of familiarity, the need to explore the other physically and emotionally, the difficulty of letting go, and the playful experimentation. Although there appears a pleasurable wish for security and permanence, this seems modified sometimes by feelings of anxiety, recalling Main and Solomon's (1990) Type D (disorganized/disorientated) attachments; despite the affinities between attachment bonds and everyday adult romantic love (Sternberg and Barnes 1988), it would be unwise to push the homology further.

59   Parker and Parker 1986.

60   Shepher 1983; Fox 1980.

61   La Fontaine 1990.

62   Erickson 1993; Roscoe 1994.

63   Count 1967.

64   McClelland *et al.* 1986.

65   Cf. *ibid.*

66   Holland 1992.

67   Vidal 1985.

68   Compare the standard social anthropological position: Fortes 1983.

69   Erickson 1989; Hayashi and Kimura 1978.

70   Though smell appears less significant in the phenomenological world of primates than of other animals, it is closely related to the MHC complex of genes involved in the immune system, and thus with the body's recognition of self and other.

71   Clark 1977.

72   Vidal 1985; cf. Roscoe 1994.

73   Although the 'optimal non-resemblance' model would suggest that in the absence of appropriate bonding, 'biological incest' is more likely than 'social (step or adoptive) incest'. The sexual attraction of stepfathers to their stepdaughters is perhaps in part because the young girl resembles her mother.

74   Shaw 1992.

75   La Fontaine 1990.

Chapter 9

1 Skultans 1987.
2 Littlewood 1986.
3 See Chapter 1, note 33.
4 Heelas and Lock 1981; Marsella and White 1982; Carrithers *et al.* (1986); Wilkes 1988.
5 Taussig 1980.
6 E.g. Shweder and Bourne 1982.
7 Metzger 1981.
8 Wu 1982.
9 Harré 1986.
10 DeVos 1985; Doi 1971.
11 Leff *et al.* 1987.
12 Bharati 1985.
13 Gaines 1979.
14 Ritenbaugh and Simons 1985.
15 Langness and Levine 1986.
16 Kleinman 1988a; Scambler and Hopkins 1986; Estroff 1981; Johnson and Johnson 1983.
17 Myers 1976; White 1982.
18 Eckman 1980.
19 Heelas and Lock 1981.
20 See p. 27; Littlewood 1988.
21 Vitebsky 1992.
22 Ellenberger 1970: 171; Harris 1985.
23 Gauld 1992; Micale 1995. The Nancy School argued clinical suggestion led to physiological trance, the Parisians the converse. Similarly, colonial officers in the Malay Peninsula wondered if latahs were induced by others to commit murder (Winzeler 1995).
24 Matthews 1992; Ellenberger 1970: 126–7.
25 Devereux 1953: *passim.*
26 In a number of recent publications the classicist Helen King has queried the antiquity of hysteria as a distinct category.
27 The French noun *conscience* denotes psychophysiological state or entity (consciousness) as well as moral accountability (conscience), aspects which were more likely to be distinguished by the anglophone investigators leaving a gap in which spiritualism entered (p. 154). There were a number of similar terms for the more developed instances (*conscience dissociée*) involving idioms of doubling and multiplicity, alternation, narrowing, dissociation, fragmentation, disintegration, decomposition, de-aggregation, splitting-off or variation, depending on the extent of one-way or mutual amnesia (Campbell *et al.* 1925: 195; Ellenberger 1970: *passim*).
28 Ellenberger 1970: 129–31; Micale 1995: Ch.1.
29 Kenny 1986: 150.
30 (i) spontaneous multiple personality, each of whom (or each of which for those who preferred states to personalities) has a sense of complete individuality which excludes the others; (ii) successive multiple personalities who are

cognizant of each other; (iii) successive multiple personalities mutually amnesic yet who for the clinical observer seem to have some awareness of the other stages, giving the whole pattern a motivated quality; (iv) successive multiple personalities with one-way amnesia, the most common form, the second personality characteristically being the 'inverse' of the first; (v) less discrete and enduring personality clusters which emerge in the course of treatment (Ellenberger 1970). For current equivalents, see Brown's (1988) schema.

31 Prince 1905: 7.

32 The family comprises: B1, the woman who consulted, is controlled, educated, prim and proud; B2 (The Saint) is B1 heightened under hypnosis; B3 (The Devil) who comes unbidden is jokey, indulgent, flirtatious and ignorant yet sympathetic; B4 (The Woman) is stable, serious and practical, an early but abandoned choice for 'the real Miss B.'; together with other clusters and partial manifestations of these four. Prince's designations recall those of the stock characters of the silent cinema. He becomes rather attached to B3, whom he names Sally, and then unhappy as he realizes he must kill her off. Sally protests she will not be 'squeezed' but then starts to fade away.

33 Kenny 1986: 155. Showalter (1990) shows how hysteria was manifest in countless Victorian plays and novels.

34 Geertz 1983: 59.

35 Janet 1925; Ellenberger 1970: Chapter 3.

36 *Ibid.* Not that these two, any more than the physiological process and its ideational content, were easily distinguished in the neurologists' materialist psychology. Nor are they now, given the 'sincere' denial of blindness in Anton's syndrome or the continued experience of an amputated 'phantom limb'. A third explanation, that of feigning – what we might now term role-playing (Spanos and Gottlieb 1979) – was put forward by Flournay and Benedikt and later advanced by Charcot's critics and envious colleagues. Charcot himself was generally a materialist in the French anticlerical style but remained ambivalent about the significance of volition and habit (Williams 1994).

37 Harrington 1987. 'Nervous energy' was a naturalistic reading of human volition as a function of the number of brain cells: a weak nervous constitution resulted in a weak will (Campbell *et al.* 1925: 91). Indeed Beard (1881: 12) likened man to an electric battery. In his unpublished *Project for a Scientific Psychology* Freud attempted to reconcile the (motivated) physical passage of energy through neurones with their consequent organization into structured channels which then facilitated the same mental patterns (an idea that is also found in Prince's 'nets' or 'neurograms' and that goes back to Lamarck and to Descartes' 'canalization' and is analogous to our popular understandings of 'vice' or 'addiction' as initially volitional but increasingly compulsive (Little-wood 1993b)). Freud's abandonment of the manuscript in 1895 is often taken as his move from the physicalism of Helmholtz and Brucke towards a more purely interpretive and dynamic (purposive) psychology. Edelman's recent (1992) 'neural Darwinism' proposes something similar: rather than simply enacting a genetic programme to provide a mirror of external reality, the

connections between cells in the developing post-natal brain are influenced by inputs from their environment and respond correspondingly, actively competing against and colonizing the organization of other groups of cells in relation to their outside world. To an extent then their 'design-fixing repertoires' approach what may be termed representation – intentionality in the philosopher's sense. Putting Edelman's theory together with Dennett's (1991) and Dawkins' (1982) suggestion that the brain is colonized by memes (the anthropologist's collective representations) argues for one way into the naturalistic–personalistic antinomy (p. xiii). Compare Sperber 1985.

38   Ellenberger (1970) points out that many of these ideas have been credited to Freud. Janet, like other members of the 'first dynamic psychiatry' such as Prince and James who argued variously for a purposive unconscious, did not accept Freud's suggestion that psychic energy and its hydraulic transformations were essentially sexual (libido).

39   Hacking 1995.

40   Hacking 1992b. A philosophical replay: Kant had criticized the British empiricists for maintaining that mentation is grounded in experience, Locke having argued that memory was 'recovered sensations'.

41   Ellenberger 1966.

42   Panpsychism: mind being variously elided with or distinguished from spirit. Although the French neurologists might recognize 'nervous energy' in telepathy and precognition (as did Freud and Jung), neither phenomenon was significant in their account of the mechanism of double consciousness. By contrast, the British psychiatrist and anthropologist William McDougall (Rivers' colleague on the Torres Straits expedition) regarded the subselves as only held together by continual telepathy, and took one of Miss Beauchamp's personalities for an autonomous spirit (McDougall 1911: 367). A variant of panpsychism has recently been revived on the basis of quantum theory by Roger Penrose; the less determined your particles, the less material they seem.

43   Owen 1989; Gauld 1992.

44   Kenny 1986; Owen 1989.

45   Or rather who attributed it to Malicious Animal Magnetism. Henry James' *The Bostonians* captures well the local preoccupations through which his brother's clinical practice developed.

46   Fuller 1982.

47   Ellenberger 1970: 101. Micale (1995: 199) details the explosion of novels, plays and pornography based on Charcot's Salpêtrière, a prefiguring of our recent dramatizations of Victorian psychiatry.

48   A fact psychoanalysts, themselves often women, attributed to a lessening repression of women's sexuality (Showalter 1993: 326–7), to sex education and a greater 'openness' about sexual matters (Kenny 1986); what Micale (1995: 170) terms de-Victorianization.

49   Campbell *et al.* 1925: 200.

50   *Ibid.*: 293.

51   Anna O., 'the first psychoanalytic patient', had manifested something like a second, sick self who lived exactly 365 days before the well self, events recapitulating each other in a day-to-day correspondence. She spoke to her

doctors in English, at times apparently ignorant of German.

52 Campbell *et al.* 1925: 300.

53 Masson 1984. Freud's own justification was lack of empirical evidence and sheer implausibility; critics have argued rather that he suppressed the clear evidence of child sexual abuse because he was a male doctor, or because it would have been politically disadvantageous for his career, or because he himself had to repress his incestuous desires and replace them by those of the child, or because as a Jew with many Jewish patients he was distancing himself from Austrian medical anti-Semitism which argued incest was common amongst Eastern European Jews.

54 Janet 1925.

55 As opposed to 'involuntary' possession trance which is regarded both locally and by psychiatrists as undesired and undesirable (Lewis 1969; Boddy 1989); our ascription of volition, however, is as culturally determined as the participant's own experience of loss of agency. We might recall the debunking legacy of medical modernism which, if it no longer attempted to unmask all non-medical healers as charlatans, nevertheless sought some explanation more essential – whether physiological, psychological or sociological – which structured the participant's experience.

56 See p. 16. As they apparently did in latah. Magical thinking – a projection of personal wishes and fears, and a confusion between fantasy and reality, between self and other, with coexistence of contraries and a continued association of objects once in contact, dominated by the power of resemblance and a compulsion to repeat – was identified in women and children who, like tribal peoples, had still to develop beyond the earlier evolutionary stage of (in psychoanalytical terminology) the primary process of the unconscious mind. With civilization, there was a depersonification and internalization of the spirits from the possessing demons of early modernity (Clarke 1975: 256), via the 'natural spirits' of Renaissance physiology to the imponderable fluids and magnetic humours of the Enlightenment, and thence to the psychological faculties of Cognition, Affect and so on.

57 E.g. Spanos and Gottlieb 1979. (Cf. Nadel, Field, Fortes, Turner, Lewis, Needham, Kapferer.) Sperber, Crapanzano and the American cognitive anthropologists (Shweder, D'Andrade, Holland, Quinn, Levine, Schwartz, Lutz, White) emphasize fairly autonomous inter-subjective cognition, while the older psychoanalytical determinism is maintained by Obeyesekere and Spiro.

58 Bourguignon 1973; Littlewood and Lipsedge 1987; Laughlin *et al.* 1993.

59 For example: Hilgard 1977; Spiegel 1994.

60 Campbell *et al.* 1925; Schrödinger 1944; Ornstein 1985; cf. Dennett 1991.

61 Jaynes 1990; Laughlin *et al.* 1993; Spiegel 1994; cf. Byrne and Whiten 1988.

62 Similar to Johnson's (1987) 'bodily metaphors' like the experience of gravity, laterality or containment.

63 As 'passiones' (Lienhardt 1961: 151): 'A diviner is a man in whom the division is permanently present; a Power, or Powers, are always latent within him but he has the ability to dissociate them in himself at will, letting them manifest themselves in him. While thus dissociated, the diviner *is* a Power, for which his

body is host' (emphasis in the original; see also Krippner 1987, Stoller 1989). And, if dissociation provides an available model for multiplicity, then also in psychosis – particularly where there seems a phasic shift of the 'whole personality' as in manic-depressive or toxic psychoses (Littlewood 1993b). Less so with the fragmentation of psychological experience held to be characteristic of schizophrenia where our bounded identity may become elusive, though doubling or spirit intrusion may still be an accessible explanatory model: indeed hospital psychiatrists repeatedly complain of the popular idea of schizophrenia as Jekyll and Hyde dualism. (A 1980s horror film, *Schizo*, was advertised by a poster showing two hands, one open, one clenching a knife, with the legend 'His right hand didn't know what his left hand was doing'; recalling the competing angels sitting on each shoulder of medieval ascetics or the self-tattooing on the knuckles of certain men – assumed to be suffering from psychopathy or Tourette's syndrome, or else members of a delinquent subculture – on the right hand HATE, on the left LOVE.) I recall as a young psychiatrist brushing aside a psychotic patient's tentative suggestion of his dual personality – 'No, that's hysteria, you've got schizophrenia.'

64 Tart 1980: 249.

65 Bourguignon (1973) distinguishes between T (trance, altered state of consciousness), P (the local ascription of possession) and PT (both occurring together), thus recalling the binarism of physiology:concept – *res extensa:res cogitans*. On the whole British anthropology with its suspicion of empirical psychology ducks the naturalistic approach to emphasize 'dissociation' as purely conceptual (as does e.g. Lienhardt, note 63). The idea that the relationship between the moral and the physical is illustrated best where the physical dominates goes back at least to the Enlightenment physician Alibert, who urged the study of dreams, madness and animal instinct as a route to understanding everyday mental processes.

66 Needham 1981; Lakoff 1987; Littlewood 1993c.

67 *Habitus* (Mauss 1950: 111); similarly Johnson 1987; Bloch 1991. Cognitive psychologists have generally accepted that perception is enacted in a sensorimotor process, an engagement in the world which creates its objects.

68 Young 1984; Littlewood 1996b.

69 I am grossly simplifying Horton's instances for which McDougall's 'animism' offers an academic psychology closer than Freud's hierarchy, the components each having a greater personified autonomy, more of a 'vertical' split recalling Plato's distinction between appetite, spirit and reason as fairly autonomous agencies (Price 1995).

70 Mauss 1950: 61. Mauss restricted the term *moi*, conventionally translated as 'self' (or 'person'), to the social and moral representation, not as I have done here to the operational and embodied 'I': cf. William James' 'empirical me', the 'private self' of Lienhardt and the 'biological individual' of La Fontaine (both in Carrithers *et al.* 1986), or the 'individual body' of Scheper-Hughes and Lock (1987). Yet in cognized experience these must generally be fairly isomorphic, or at least not too disconsonant, with the representation of the

self. Patients in psychoanalysis are not encouraged to personify the analytic mechanisms (which are anyway objectified more in the professional literature than in the consultation), nor does the contemporary psychologist generally wonder if someone at any one moment should be distinguished as either a cognitive or an affective being. In Creole Trinidad, where different individuals may describe themselves as comprising a physical body to which are added quite various combinations of a soul, a spirit, a mind, a shadow and a guardian angel, they do not recognize themselves as fragmented except in certain crises where everyday unity is called into question (generally moral responsibility for otherwise unintelligible or antisocial actions) or during personal cogitations on how to diminish physical pain or discard undesirable vices (Littlewood 1993b). No more does the European Christian generally worry about whether her mind or her soul is in charge except for moments of temptation, guilt, religious doubt or conversion.

71 Laughlin *et al.* 1993; Dennett 1989.
72 Schutz 1976. Or more modestly, the self at dinner, at war, making love.
73 Such as a male (for women), or colonial officer, foreigner or enemy: an idea emphasized in the so-called strategic and deprivation theories of spirit mediumship (Lewis 1969; Wilson 1967; cf. Boddy 1989).
74 Harré 1983.

Chapter 10
1 Gabbard and Gabbard 1987: we might recall Dennett's (1991) Joycean machine, spontaneous parallel processes being interpreted serially as a Jamesian stream of consciousness. Basinger (1994) argues that the continuing popularity of Hollywood's bad twin or double (from *The Twin Pawns* (1919), *The Twins' Double* (1914)) allowed the female audience to have their narrative cake and eat it, a resistance to male demands for a submissive female yet one ultimately reconciled in the good twin's voluntary submission to husband or father. The tragic converse, dissolution of the individual personality through alien penetration, has remained the staple cinematic horror (*Hands of Orlac*, *The Invasion of the Body Snatchers*, *Rosemary's Baby*, *Westworld*, *Alien*, the 1980s cyberpunk films).
2 *Sybil* (Schreiber 1973) was followed by other popular accounts: *The Five of Me* (1977), *Tell Me Who I Am Before I Die* (1977), *The Flock* (1991), and a male case, *The Minds of Billy Milligan* (1981). The first published case of satanic abuse was *Michelle Remembers* (1980).
3 Thigpen and Cleckley 1957.
4 Burne 1993.
5 Spanos 1989; Ross 1994.
6 On which, see Kenny 1981.
7 Aldridge-Morris 1989; Friesen 1991; Merskey 1992; Loftus and Ketcham 1994. MPD (renamed Dissociative Identity Disorder, apparently to reduce the consequences of giving the emergent states proper names (Hacking 1995)), is now recognized as a disease by the American Psychiatric Association (DSM-IV) and, less certainly, by the World Health Organization (ICD-10). Its 'cultural' context is briefly addressed in the revisions for the

DSM-IV manual (Lewis-Fernández *et al.* 1993) and in some of the reviews in Kirmayer 1992b.

8   Casey 1991; Jaroff 1993.

9   Brown 1991; Crabtree 1988.

10   Piper 1994; Putnam 1989; Friesen 1991.

11   Armstrong and Loewenstein 1990; Friesen 1991.

12   Putnam 1989; Brown 1991. These are all characteristics of the notoriously vague British category of personality disorder (character disorder and oppositional defiant disorder in the USA), which has been variously described as a discrete illness or else as just the extreme end of certain 'personality dimensions' elicited by psychologists (inadequate, psychopathic, hysterical and so on) which leads individuals into an adversarial relationship with Euro-American values of self-reliance and responsibility while providing rich and dramatic fantasy lives. I recall a self-mutilating patient I saw in University College Hospital after she 'took an overdose', who told me of the recent murder of her boyfriend, the deaths in car accidents the previous week of both her identically named twin sister and her nephew, and a gripping life history of sibling incest, mistaken identity, family diabolism and a millionaire father who was a well-known 'television personality'.

13   Frequently prostituting, drug-dealing and forging cheques, for example the cases reported by Ross (1994) who points out the parallels between his own patients and Prince's Miss Beauchamp.

14   Kenny 1986; Merskey 1992. A recent court case involves a woman accusing a man of inducing one of her alters, a naive young girl, to emerge so he could rape their body more easily.

15   The earlier private repression of trauma is translated into the late twentieth century's public repression of the abuse of innocent children (cf. Hacking 1991a; Crews 1994).

16   Or indeed, judging from Ross' accounts, a popular television soap opera. Like the spirits of vodun, an individual's alters may constitute a society: one patient manifested two 'communities' plus cadet subcommunities, each of the two larger groups itself containing three sets of 'families', and within each family three sets of paired alters known as 'sisters' (Ross 1994: 143). Other recent variants are that the person who had raped the physical patient was really an alter of her father, or that a continued incestuous relationship with the father involved only one of the patient's alters (*ibid.*: 170, 173). Less personified alters can be recognized by the patient as simply consolidations of her free-floating attitudes or emotions such as self-hatred and depression, which can thus be 'exorcised' out of her through specific psychological therapies or pharmaceutical drugs: 'The Stranger Within was very scared of clomipramine' (*ibid.*: 282).

17   Kenny 1981: 343.

18   Victor 1993; La Fontaine 1994, 1998.

19   Jaroff 1993; Sinason 1994.

20   Csordas 1992; Victor 1993; e.g. Koch 1972. Such as the Institute for Pregnancy Loss and Child Abuse Research and Recovery (*The Times*, London, 4 March 1994, p. 17). Why teaching and social work? Both are low-status,

poorly paid professions, with a high proportion of women, and a good deal of publicly defined responsibility and personal commitment to young children, yet with little independent authority, no consistently accepted intellectual rationale or body of accepted practice, and vulnerable to sudden swings of public policy and professional justification. Their practitioners are constantly faced with balancing their client's wishes and capabilities against (in the earlier socialist social work, malevolent) state institutions. La Fontaine (1994: 31) argues that they 'are reluctant to accept that parents, even those classified as social failures, will harm their children ... Demonising the marginal poor and linking them to unknown satanists turns intractable cases into manifestations of evil.' MPD itself has been identified as especially common among social workers and nurses (e.g. O'Dwyer and Friedman 1993), who are also identified with the not unrelated pattern of Munchausen's Syndrome by Proxy: the induction of symptoms in their children by isolated mothers in establishing a parenting relationship together with a male hospital doctor (Chapter 4). (Here again issues of verification have dominated.) And we can note a similarity with other illnesses commonly reported amongst nurses, particularly eating disorders and deliberate self-harm (Chapters 3 and 5); the extent to which these too involve some new dissociated identity is currently argued by therapists, while parallels between self-denial in eating disorders and in women's religious experience have frequently been argued (Chapter 5). (Compare *trumba* spirits in Mayotte who may either barely eat or else eat excessively and then purge their host's body (Lambek 1981).)

21   Described in Tate 1991 and Thomas 1993.
22   Sinason 1994.
23   Similarly Ross 1994: 137.
24   Sinason 1994: 8, 3.
25   *Ibid.*: 63. (Similarly Ross 1995: *passim*).
26   *Ibid.*: 204, 208.
27   Ross 1994: 109.
28   Sinason 1994: 278, 290.
29   Transcript of Fourth Annual Eastern Regional Conference on Abuse and Multiple Personality, Virginia, USA, 1993.
30   Jaroff 1993; Mack 1994; Bryan 1995.
31   Schnabel 1994.
32   Bryan 1995.
33   Schnabel 1994.
34   Hacking 1995.
35   Crews 1994.
36   Mack 1994: 4.
37   Schnabel 1994.
38   Simons and Hughes 1985.
39   Schnabel 1994; Foreward and Buck 1981; Ross 1994; Crabtree 1988.
40   Horn 1993; Young 1995. Or indeed as induced by witches trained in hypnotherapy who 'lay down' (Hacking 1995) 'cultified multiples' (Mulhern 1994) programmed both to interfere with any future therapy and to relay information about the therapists back to the cult.

41 E.g. Mack 1994; Ross 1994: 125. Professor Ross, who proposes coercive exorcism, notes that 'The reductionist, atheistic bias of modern psychiatry which dismisses the reality of demons is just that, reductionism. It is not science.'

42 Jaroff 1993.

43 Horn 1993.

44 *Ibid.*; Loftus and Ketcham 1994; Wright 1993. (Compare self-accusations of witchcraft in Ghana: Field 1960.) In one case resulting in a 20-year prison sentence, the self-accusation issue generated a multitude of books in 1993 (Crews 1994); the abuse therapist Ross (1994: ix) argues that the study of dissociation alone is far too extensive for anyone to have read the literature.

45 Herman 1992; Jaroff 1993; Piper 1994; Loftus and Ketcham 1994; Terr 1994; Ross 1995.

46 Hacking 1992b. His more recent book, somewhat more sympathetic to the movement, nevertheless offers a powerful argument against 'retroactive application' of new explanations like MPD to earlier life events (Hacking 1995).

47 What neurobiologists refer to as the 'binding problem'. Paragraph references: Wilkes 1988; Braude 1991; Dennett 1991, 1992; Hacking 1991b.

48 Cf. Hacking 1995. By the 1920s 'personality' had become virtually synonymous with 'consciousness' (e.g. Campbell *et al.* 1925: 246), perhaps as a particularly American elision of the self as simultaneously social actor, natural type, psychological mechanism and moral character: something like the popular idea of 'charisma' or its predecessor 'magnetism'. 'Personality', the narrator in *The Great Gatsby* remarks, may be 'an unbroken series of successful gestures'. It has long been associated with individual agency: 'For a time he loses the sense of his own personality, and becomes a mere passive instrument of the deity' (1655: cit. OED).

49 The distinctive characteristics of the second wave, the multiplicity of personalities of both sexes (Dr Jekyll's 'multifarious, incongruous and independent denizens') and their appeals for life, both had precedents in the 1890s (Ellenberger 1970, Ch. 3; Kenny 1986; Showalter 1987b; Hacking 1995).

50 Crews 1994. Turning 'a $2,000 eating disorder patient into a $200,000 multiple-personality disorder' (an American lawyer quoted in Horn 1993: 55); '. . . a highly lucrative enterprise not just of therapy and publishing but also of counselling, workshop hosting, custody litigation, criminal prosecution, forced hospitalization, and insurance and "victim compensation" claims' (Crews 1994: 49). See also *The Times*, London, 6 January 1994, p. 11.

51 Reviewed in Piper 1994. While post-abuse counselling, like therapies for rape and post-traumatic stress disorder, may accept the psychoanalytical understanding of an illness as a potential avoidance of other dilemmas, counsellors in the 'recovery movement' are trained to emphasize one particular trauma. To understand the process by which memories are banished from awareness they retain, however, like the Scientologists and other religious therapeutic groups, the Freudian term 'repression' (on the popularization of which see Moscovici 1976, Crews 1994, Loftus and Ketcham 1994). These therapies are

open to the criticism made against social workers of too readily accepting the reality of reported incidents which may be exaggerated, imagined, fabricated or induced (Campbell 1988; Loftus and Ketcham 1994). Repressed memories of sexual trauma are revealed to the expert by too soft or loud a voice, by starvation or by obesity, by avoidance of the dentist, by an increased interest in sex or by a decreased interest (cited in Crews 1994): 'If you think you have been abused you probably have' (a therapist quoted in Horn 1993). Querying the veracity of one's memories is simply a denial of one's trauma, leaving the issue, like that of alternative medicine, in the usual circular debates on consensual reality – for the very justification of the therapy is that there has indeed been an observable trauma potentially accessible at some point to empirical validation.

52 Three cases by 1992 (O'Dwyer and Friedman 1993) as against an estimated one million in the United States (Crews 1994). For continental Europe, see Lewis-Fernández *et al.* 1993. American psychiatrists argue that their British colleagues have simply failed to diagnose clear cases (*British Journal of Psychiatry*, corr., 1992, 16, 415–20).

53 Cited in Burne 1993.

54 La Fontaine 1990.

55 Compared with 40,000 in the United States, where there are more than 250,000 lay psychotherapists.

56 Hacking 1992b.

57 Kenny 1986.

58 As in the Durkheimian approach of Mary Douglas, in which loosely organized polities (the United States?) parallel and somehow facilitate individual dissociation and spirit intrusion. Both psychologically orientated anthropologists and cultural critics (e.g. Kenny 1986; Lasch 1978) commonly take individual conflicts as the microcosm of wider social fragmentations. And thus an organization's fault lines illuminate the quotidian, whether in the justifications of cultural psychiatry (culture-bound syndromes), anthropology (social dramas) or neuropsychology (head injuries).

59 Young 1995.

60 Micale 1993.

61 In Pierce's semiotics, as an index rather than an icon. In either case, taken by the social theorist as emblematic of a society's preoccupations or representative of its structure (or somehow both: Showalter 1987a).

62 Moscovici 1976; Young 1993a. The late nineteenth century has become the focus in a multitude of recent historical studies on the social resonance of hysteria, degeneration, race and eugenics as the 'master pathologies' of the fin-de-siècle (Nye 1984: 140).

63 Spiegel 1994; Brown 1991. Ross (1994) argues that MPD and PTSD are the new paradigm by which we must now recognize virtually all psychiatric illnesses as caused by an external trauma.

64 Young 1995.

65 Hughes 1992.

66 Or transformed into a 'second self' (Stearns 1994). Schwartz (in Crary and Kwinter 1992) details how once graphology became established as a measure

of character, those failing in business were advised 'you can change your character by changing your writing'.

67 *The Times*, London, 11 September 1993; for example Martin 1993.

68 A British newspaper sardonically comments that contemporary 'Americans seem increasing incapable of having normal personal relationships' and cites date rape and the provision of legal contracts before entering sexual relationships (*The Times*, London, 11 September 1993, Magazine, p. 16).

69 Kenny 1986: 2. And Lasch 1978; Rieff 1966; Bellah *et al.* 1985.

70 Cf. Renaissance self-fashioning or the eighteenth-century 'project'.

71 A common modernist image is the empty self (Lasch 1978); the American poet Anne Sexton developed a second personality, Elizabeth, in the course of her psychoanalysis, whose appearance was discouraged by her therapist, to whom Sexton then wrote plaintively 'I suspect I have no self so I produce a different one for different people' (Ross 1994).

72 Cf. German and Russian nineteenth-century literary concerns with the *doppelgänger* (Hawthorn 1983, Miller 1985, Showalter 1990, Tanner 1993): James Thompson's *City of Dreadful Night* – 'I was twain, two selves distinct that cannot join again'; Dickens' *Edwin Drood* – 'two states of consciousness which never clash, but each of which pursues his separate ways as though it were continuous instead of broken'; Stevenson's *Dr Jekyll and Mr Hyde* – 'man is not truly one but truly two'; or Poe's *William Wilson*. Inspired by the literature on hypnotism, modernism developed a more fractured individual (Dostoyevsky) whose apparent linear consciousness either congealed into temporary consistences (Joyce, Woolf) or was accessible to an enduring self (Pirandello). Descartes' proposition that one cannot think there is no 'I' has become increasingly implausible.

73 Giddens 1992. Schwartz (1996) describes the pervasive Western image of multiplicity in recent years.

74 Wilson 1988; Beck 1992.

75 Lears 1983.

76 Warhol's ('I want to be a machine') and Oldenberg's multiples, body counts and mass disaster statistics, serial killers, serial monogamy, embryo banks and multiple births: the sheer absurdity of multiplication as Walter Benjamin put it.

77 Ellenberger 1970: 279–83; Nye 1984.

78 Ellenberger 1970; Lears 1983; Micale 1995: 200–20. Particularly of a manipulationist and thaumaturgical bent (to use Bryan Wilson's typology). The dynamic psychiatries which appeared in the early twentieth century have been argued by many, including Stuart Hughes and Henri Ellenberger, to be attempts to incorporate such angst into scientific positivism, co-opting Romanticism into the Enlightenment, heart into head. 'And we might argue similarly for the archaeological deductions of the detective novel (appropriated for psychiatric histories by Prince and Freud, and for a topological neurology by Hughlings-Jackson, Rivers and Lewin) which sought to locate and discipline the irrational structures which lurked beneath the even tenor of bourgeois life – an 'unmasking psychiatry' (Ellenberger 1970). De Man (1979) notes the pervasive Romantic topology of depth as true, elemental and

determining: as Coué's Law of Reversed Effort put it, 'When the will and the imagination are in conflict, the imagination always wins' (Campbell *et al.* 1925: 309).

79 Authenticity rather than sincerity; experience not action. And there were born-again Catholics and Jews in the New Right as public officials and Presidents Reagan and Bush rather unconvincingly attested to born-again experience. Strozier (1994) notes the convergence between the alien abductions and the Christian Right's rapture (faithful individuals plucked from the earth before the 'end time tribulation' to meet Christ in the air: following 1 Thessalonians 4.17). Some doctors propose that the Satanic and UFO breeding programmes are the same experiment (e.g. Ross 1994): what cyberaesthetics plausibly lauds as technology's 'harvesting of humans' (Kroker 1992).

80 For what it is worth: the 'end of history' in the triumph of market rationalism (consolidation of colonial power: economic victory in the Cold War) yet with foreboding over the nascent power of the East (the Russo–Japanese War: Japanese technology); the quest for inviolable boundaries (Entente: Star Wars); incorporation of the defeated radical left (1871: 1968); military incompetence and betrayal, and their consequences for national identity (Sedan: Vietnam); the loss of social morality in the encouragement of personal achievement and managerial self-creation; public secularization yet the growth of self-proclaimed irrationalism and religious revivalism (Theosophy: New Age; Huysman: Burroughs; Baudelaire: Leary); frustrated expectations of the emancipation of women; incorporated 'foreigners within' (Jews: Hispanics); variant sexualities enhanced, particularly in a plethora of popular medical textbooks, only to be denied as dangerous (epicene: camp; syphilis: AIDS); the promise of eugenics and the Human Genome Project; the prominence of psychiatrists in debates on criminal and medical accountability; dissatisfaction with naturalistic representation (symbolism: deconstruction); technological success but long-term biological pessimism (race: environment; primitivism: deep ecology). All these could be argued as 'causes of anxiety', as narcissistic symptoms of the dissolution of an earlier unity, should we favour such an idiom – as did the nineteenth-century pathologist Virchow in taking the 'psychic epidemics' (mass hysteria) of the mid-century as *formes frustes* of the revolutionary impulse of 1848 (Littlewood 1993b) or the physician Nordau when characterizing his century's end as a veritable epidemic of hysteria (Micale 1995).

81 Falk 1994. Lears (1983) argues a concomitant shift from 'scarcity therapies' (treatment as a supplement) to 'abundance therapies' (treatment for excess).

82 Ellenberger 1970; Ronell 1989. The phonograph was a common model for the unconscious (Campbell *et al.* 1925: 318), the telegraph for the medium (Kenny 1986). Clinical engagement with the elusive secondary personalities recalls not only the practice of the medium but of the telephone operator: 'Later in the course of the same interview Chris [another personality] was obtained. The same questions were put to her' (Prince 1905: 32). Telephones, X-rays and, more recently, 'sound systems' and computers have generally replaced intruding spirits, 'influencing machines' and the voice of God as the defining technologies for alien dislocations of the self: my colleague,

Maurice Lipsedge, asks a young man diagnosed with schizophrenia how he can hear through his ears a voice that originates from inside his head; the patient explains it is like the doctor using his stereo headphones.

83 Kroker and Kroker 1987; Benedict 1991; Woolley 1993; Heim 1994; Crary and Kwinter 1992.

84 Young 1984; Boddy 1989; Littlewood 1996b.

85 Margulis 1982. And also, as might have been expected from Edelman's neural Darwinism (note 37, Chapter 9), that representations of the body on the cerebral cortex are multiply mapped.

86 Hans Moravec (1989), the director of the Carnegie Mellon University robotics centre, proposes a 20-year programme of transferring human personalities onto hard discs in preparation for our ultimate dissolution as biological beings. Dennett (1991: 430) appears mildly sympathetic to not dissimilar possibilities. In the hard AI view (function equals purpose), thermostats 'think' in that they are 'goal-directed', and mentation is no longer limited to biological organisms; similar to the hylozoic interpretation by deep ecologists of Lovelock's Gaia Hypothesis or to Sheldrake's deity as an 'evolving morphogenic field'. Haraway (1991) argues that biology as the study of material organisms has 'ceased to exist' in favour of the cybernetics of ecosystems and population genetics.

87 Kelly 1994; Emmerche 1994; Levy 1994. The physicist Stephen Hawking claimed in a lecture in 1994 that malevolent computer viruses fulfill all the criteria for life (cf. Schrödinger 1944).

88 Benedict 1991: 124, 140, 141; cf. Martin 1992.

89 Emmerche 1994: the 'self mutates into a classless cyborg' (Kroker 1992: 18).

90 Kelly 1994. Dawkins has proposed that our embodied selves are simply the mechanical replicators for genes, 'survival machines'.

91 (Although Eliot chose to locate that in the sixteenth century.) An alienation from our agency leading to what Jameson (1991: 44) terms postmodern hyperspace – an 'alarming disjunction between the body and its built environment'.

92 Martindale, Chomsky, Fodor, Pinker, Sperry, Minsky, Gardner, Dennett, Edelman. And in the cybernetic and field models of 'systemic family therapy' which replace selves with flexible control systems akin to those of contemporary 'matrix management', 're-engineering' and 'total human resource management'.

93 As internalized parents or children, as underdogs, types, archetypes, potentials, personalities, sub-personalities, voices, selves, subselves, possible selves, ego states, images, imagos, doubles, clusters, roles, parts, scripts, actors, figures, prototypes, polarities, schemas, subsystems (to take a few from Rowan 1990; compare Watkins and Johnson 1982, Crabtree 1988 or the homunculi of the *Beano* comic's Numskulls).

94 Rowan 1990: 89.

95 *Ibid.*: 44, 80

96 From Number Six and The Stranger Within to the more personalized Little Monica and Charlene, etc. (Ross 1994). (Compare the earlier Jungian archetypes: The Shadow, The Trickster, The Wise Old Woman.)

97 Bourdieu 1984. Akin to therapeutic interpretations of 'eating disorders' (Chapter 5, this volume), 'obesity' is recognized as a regressive psychological defence against MPD which can only prevent full exploitation of one's variant identities (e.g. Ross 1994).

98 Brown 1997; Heelas 1997.

99 Micale 1995: 238. He favours 'a model of influence that is neither one- nor two-directional but *circular*. In France during the nineteenth century in particular, the three primary cultures of hysteria were medical, literary and religious. To stress the isolation and exclusion of these cultures in the public sphere is to ignore deeper, underlying cultural and discursive continuities ...' (*ibid.*: 238–9, his emphasis). Not merely did decadent and positivist literature both draw on the pervasive image of the hysteric in the Salpêtrière but the current biomedical category of the hysterical personality (note 12) perhaps owes less to empirical observation than to *Madame Bovary*, in which Flaubert explored his own identification with 'male hysteria', the diagnosis he had himself been offered by his physicians for his physical complaints (*ibid.*).

100 For example, Terr 1994, Ross 1994. The cover of Terr's book offers a photomontage of a woman grotesquely spreadeagled across railway tracks as a malevolent dark engine speeds towards her open body.

101 'Penelope' fights back against a critical review of her therapist's book: '... belittling, sarcasm and a snide one-sentence summary of 15 years of my hard work on my dreams ... weight loss, exercise regimens I still adhere to, a major promotion and success as a superior at work, and a dramatic decrease in depression are all the proof I need ... ' (*New York Review of Books*, corr., 12 January 1995: 44).

102 Ellenberger 1993: 239–305.

103 Many of which (law in cyberspace, cyberterm, cyberpunk) are concerned with the problems of netlaw, netpolice, 'the migration of "real" world persons into the matrix', 'new laws will have to be specially created for cyberspace and its inhabitants' (downloaded 18/1/1994 texts). A recent scandal involved a man adopting a female identity on the Web to offer advice to sexually traumatized females (Ess 1996), while some apparent 'participants' in MUDs (Multiple User Domains) are only computational 'chatterbots', i.e. programs. Conceptualizations of cyberspace vary from simply 'being in' a particular directory in a file system to the consensual virtual reality of head-mounted stereographic displays, haptic datagloves, 3-D Rooms, MUDs and so on: 'a parallel universe created and sustained by the world's computers and communication lines [of] alter-human agency' (Benedict 1991: 1); 'wherever electricity runs with intelligence' (*ibid.*: 2). Cyberpunk literature offers cyberspace as a parallel world occupied simultaneously by the undead, wraiths, shades, androids, clones and orishas, entered in dreams or through VR technology, psychoactive drugs or spirit possession (Tomas 1989). Its global matrix is the sum of all human culture, the world of disembodied memes, Karl Popper's World 3. Artificial Life proposes a not dissimilar *hyperlife* – 'that library which contains all things alive, all vivisystems, anything bucking the second law of thermodynamics, all future and all past arrangements of matter capable of open-ended evolution' (Kelly 1994). Beyond epistemological fancy, there are

commercial proposals for transgressing body forms in prosthetic *netsex* when VR technology enters the Net around 2002.

104 Presaged in Charles Reich's 'consciousness III', Lifton's 'Protean Man' (Peacock 1975).

105 Castel 1986.

106 Ross 1994:148.

107 Marx's *Eighteenth Brumaire* exemplifies the transformation of industrial power into individual power.

108 Interview on *Complete Obsession*, BBC2 television, 17 February 2000.

109 Hausman 1997.

110 Dyer 2000.

Chapter 11

1 Cf. Berger and Luckmann 1966: 1; Merskey 1992.

2 Merskey 1992.

3 AA and ME groups argue that alcoholism and myalgic encephalomyelitis are biological diseases whose causation is independent of moral agency. (Indeed something resembling aboulia is recommended in the various '12-step programmes' such as AA in which past actions are exposed as compelled by the addictive power: the first step acknowledges one's complete powerlessness over the disease, the second affirms the existence of an external Higher Power, the third turns your will over to Him: a psychology which is effective through denying it is a psychology.) The rigid dualism of self-help therapies cuts across the psychodynamic recognition of unconscious motivations, and thus rather offends therapists who work with 'psychosomatic' illness; but it is probably acceptable to most hospital doctors for whom psychological explanations come close to a personalistic explanation of frank 'malingering' or at least some slightly more sympathetic but still pejorative notion of 'hysteria', 'functional overlay', 'supratentorial', 'subjective', 'self-deception' or even – since medical students now study sociology – 'abnormal illness behaviour'. In any event, not real in that the phenomenon cannot be naturalistically specified.

4 Or indeed spirit possession if we favour a robust materialism, although here, until the 1980s, claims to physical reality were seldom advanced excepting biblical fundamentalists and some enthusiasts for extra-sensory perception. Hypnosis and other altered states of consciousness cannot be specified (Needham 1981) by any characteristic physiological pattern, although there appear some consistent changes in cortical and subcortical activity and in endorphin regulation. Physical and sexual abuse have both been associated with fairly non-specific changes in endocrine response (Brown 1991).

5 Although this was the clinical understanding appropriate at *that* moment; in Dennett's (1991) terms perhaps an Orwellian (retrospectively reconstructed) rather than a Stalinist (contemporaneously reconstructed) memory. Similarly, advocates of the idea of 'false memory' now argue they were previously mistaken in having once recognized their experience of MPD as spontaneous (Jaroff 1993; Hacking 1995). Or as both Young (1995) and Hacking (1995) put it in the terminology of American pragmatism (cf. my own text), they were 'real' but not 'true'. Hacking notes that both protagonists and antagonists of

MPD take memory as a direct mirror of the actual experiences of a body and its mind. Yet 'memory' is also a social practice in what is selected, prohibited or fantasized.

6 As Kenny (1981) puts it.

7 Reviewed in Spanos 1989.

8 Kenny 1986; Needham 1981.

9 The 'strong programme' in the sociology of science, but see Bloor's position.

10 Wittgenstein 1958.

11 E.g. Friesen 1991; Kenny 1986.

12 And society may be either an organism or just a convenient grouping of human subjects.

13 An ironic dualism (Littlewood 1993b) recalling Ribot's 'two-sided phenomenon'. The very distinction may be seen as naturalistic (the distinction in our experience and actions between the involuntary and voluntary nervous system, as Merleau-Ponty noted, or in rather different cognitive domains distinguishing animate from inanimate) or else as personalistic (given by cultural history as, for example, the dualism of Judaeo-Christianity refined in the mechanical science of the Renaissance). The antinomy in the form I have expressed it may be traced to Kant (or indeed to Descartes' *First Meditation*).

14 Baconian and eighteenth-century medicine proposed fluid reciprocity or 'rapports' between the physical and the moral (Williams 1994): what Mauss (1950: 121) called connecting cogs, Searle's (1984: 4) gap-filling efforts; currently towards one side, Dennett's (1991) multiple drafts, Edelman's (1992) neuronal group selection, Churchland's eliminative materialism or Crick's recent claim to locate free will in the anterior cingulate sulcus; towards the other perhaps Fodor's (1992) intentional realism, Penrose, Davidson, Lakoff, Hacking, McGinn, Nagel and Eccles. The monistic claims of 'embodiment' by moral philosophers and phenomenologists in practice follow a personalistic line; as do feminist assertions of a potential affinity between the new information technologies and women's lives (e.g. Haraway 1991: Ch. 8, although in a later chapter she appears to argue for a situated and embodied objectivism). There is no shortage of gushing popular religious or philosophical claims to 'holistically' transcend what is taken as an arid Western dichotomy (such as the proposed 'unity of techne and logos' in the cyberaesthetics of Kroker (1992)) but inter-theoretical reductionism has proved unconvincing here except perhaps in the field of Artificial Life. Similarly, anthropological objections to dialectic and interactionist solutions tend to replicate something very similar (e.g. Toren 1993: 462); as do our critiques of a biomedical rationality opposed to the 'life worlds' of patients. Rather, I would argue that both biomedicine and the idiom of 'experience' currently favoured in anthropology are simply systematizations of our two everyday modes of thought; whether these are to be considered 'additive' or discrepant remains a continuing problem for anthropology and psychiatry (Littlewood 1991, 2001) as for jurisprudence (see Eigen 1985).

15 See note 36, Chapter 9.

16 Cf. Jameson 1991. And recently on the physical reality of possessing spirits and extraterrestrial life forms (Ross 1994; Mack 1994), although some

enthusiasts have now retreated to an idea of psychological truth (Ross 1995).
17 And on the rights (if not yet responsibilities) of children, animals and the
    natural world (Littlewood 1993b). Andrea Dworkin has recently proposed
    that sexually abused women should sue pornographers for damages. A unitary
    and contractual individual taken as the given entity is one without an inherent
    social identity (Etzioni 1994), and empirical psychology has of course pursued
    its contrary project of delineating a Nature that exists independently of
    immediate sense perception.
18 (Or one's own body as other: Heelas 1981: 50.) Similarly from feminism
    (Haraway 1991) and computer simulations of the development of hierarchical
    social institutions (Doran *et al.* 1994). The alter of MPD seems to have shifted
    from an external to an increasingly internal locus, yet Brazilian psychiatrists
    sympathetic to Kardecism treat MPD with exorcism (as do some American
    psychiatrists: e.g. Ross 1994) or even by encouraging the individual to become
    a spirit medium (Krippner 1987). American alters may on occasion gain some
    sort of concrete existence as separate physical beings yet *within* the host body:
    'Several times Jed [an alter] was beaten up inside by the Evil One [another
    alter], and told us that his face was bruised and swollen' (Ross 1994: 129). We
    might map these shifting locations along the parameters of aboulia versus
    intentional agency, and self versus other (cf. Heelas 1981):

                                    O
          Aliens   Social roles
          Twins   Accessed computers
          Spirits   'Faces',
                                      'Masks'
A ──────────────────────────┼────────────────────────── **I**
          Souls   Virtual reality
          Sub-personalities   Personality
          Archetypes
          Faculties, Emotions
                                    S

And plot contemporary medical evaluation of the traumatic memory along the
aetiological dimensions of naturalistic–personalistic and internal–external:

                                    E
          Mistaken   Induced
N ──────────────────────────┼────────────────────────── **P**
          True   Fabricated
                                    I

19 Hofstadter (1995), Mulhern's (1994) 'conspiracy thinking', Kenny's (1986:
    26) 'paradoxes of liberty' (presaged in Augustinian psychology's opening to
    the reality of witchcraft (Matthews 1992)). Enhanced competitive individu-
    alism is the bedfellow of paranoia, whether we understand this competition in

terms of psychology (Kluckholn, Field) or social action (Lienhardt, Macfarlane). Underlying this the phenomenologists' pursuit of how the flux of pre-objective experience becomes congealed into hypostasized entities – a process surprisingly ignored by anthropologists interested in cognition but which has been variously addressed by Marxists, Kleinians and Buddhists through the idea that nominal categories are less ambiguous than experiencing, and under problematic circumstances we essentialize a fetishized world following our own objectification of ourselves as physical entities (Mead 1934); early in life we start to perceive the world as nominalized – as composed of entities of recurrent invariance (Schutz 1976; Laughlin *et al.* 1993) whose interaction then inevitably becomes problematic (Lukacs); such reification is fundamental to social categorization, giving ontological status to the experienced world (Lakoff 1987). And in the same way, since Kant we reify our awareness and action in the world as consciousness, as something like an entity.

20 Strozier 1994.

21 And there are a number of psychophysiological studies which demonstrate consistent differences in 'suggestible hypnotic subjects' in their predisposing personality, cerebral evoked potentials, proneness to sleepwalking, daydreaming, fantasy-induced orgasm and so on (Wilson and Barber 1981; Brown 1991). Trance and other altered states of consciousness have been likened to temporal lobe epilepsy, with similar alterations in limbic and adrenal function (Erwin *et al.* 1988).

22 Kenny 1986: 17. 'Multiple personality disorder is a little girl imagining the abuse is happening to someone else' (Ross 1994: vi).

23 Who may have the same (late dynastic Egypt) or very similar (contemporary Afro-Caribbean) names. As Dennett (1991: 422) puts it, a situation of one mind in two bodies: like incest or nationalism, an elision of personal identities, the inverse of multiple personality. As the structuralist might observe, incest (not enough differentiation) is the classic trauma for multiple personality (too much differentiation).

24 Boureau (1991) argues that fourteenth-century witch-finding enthusiasms were facilitated by a theological debate on somnambulism which favoured a post-Thomist idea of something like moral dissociation – and thus a potential vulnerability to daytime displacement of aspects of the self in frank possession.

25 Akin to the projective identification of psychoanalysis. Bloch (1993), employing Lienhardt's (1961) Dinka material, argues that an initial experience of something like alien penetration may be followed by an attempt at catharsis which, if unsuccessful, then leads to identification with the intrusion as 'possession' or assimilation.

26 Parfit 1984. Or whether the American convict executed for a murder after twenty years in prison is the 'same person'.

27 Well illustrated in Firth's account of Tikopian responses to solitary canoe trips: heroic self-transformations by men, dangerous cries for help by women (p. 41). We might argue more embodied analogies between subjectivity and experienced 'space' and 'constraint': Bourguignon (1973: Intro.) describes trance and vision quests (Chapter 9, note 65) as more plausible for nomadic

societies, possession trance for settled communities; and the cognitions of female sexuality and pregnancy make possible idioms of spirit penetration and an unfolding cosmology (Littlewood 1996b). Compare cyberspace: male surfing but female occupation of MUDs and other habitats (Ess 1996).

28   Spanos 1989; Hacking 1992a.

29   Kirmayer 1992a.

30   Littlewood 1991.

31   Geertz 1968; Lewis 1969; Chapter 3, this volume; cf. Kapferer 1979.

32   I have never seen a patient with Munchausen's Syndrome (p. 66, where the individual is recognized by others as deliberately inducing illness through self-mutilation, opening scabs, swallowing metal objects) who was not in some way 'genuinely hurt' at being accused of malingering; and contrariwise in every patient with a non-psychotic illness, the illness comes over to me as, in a sense, 'motivated'.

33   Ellenberger 1966.

34   Ardener 1975.

35   Lewis 1970.

36   Of the sort suggested in Giddens 1992. The litigiousness of both protagonists and antagonists in the MPD drama seems to have prevented any serious ethnography. Beyond the therapists' own reports we know little of the clinical encounter, the everyday life of the patient, their changes in domestic or social circumstances of the sort of detail so well presented for women's possession in Northern Sudan by Boddy (1989).

37   Walker 1993; Ross 1994; Wright 1993; Wyllie 1973. I forget who first proposed the canard that the history of Western psychotherapy is that of the increasing attribution of malevolence to parents.

38   E.g. Walker 1993. A common justification of MPD is that any sort of sexual abuse was once disbelieved yet the phenomenon is now clinically accepted: therefore Satanic abuse similarly (e.g. Sinason 1994). 'The study of trauma in sexual and domestic life becomes legitimate only in a context that challenges the subordination of women and children. Advances in the field occur only when they are supported by a political movement powerful enough to legitimate an alliance between investigators and patients and to counteract the ordinary social processes of silencing and denial' (the American protagonist of 'recovered memories' Judith Herman (1992) quoted in Crews 1994: 54). The accusations of the MPD therapists are directed not only at the sexual abuser but at any denier of the act: as with witchcraft accusations, restitution necessitates public repentance by the perpetrator who must be named by the victim to ensure full recovery (e.g. Herman 1992).

39   Larose 1977; Boddy 1989; similarly Stoller 1989.

40   Ellenberger 1970. Nineteenth-century double consciousness – the bland innocent girl revealing her capricious secondary personality – recalls Romantic moral dualism. (Reading clinical accounts such as those of Prince suggests that it was only in the course of extended hypnotic interventions that the vaguer third or fourth personalities began to emerge as the doctor tried to isolate the real self.) By contrast, Ross notes approvingly that 29 per cent of North American alters are now immediately diagnosed as demons, this in a

society where more than 2 per cent of the population currently report that they have been demonically possessed, half accept the existence of angels, and a third anticipate being raptured by Jesus into the skies (Ross 1994: 124; Strozier 1994: 5).

41 Recognized by MPD therapists as 'polyfragmentation' (Ross 1994). As if, pursuing our overinterpretation, with the 'self as a reflexive project' (Giddens 1992), late modernity cannot sustain the attempt to unify time, place and action, yet cannot cope with flux alone, and retreats to concretized but inconstant simulacra of an embodied individual: akin to what Felix Guattari termed the 'reterritorializations' of post-colonial consciousness. Participants in electronic conferencing still tend to act as if in Cartesian space, and place considerable importance on establishing the sex and other physical character-istics of their fellow participants.

42 In their terms, no longer as sufferers or even victims but as witnesses: cf. the politics of Survivor Syndrome in Israel or of therapy groups for the survivors of torture, or of the post-Soviet group Memorial. Similarly in the literature of a number of survivors' groups, the problem is presented as real but falsely 'contained' by powerful interests, including medicine, and the group's task is to enable the survivor to 'find a voice' – public expression and accusation. (The now common term 'survivor' was popularized in psychotherapy by Bruno Bettelheim to refer to the people liberated from Nazi concentration camps.)

43 On Western sickness as counterhegemonic see Littlewood 1991. Showalter (1993) details our strange 'modern marriage of hysteria and feminism', hysteria now affirmed as a proto-feminism, a bodily and linguistic resistance to male power: an image perhaps not so dissimilar from that offered by nineteenth-century medicine itself (and later, Surrealism: Breton 1964) which took the hysteric as the quintessential female, neurasthenia being the consequence of, if not the impetus for, female emancipation (Kenny 1986: 136: see also Micale 1995: 66–88). Bryan Turner (1984) argues that hysteria provided the Victorian bourgeoisie with a 'solution' for the sexuality of their unmarried women in a period of delayed marriage: as with MPD or other illnesses, I think a deprivation model which takes women's bodies simply as objects of (and resistance to) male commodification is inadequate but we might consider the very material consequences of serial monogamy for contemporary working-class women in America. Boddy (1989) notes that to read Northern Sudanese possession trance simply as women's symbolic 'resistance' to men misses very real bodily insults which are readily recognized by the women themselves (cf. Kapferer 1979), yet their trancing is primarily an ambiguous accommodation and a self-sustaining aesthetic. Her account of the zár spirits entering a body 'sealed' earlier through the scarring of infibulation recalls MPD's interesting elision of Christian fundamentalism with feminist politics in affirming American women's control over their body entrances and margins (*Our Bodies, Ourselves*). Double consciousness and hysteria have certainly been portrayed as a battle between woman and doctor, both in the military metaphors of the clinician and in recent feminist revisions. The doctor triumphed only partially with the triumph of psychoanalysis: as

hysteria's elusive mimesis of physical disease was banished to a realm of unconscious fantasy, the patient was left to string out her 'resistances' for as extended a period of combative therapy as possible. On the gender conflict model, the recovery of lost memories of abusive power, now validated by courts and scientists, seems to reframe and challenge the terrain towards a closer mimesis of the actual dominance itself. Mulhern, however, has argued that MPD initially represented a depoliticization of feminist social work in which during the 1980s socialism was discarded in favour of therapy.

44 Compare Lewis 1969, Janzen 1978, Sharp 1993. And who then attract recruits who had not previously regarded themselves as sufferers but who now revise their biographies. I recall Trinidadian doctors' complaints that AA in Port-of-Spain was an Asian business fraternity whose members had no real drink problems (similarly Britain: Anon. 1994).

45 Owen 1989. Cf. the current term for a New Age medium whose profession emerges out of her affliction with MPD – *trance channeller*; similarly among contemporary groups for survivors of civil disasters or for relatives of the victims, who transcend their suffering through advocating greater safety controls and public accountability.

Bibliography

Aber, S. M. and Higgins, P. M. (1982) The natural history and management of the loin pain/haematuria syndrome. *British Journal of Urology*, *54*, 613–15

Ackernecht, E. (1943) Psychopathology, primitive medicine and primitive culture. *Bulletin of the History of Medicine*, *14*, 30–68

Adams, A. E. (1993) Dyke to dyke: ritual reproduction at a U. S. men's military college. *Anthropology Today*, *9*, No.5, 3–6

Adler, M. (1986) *Drawing down the Moon*. 2nd rev. edn. Boston: Beacon Press

African Rights (1993) *The Nightmare Continues . . . Abuses Against Somali Refugees in Kenya*. London: African Rights

African Rights (1995) *Rwanda: Death, Despair and Defiance*. Rev. edn. London: African Rights

African Watch Women's Rights Project (1993) *Seeking Refuge, Finding Terror: The Widespread Rape of Somali Women Refugees in North Eastern Kenya*. New York: Africa Watch

Ainsworth, M. D. S., Blehar, M., Waters, E. and Wall, S. (1977) *Patterns of Attachment: Observations in the Strange Situation and at Home*. Hillsdale, NJ: Erlbaum

Aldridge-Morris, R. (1989) *Multiple Personalities: An Exercise in Deception*. London: Erlbaum

Alexander, Y. (1979) Terrorism, the media and the police. In D. Kupperman and D. Trent, *Terrorism: Threat, Reality and Response*. Stanford: Stanford University Press

Al-Issa, I. (1980) *The Psychopathology of Women*. New Jersey: Prentice Hall

Allen, H. (1984) Psychiatry and the construction of the feminine. In P. Miller and N. Rose (eds), *The Power of Psychiatry*. Cambridge: Polity Press

Allison, D. and Roberts, M. (1998) *Disordered Mother or Disordered Diagnosis? Munchausen by Proxy Syndrome*. London: Academic Press

Allodi, F. (1988) Your neighbour's son. *Social Science and Medicine*, *26*, 1173–4

Alloway, R. and Bebbington, P. (1987) The buffer theory of social support: a review of the literature. *Psychological Medicine*, *17*, 91–108

Ammar, S., Attia, S., Douki, S., Tabone, B. and Hamoyda, C. (1980) A propos de la recrudescence des délires mystiques en Tunisie. *Information Psychiatrique*, *56*, 711–15

Amnesty International (1993a) *India: Reporting of Rape in 1993*. London: Amnesty International

Amnesty International (1993b) *Rape and Sexual Abuse by Armed Forces*. London: Amnesty International

Amnesty International (1993c) *Bosnia-Herzegovina: Rape and Sexual Abuse by Armed Forces*. London: Amnesty International

Amnesty International (1996) *Prescription for Change: Health Professionals and the Exposure of Human Rights Violations*. London: Amnesty International

Amnesty International Medical Commission (1989) *Doctors and Torture*. London: Bellew

Andrews, J. D. W. (1966) Psychotherapy of phobias. *Psychological Bulletin*, 66, 455–80

Anon. (1993) The psychiatrist and the siege. *Psychiatric Bulletin*, 17, 129–34

Anon. (1994) AA's potent network. *The Times*, supplement, 5 February, 1

Apter, M. J. (1982) *The Experience of Motivation: The Theory of Psychological Reversals*. London: Academic Press

Ardener, E. (1989) The problem of dominance. In E. Ardener, *The Voice of Prophecy and Other Essays*, (ed.) M. Chapman. Oxford: Blackwell. (Orig. pub. in 1981)

Ardener, S. (1975) Sexual insult and female militancy. In S. Ardener (ed.), *Perceiving Women*. London: Dent

Ardener, S. (1981) The nature of women in society. In S. Ardener (ed.), *Defining Females*. London: Croom Helm

Arens, W. (1986) *The Original Sin: Incest and Its Meaning*. New York: Oxford University Press

Armstrong, D. (1987) Theoretical tensions in biopsychosocial medicine. *Social Science and Medicine*, 25, 1213–18

Armstrong, J. G. and Loewenstein, R. J. (1990) Characteristics of patients with multiple personality and dissociative disorders on psychological testing. *Journal of Nervous and Mental Disease*, 178, 448–54

Aronowitz, R. A. (1998) *Making Sense of Illness: Science, Society and Disease*. Cambridge: Cambridge University Press

Arya, D. K. (1992) Anorexia nervosa: is the conflict hypothesis valid? *British Journal of Psychiatry*, 100, 131–2

Ashton, J. R. and Donnan, S. (1981) Suicide by burning as an epidemic phenomenon: an analysis of 82 deaths and inquests in England and Wales in 1978–79. *Psychological Medicine*, 11, 735–9

Asia Watch and Physicians for Human Rights (1993) *Rape in Kashmir: A Crime of War*. New York: Asia Watch

Austen, J. (1814) *Mansfield Park*. 1970 edn. London: Dent

Austin, R. (1977) *Sex and Gender in the Future of Nursing*. *Nursing Times* Occasional Papers, 4 August, 1 September

Baier, A. (1994) *Moral Prejudice: Essays on Ethics*. Cambridge: Cambridge University Press

Bailey, S. D. (1972) *Prohibitions and Restraints in War*. London: Oxford University Press

Bancroft, J., Hawton, K., Simkin, S., Kingston, B., Cumming, C. and Whitwell, D. (1979) The reasons people give for taking overdoses. *British Journal of Medical Psychology*, 52, 353–65

Banks, C. G. (1992) 'Culture' in culture-bound syndromes: the case of anorexia nervosa. *Social Science and Medicine*, 34, 867–84

Barrell, J. (1991) *The Infection of Thomas De Quincey: A Psychopathology of Imperialism*. New Haven: Yale University Press

Barth, F. (1969) *Ethnic Groups and Boundaries*. Boston: Little, Brown.

Bartholomew, R. E. (1990) Ethnocentricity and the social construction of 'mass hysteria'. *Culture, Medicine and Psychiatry*, *14*, 455–94

Bartov, O. (1996) *Murder in Our Midst: The Holocaust, Industrial Killing, and Representation*. New York: Oxford University Press

Basinger, J. (1994) *A Woman's View: How Hollywood Spoke to Women 1930–1960*. London: Chatto and Windus

Bastide, R. (1972) *Le Reve, la transe et la folie*. Paris: Flammarion

Bateson, G. (1958) *Naven*. 2nd edn. Stanford: Stanford University Press

Beard, G. M. (1881) *American Nervousness: Its Causes and Consequences*. New York: Putnam

Beattie, J. (1977) Spirit mediumship as theatre. *Royal Anthropological Institute News*, No.20, 1–6

Beck, V. (1992) *Risk Society: Towards a New Modernity*. London: Sage

Bell, C. and Newby, H. (1976) Husbands and wives: the dynamics of the differential dialectic. In D. L. Barker and S. Allen (eds), *Dependence and Exploitation in Work and Marriage*. London: Longman

Bell, R. M. (1985) *Holy Anorexia*. Chicago: University of Chicago Press

Bellah, R. N., Madsen, R., Sullivan, W. M., Swidler, A. and Tipton, S. M. (1985) *Habits of the Heart: Individualism and Commitment in American Life*. Berkeley: University of California Press

Bemporad, J. R., Ratey, J. J., O'Driscoll, G. and Doehler, M. L. (1988) Hysteria, anorexia and the culture of self-denial. *Psychiatry*, *51*, 96–103

Benedict, M. (ed.) (1991) *Cyberspace: First Steps*. Cambridge, MA: MIT Press

Benedict, R. (1935) *Patterns of Culture*. London: Routledge and Kegan Paul

Benedict, R. (1946) *The Chrysanthemum and the Sword: Patterns of Japanese Culture*. Boston: Houghton Mifflin

Berger, J. (1971) *Ways of Seeing*. Harmondsworth: Penguin

Berger, P. and Luckmann, T. (1966) *The Social Construction of Reality*. New York: Doubleday

Best, G. (1994) *War and Law since 1945*. Oxford: Oxford University Press

Bharati, A. (1985) The self in Hindu thought and action. In A. J. Marsella, G. DeVos and F. L. K. Hsu (eds), *Culture and Self: Asian and Western Perspectives*. London: Tavistock

Bhattacharyya, D. P. (1986) *Pagalami: Ethnopsychiatric Knowledge in Bengal*. New York: Syracuse University Press

Birnbaum, K. (1923) Der Aufbau der Psychosen. Trans. as 'The making of a psychosis'. In S. R. Hirsch and M. Shepherd (eds), *Themes and Variations in European Psychiatry*. Bristol: Wright

Bleuler, E. (1911) *Dementia Praecox*. New York: International Universities Press

Bloch, M. (1991) Language, anthropology and cognitive science. *Man* (n.s.), *26*, 183–98

Bloch, M. (1993) *Prey into Hunter: The Politics of Religious Experience*. Cambridge: Cambridge University Press

Bloch, M. and J. (1980) Women and the dialectics of nature. In C. MacCormack and M.

Strathern (eds), *Nature, Culture and Gender*. Cambridge: Cambridge University Press

Blovin, S. F. and Blovin, M. (1988) Inbreeding avoidance behaviours. *Trends in Ecology and Evolution*, 3, 230–3

Boddy, J. (1989) *Wombs and Alien Spirits: Women, Men and the Zar Cult in Northern Sudan*. Madison: University of Wisconsin Press

Boehm, C. (1983) *Montenegrin Social Organisation and Values*. New York: AMS Press

Bolter, J. D. (1986) *Turing's Man: Western Culture in the Computer Age*. Harmondsworth: Penguin

Boorse, C. (1975) On the distinction between disease and illness. *Philosophy and Public Affairs*, 5, 49–68

Boskind-Lodahl, M. (1976) Cinderella's stepsisters: a feminist perspective on anorexia nervosa and bulimia. *Signs (Journal of Women in Culture and Society)*, 2, 342–56

Boudin, J. (1857) *Traité de géographie et de statistiques médicales et des maladies endémiques*. Paris: Baillière

Bourdieu, P. (1977) *Outline of a Theory of Practice*. Cambridge: Cambridge University Press

Bourdieu, P. (1984) *Distinction: A Social Critique of the Judgement of Taste*. London: Routledge and Kegan Paul

Boureau, A. (1991) Satan et le dormeur: une construction de l'inconscient au Moyen Age. *Chimère*, 14, 41–61 (Cited in Mulhern 1994)

Bourguignon, E. (ed.) (1973) *Religion, Altered States of Consciousness and Social Change*. Colombus: Ohio State University Press

Bourguignon, E. (1978) Spirit possession and altered states of consciousness: the evolution of an enquiry. In G. D. Spindler (ed.), *The Making of Psychological Anthropology*. Berkeley: University of California Press

Bowlby, J. (1982) *Attachment and Loss, Vol.1. Attachment*. Rev. edn. Harmondsworth: Penguin

Boyers, R. and Orrill, R. (eds) (1972) *Laing and Anti-Psychiatry*. (Orig. pub. in *Salmagundi*, special issue 1971) Harmondsworth: Penguin

Bradbury, J. (1992) *The Medieval Siege*. Woodbridge: Boydell

Bradford, J. and Balmaceda, K. (1983) Shoplifting: is there a specific psychiatric syndrome? *Canadian Journal of Psychiatry*, 28, 248–53

Braude, S. (1991) *First Person Plural: Multiple Personality and the Philosophy of Mind*. London: Routledge

Breton, A. (1964) *Nadia*. Rev. edn. Paris: Gallimard

Brigham, A. (1832) *Remarks on the Influence of Mental Cultivation upon Health*. Hartford: Huntingdon

British Medical Journal (1970) Correspondence: 17, 31 January, 7, 21 February, et seq.

British Medical Journal (1971) Editorial: Suicide Attempts, 2, 483

Broverman, I. D., Broverman, D. M., Clarkson, F. E., Rosenkrantz, P. S. and Vogel, S. R. (1970) Sex role stereotypes and clinical judgements of mental health. *Journal of Consulting and Clinical Psychology*, 34, 1–7

Brown, B. G. (1988) The BASK model of dissociation. *Dissociation*, 1, 4–18

Brown, J. C. (1986) *Immodest Acts: The Life of a Lesbian Nun in Renaissance Italy*. New York: Oxford University Press

Brown, M. F. (1997) *The Channeling Zone: American Spirituality in an Anxious Age.* Cambridge, MA: Harvard University Press

Brown, P. (1991) *The Hypnotic Brain: Hypnotherapy and Social Communication.* New Haven: Yale University Press

Brown, P. J. and Konner, M. (1981) An anthropological perspective on obesity. *Annals of the New York Academy of Sciences,* 499, 29–46

Brown, T. M. (1985) Descartes, dualism and psychosomatic medicine. In W. F. Bynum, R. Porter and M. Shepherd, *The Anatomy of Madness,* Vol.1. London: Tavistock

Brownmiller, S. (1975) *Against Our Will: Men, Women and Rape.* London: Secker and Warburg

Brumberg, J. J. (1988) *Fasting Girls: The Emergence of Anorexia Nervosa as a Modern Disease.* Cambridge, MA: Harvard University Press

Bryan, C. D. (1995) *Close Encounters of the Fourth Kind: Alien Abduction and UFOs: Witnesses and Scientists Report.* London: Weidenfeld and Nicolson

Buckle, H. T. (1856) *The History of Civilisation in England.* London: J. W. Parker and Son.

Buglass, D. D., Clarke, J., Henderson, A. S., Kreitman, N. and Priestly, A. S. (1977) A study of agoraphobic housewives. *Psychological Medicine,* 7, 73–86

Bulik, C. M. (1987) Eating disorders in immigrants. *International Journal of Eating Disorders,* 6, 133–41

Burne, J. (1993) One person, many people. *The Times,* 4 March

Bynum, C. W. (1987) *Holy Feast and Holy Fast: The Religious Significance of Food to Medieval Women.* Berkeley: University of California Press

Bynum, C. W. (1988) Holy anorexia in modern Portugal. *Culture, Medicine and Psychiatry,* 12, 239–48

Byrne, R. and Whiten, A. (eds) (1988) *Machiavellian Intelligence: Social Expertise and the Evolution of Intellect in Monkeys, Apes and Humans.* Oxford: Clarendon Press

Campbell, A. and Gibbs, J. J. (eds) (1986) *Violent Transactions: The Limits of Personality.* Oxford: Blackwell

Campbell, B. (1988) *Unofficial Secrets: Child Sexual Abuse – the Cleveland Case.* London: Virago

Campbell, C. M., Langfield, H. S., McDougall, W., Roback, A. A. and Taylor, E. W. (eds) (1925) *Problems of Personality: Studies Presented to Dr Morton Prince.* London: Kegan Paul, Trench and Trubner

Canning, H. and Meyer, J. (1966) Obesity – its possible effect on college acceptance. *New England Journal of Medicine,* 275, 1172–4

Caramagno, T. C. (1992) *The Flight of the Mind: Virginia Woolf's Art and Manic-Depressive Illness.* Berkeley: University of California Press

Carothers, J. C. (1953) *The African Mind in Health and Disease.* Geneva: World Health Organization

Carothers, J. C. (1954) *The Psychology of Mau Mau.* Nairobi: Government Printers

Carpenter, M. (1978) The new managerialism and professionalism in nursing. In M. Stacey, M. Reid, C. Heath and R. Dingwall (eds), *Health and the Divisions of Labour.* London: Croom Helm.

Carr, J. E. (1978) Ethno-behaviourism and culture-bound syndromes: the case of amok. *Culture, Medicine and Psychiatry, 2,* 269–93

Carr, J. E. and Tan, E. K. (1976) In search of the true amok: amok as viewed within the Malay culture. *American Journal of Psychiatry, 133,* 1295–9

Carrithers, M., Collins, S. and Lukes, S. (1986) *The Category of the Person: Anthropology, Philosophy, History.* Cambridge: Cambridge University Press

Casey, J. F. (1991) *The Flock.* London: Abacus

Caskey, N. (1986) Interpreting anorexia nervosa. In S. R. Suleiman (ed.), *The Female Body in Western Medicine.* Cambridge, MA: Harvard University Press

Cassell, J. (1986) Dismembering the images of God: surgeons, heroes, wimps and miracles. *Anthropology Today, 2,* No.2, 13–15

Cassell, J. (1987) Control, certitude and the 'paranoia' of surgeons. *Culture, Medicine and Psychiatry, 11,* 229–49

Castel, R. (1986) *Advanced Psychiatric Society.* Berkeley: California University Press

Chagnon, H. A. (1990) Reproductive and somatic conflicts of interest in the genesis of violence and warfare among tribesmen. In J. Has (ed.), *The Anthropology of War.* Cambridge: Cambridge University Press.

Chakraborty, A. and Banerji, G. (1975) Ritual, a culture-specific neurosis and obsessional states in Bengali culture. *Indian Journal of Psychiatry, 17,* 211–16

Chapman, S. (1979) Advertising and psychotropic drugs: the place of myth in ideological reproduction. *Social Science and Medicine, 13,* 751–64

Chernin, K. (1985) *The Hungry Self: Women, Eating and Identity.* New York: Times Books

Chesler, P. (1974) *Women and Madness.* London: Allen Lane

Cheyne, G. (1734) The English Malady. In V. Skultans (1979), *English Madness: Ideas on Insanity 1580–1890.* London: Routledge and Kegan Paul

Chiles, J. A., Strosahl, K. D., McMurtray, L. and Lineham, M. M. (1985) Modelling effects on suicidal behaviour. *Journal of Nervous and Mental Disease, 173,* 479–81

Chodoff, P. and Lyons, H. (1955) Hysteria, the hysterical personality and hysterical conversion. *American Journal of Psychiatry, 114,* 734–40

Choudry, I. Y. and Mumford, D. B. (1992) A pilot study of eating disorders in Mirpur (Pakistan) using an Urdu version of the Eating Attitudes Test. *International Journal of Eating Disorders, 11,* 243–51

Chrisman, N. J. (1982) Anthropology and nursing: an exploration of adaptation. In N. J. Chrisman and T. W. Maretzki (eds), *Clinically Applied Anthropology.* Dordrecht: Reidel

Chrisman, N. J. and Maretzki, T. W. (eds) (1982) *Clinically Applied Anthropology.* Dordrecht: Reidel

Christensen, S. M. and Turner, D. R. (eds) (1993) *Folk Psychology and the Philosophy of Mind.* Hillsdale: Erlbaum

Ciba Foundation Symposium (1993) *Chronic Fatigue Syndrome.* Chichester: Wiley

Cicchetti, D., Cummings, E. M., Greenberg, M. T. and Marvin, R. S. (1990) An organisational perspective on attachment beyond infancy. In M. T. Greenberg, D. Cicchetti and E. M. Cummings (eds), *Attachment in the Preschool Years.* Chicago: University of Chicago Press

Clark, C. B. (1977) A preliminary report on weaning among chimpanzees of the

Gombe National Park. In S. Chevalier-Skolnikoff and F. E. Poirier (eds), *Primate Biosocial Development*. New York: Garland

Clarke, B. (1975) *Mental Disorder in Earlier Britain*. Cardiff: University of Wales Press

Clarke, W. C. (1973) Temporary madness as theatre: wild-man behaviour in New Guinea. *Oceania*, *43*, 198–214

Coburn, J. and Ganong, L. (1989) Bulimic and non-bulimic college females' perceptions of family adaptability and family cohesion. *Journal of Advanced Nursing*, *14*, 27–33

Cohn, N. (1993) *Cosmos, Chaos and the World to Come: The Ancient Roots of Apocalyptic Faith*. New Haven: Yale University Press

Coker, C. (1994) *War and the Twentieth Century: A Study of War and Modern Consciousness*. London: Brassey's

Collingwood, R. G. (1945) *The Idea of Nature*. Oxford: Clarendon Press

Cooper, D. (1967) *Psychiatry and Anti-Psychiatry*. London: Tavistock

Cooper, J. E. and Sartorius, N. (1977) Cultural and temporal variations in schizophrenia: a speculation on the importance of industrialisation. *British Journal of Psychiatry*, *130*, 50–5

Cooperstock, R. (1971) Sex differences in the use of mood-modifying drugs: an explanatory model. *Journal of Health and Social Behaviour*, *12*, 238–44

Cooperstock, R. and Sims, M. (1971) Mood-modifying drugs prescribed in a Canadian city: hidden problems. *American Journal of Public Health*, *61*, 1007–16

Corin, E. (1978) La possession comme langage dans un contexte de changement socio-culturel. *Anthropologie et Société*, *2*, 53–74

Corin, E. and Bibeau, G. (1980) Psychiatric perspectives in Africa: 2. *Transcultural Psychiatric Research Review*, *17*, 205–34

Count, E. W. (1967) The lactation complex: a phylogenetic consideration of the mammalian mother–child symbiosis. *Homo*, *18*, 38–54

Crabtree, A. (1988) *Multiple Man: Explorations in Possession and Multiple Personality*. New York: Praeger

Cranshaw, R. (1983) The object of the centrefold. *Block*, No.9, 26–33

Crapanzano, V. (1973) *The Ḥamadsha: A Study in Moroccan Ethnopsychiatry*. Berkeley: University of California Press

Crapanzano, V. and Garrison, V. (eds) (1977) *Case Studies in Spirit Possession*. New York: Wiley

Crary, J. and Kwinter, S. (1992) *Zone 6: Incorporations*. Boston: MIT Press

Crawford, M. and Wessely, S. (1998) The changing epidemiology of deliberate self-harm: implications for service provision. *Health Trends*, *30*, No.3, 66–8

Crews, F. (1994) The revenge of the repressed. *New York Review of Books*, 17 November, 54–60; 1 December, 49–58; corr. 12 January, 1995, 44–8

Crisp, A. H. (1980) *Anorexia Nervosa: Let Me Be*. London: Academic Press

Csordas, T. J. (1992) The affliction of Martin: religious, clinical and phenomenological meaning in a case of demonic oppression. In A. D. Gaines (ed.), *Ethnopsychiatry: The Cultural Construction of Professional and Folk Psychiatries*. New York: SUNY Press

Culpin, M. (1953) Neurasthenia in the tropics. *The Practitioner*, *85*, 146–54

Daily Express (1984) Wives hooked on illness are giving GPs a headache. 27 March

Daily Telegraph (1984) Waitresses told 'Slim or lose jobs'. 13 August

Das, V. (1996) Language and body: transactions in the construction of pain. *Daedalus*, Winter, 67–92

Davidson, P. and Jackson, C. (1985) The nurse as a survivor: delayed post-traumatic stress reaction and cumulative trauma in nursing. *International Journal of Nursing Studies*, 22, 1–13

Davis, C. and Yager, J. (1992) Transcultural aspects of eating disorders: a critical literature review. *Culture, Medicine and Psychiatry*, 16, 377–94

Dawkins, R. (1982) *The Extended Phenotype*. San Francisco: Freeman

De Jong, J. T. V. M. (1987) *A Descent into African Psychiatry*. Amsterdam: Royal Tropical Institute

De Man, P. (1979) *Allegories of Reading*. New Haven: Yale University Press

De Salvo, L. A. (1989) *Virginia Woolf: The Impact of Childhood Sexual Abuse on Her Life and Work*. Boston: Beacon Press

De Swaan, A. (1981) The politics of agoraphobia. *Theory and Society*, 10, 359–85

Deleuze, G. and Guattari, F. (1984) *Anti-Oedipus: Capitalism and Schizophrenia*. London: Athlone

Dennett, D. (1989) *The Intentional Stance*. Cambridge: MIT Press

Dennett, D. C. (1991) *Consciousness Explained*. New York: Little, Brown & Co.

Dennett, D. C. (1992) Multiple personality (corr.). *London Review of Books*, 9 July, 4

Deutsch, E. (ed.) (1991) *Culture and Modernity*. Cambridge: Harvard University Press

Devereux, G. (1951) *Reality and Dream: Psychotherapy of a Plains Indian*. New York: International Universities Press

Devereux, G. (ed.) (1953) *Psychoanalysis and the Occult*. New York: International Universities Press

Devereux, G. (1956) The normal and abnormal: the key problem in psychiatric anthropology. (Reprinted, trans. in Devereux 1970)

Devereux, G. (1970) *Essais d'ethnopsychiatrie générale*. Paris: Gallimard

DeVos, G. (1985) Dimensions of the self in Japanese culture. In A. J. Marsella, G. DeVos and F. L. K. Hsu (eds), *Culture and Self: Asian and Western Perspectives*. London: Tavistock

Di Nicola, V. F. (1990) Anorexia multiforme: self-starvation in historical and cultural context. Part 2: Anorexia nervosa as a culture-reactive syndrome. *Transcultural Psychiatric Research Review*, 27, 245–86

Diethelm, O. (1971) *Medical Dissertations of Psychiatric Interest Printed before 1750*. Basle: Karger

Doi, T. (1971) *Amae no Kozo*. Trans. as *The Anatomy of Dependence*. Tokyo: Kodansha

Dolan, B. M. (1991) Cross-cultural aspects of anorexia nervosa and bulimia nervosa: a review. *International Journal of Eating Disorders*, 10, 67–78

Dolan, B. and Ford, K. (1991) Binge eating and dietary restraint: a cross-cultural analysis. *International Journal of Eating Disorders*, 10, 343–53

Dolan, B., Lacey, J. H. and Evans, C. (1990) Eating behaviour and attitudes to weight and shape in British women from three ethnic groups. *British Journal of Psychiatry*, 157, 523–8

Donzelot, J. (1977) *La Police des familles*. Paris: Minuit

Doran, J., Palmer, M., Gilbert, N. and Mellors, P. (1994) The EOS Project: modelling Upper Palaeolithic social change. In N. Gilbert and J. Doran (eds), *Simulating Societies*. London: UCL Press

D'Orban, P. T. (1976) Child stealing: a typology of female offenders. *British Journal of Criminology*, *16*, 275–81

Dunbar, G. C., Perera, M. H. and Jenner, F. A. (1989) Patterns of benzodiazepine use in Great Britain as measured by a general population survey. *British Journal of Psychiatry*, *155*, 836–41

Durkheim, E. (1898) La prohibition de l'inceste et ses origines. *L'Année Sociologique*, *1*, 1–70

Durkheim, E. (1901) *Les Règles de la méthode sociologique*. Rev. edn. Paris: Alcan

Durkheim, E. (1951) *Suicide*. New York: Free Press (Orig. pub. 1897)

Dyer, C. (2000) Surgeon amputated healthy legs. *British Medical Journal*, *320*, 332

Easlea, B. (1980) *Witch Hunting, Magic and the New Philosophy: An Introduction to Debates of the Scientific Revolution 1450–1750*. Sussex: Harvester Press

Eastwell, H. D. (1982) Voodoo death and the mechanism for the despatch of the dying in East Arnhem. *American Anthropologist*, *84*, 5–18

Eckman, P. (1980) Biological and cultural contributions to body and facial movement in the expression of emotions. In A. O. Rorty *et al.* (eds), *Explaining Emotions*. Berkeley: University of California Press

Edelman, G. M. (1992) *Bright Air, Brilliant Fire: On the Matter of the Mind*. New York: Basic Books

Edwards. S. (2000) Will women be the losers after provocation ruling? *The Times*, 21 March, 16

Ehrenseich, B. (1997) *Blood Rites: Origins and History of the Passions of War*. New York: Metropolitan Books

Eibl-Eibelsfeldt, I. (1979) *The Biology of Peace and War*. London: Thames and Hudson

Eigen, J. P. (1985) Intentionality and insanity: what the eighteenth century juror heard. In W. F. Bynum, R. Porter and M. Shepherd (eds), *The Anatomy of Madness*, Vol.2. London: Tavistock

Eisenberg, L. (1977) Disease and illness: distinctions between professional and popular ideas of sickness. *Culture, Medicine and Psychiatry*, *1*, 9–23

Elder, G. H. (1969) Appearance and education in marriage mobility. *American Sociological Review*, *34*, 516–33

Eliade, M. (1964) *Shamanism: Archaic Techniques of Ecstasy*. Princeton: Princeton University Press

Ellenberger, H. F. (1966) The pathogenic secret and its therapeutics. *Journal of the History of the Behavioural Sciences*, *2*, 29–42

Ellenberger, H. F. (1970) *The Discovery of the Unconscious: The History and Evolution of Dynamic Psychiatry*. London: Allen Lane

Ellenberger, H. F. (1993) *Beyond the Unconscious: Essays*. Princeton: Princeton University Press

Emmerche, C. (1994) *The Garden in the Machine: The Emerging Science of Artificial Life*. Princeton: Princeton University Press

Entralgo, P. L. (1969) *Doctor and Patient.* London: Weidenfeld and Nicolson

Erickson, M. T. (1989) Incest avoidance and familial bonding. *Journal of Anthropological Research, 45,* 267–91

Erickson, M. T. (1993) Rethinking Oedipus: an evolutionary perspective on incest avoidance. *American Journal of Psychiatry, 150,* 411–15

Ernst, W. (1991) *Mad Tales from the Raj: The European Insane in British India.* London: Routledge

Erwin, F. R., Palmour, R. M., Murphy, B. E. P., Prince, R. and Simons, R. C. (1988) The psychobiology of trance: physiological and endocrine correlates. *Transcultural Psychiatric Research Review, 25,* 267–84

Ess, C. (ed.) (1996) *Philosophical Perspectives on Computer-mediated Communication.* New York: SUNY Press

Estroff, S. E. (1981) *Making It Crazy: An Ethnography of Psychiatric Clients in an American Community.* Berkeley: University of California Press

Etzioni, A. (1994) *The Spirit of Community: Rights, Responsibilities and the Communitarian Agenda.* New York: Crown

Evans-Pritchard, E. E. (1940) *The Nuer.* Oxford: Oxford University Press

Fabrega, H. (1979) Neurobiology, culture and behaviour disturbances. *Journal of Nervous and Mental Disease, 167,* 467–74

Faiola, A. (1997) Argentine teens desperate to be thin. *Washington Post,* reprinted in *Guardian Weekly,* 20 July, 17

Falk, P. (1994) *The Consuming Body.* London: Sage

Fanon, F. (1952) *Peau noire. Masques blancs.* Paris: Seuil

Fanon, F. (1965) *The Wretched of the Earth.* London: MacGibbon and Kee

Feldman, W., Feldman, E. and Goodman, J. T. (1988) Culture versus biology: children's attitudes towards thinness and fatness. *Paediatrics, 81,* 190–4

Field, M. J. (1960) *Search for Security: An Ethno-Psychiatric Study of Rural Ghana.* London: Faber and Faber

Firth, R. (ed.) (1957) *Man and Culture: An Evaluation of the Work of Bronislaw Malinowski.* London: Routledge and Kegan Paul

Firth, R. (1961) Suicide and risk-taking in Tikopia society. *Psychiatry, 2,* 1–17

Firth, R. (1967) Ritual and drama in Malay spirit mediumship. *Comparative Studies in Society and History, 9,* 190–207

Firth-Cozens, J. (1987) Emotional distress in junior house officers. *British Medical Journal, 295,* 533–6

Fisher, L. E. (1985) *Colonial Madness: Mental Health in the Barbadian Social Order.* New Brunswick: Rutgers University Press

Flint, M. (1975) The menopause: reward or punishment? *Psychosomatics, 16,* 161–3

Fodor, I. (1976) The phobic syndrome in women. In V. Franks and V. Burtle (eds), *Women in Therapy.* New York: Bruner/Mazel

Fodor, J. A. (1992) *A Theory of Content and Other Essays.* Cambridge: MIT Press

Foreward, S. and Buck, C. (1981) *Betrayal of Innocence.* Harmondsworth: Penguin

Fortes, M. (1983) *Rules and the Emergence of Society.* London: Royal Anthropological Institute

Foucault, M. (1973) *The Birth of the Clinic: An Archaeology of Medical Perception.* London: Tavistock

Fox, R. (1980) *The Red Lamp of Incest*. New York: Dutton
Frake, C. O. (1980) *Language and Cultural Description*. Stanford: Stanford University Press
Frank, J. (1961) *Persuasion and Healing: A Comparative Study of Psychotherapy*. New York: Schocken
Freud, S. (1913) *Totem and Taboo*. 1950 edn. London: Hogarth Press
Freud, S. (1946) Fragment of an analysis of a case of hysteria. *Collected Works: Vols 55–6*. London: Hogarth
Friesen, J. G. (1991) *Uncovering the Mystery of Multiple Personality Disorder*. San Bernadino: Here's Life Publishers
Fromm, E. (1977) *The Anatomy of Human Destructiveness*. London: Routledge and Kegan Paul
Fry, W. F. (1962) The marital context of an anxiety syndrome. *Family Process, 14*, 245–52
Fuller, R. (1982) *Mesmerism and the American Cure of Souls*. Philadelphia: Philadelphia University Press
Fumaroli, M. (1996) A Scottish Voltaire: John Barclay and the character of nations. *Times Literary Supplement*, 19 January, 16–17
Furnham, A. and Alibhai, N. (1983) Cross-cultural differences in the perception of female body shapes. *Psychological Medicine, 13*, 829–37
Furnham, A. and Hume-Wright, A. (1992) Lay theories of anorexia nervosa. *Journal of Clinical Psychology, 48*, 20–36

Gabbard, K. and Gabbard, G. O. (1987) *Psychiatry and the Cinema*. Chicago: University of Chicago Press
Gabe, J. and Williams, P. (1986) *Tranquillisers: Social, Psychological and Clinical Perspectives*. London: Tavistock
Gaines, A. D. (1979) Definitions and diagnoses: cultural implications of psychiatric help-seeking and psychiatrists' definitions of the situation in psychiatric emergencies. *Culture, Medicine and Psychiatry, 3*, 381–418
Gaines, A. D. (1982a) Knowledge and practice: anthropological ideas and psychiatric practice. In N. J. Chrisman and T. W. Maretzki, *Clinically Applied Anthropology*. Dordrecht: Reidel
Gaines, A. D. (1982b) Cultural definition, behaviour and the person in American psychiatry. In A. J. Marsella and G. M. White, *Cultural Conceptions of Mental Health and Therapy*. Dordrecht: Reidel
Gaines, A. D. (1992) *Ethnopsychiatry*. New York: SUNY Press
Ganser, S. J. M. (1897) A peculiar hysterical state. Trans. In S. R. Hirsch and M. Shepherd (eds) (1974), *Themes and Variations in European Psychiatry*. Bristol: Wright
Gardner, R. (1989) Psychiatric syndromes as infrastructure for intra-specific communication. In M. R. A. Chance (ed.), *Social Fabrics of the Mind*. Hillsdale: Erlbaum
Garner, D. M. and Garfinkel, P. E. (1980) Socio-cultural factors in the development of anorexia nervosa. *Psychological Medicine, 10*, 747–56
Garner, D. M., Garfinkel, P. E., Schwart, D. M. and Thompson, M. M. (1990) Cultural expectations of thinness in women. *Psychological Reports*, 483–91

Gaskell, S. (1860) On the want of better provisions for the labouring and middle classes when attacked or threatened with insanity. *Journal of Mental Science*, 6, 321–7

Gauld, A. (1992) *A History of Hypnotism*. Cambridge: Cambridge University Press

Gavish, L., Hofmann, J. E. and Getz, L. L. (1984) Sibling recognition in the prairie vole. *Animal Behaviour*, 23, 362–6

Gaze, H. (1987) Men in nursing. *Nursing Times*, 83, No.20, 25–7

Geddes, D. and Smith, I. (1986) Solicitor will not fight extradition. *The Times*, 1 October

Geertz, C. (1966) Religion as a cultural system. In M. Banton (ed.), *Anthropological Approaches to Religion*. London: Tavistock

Geertz, C. (1968) The impact of the concept of culture on the concept of man. In Y. A. Cohen (ed.), *Man in Adaptation*. Chicago: Aldine

Geertz, C. (1983) 'From the native's point of view': on the nature of anthropological understanding. In C. Geertz, *Local Knowledge*. New York: Basic Books

Geertz, C. (1984) *Local Knowledge: Further Essays in Interpretative Anthropology*. New York: Basic Books

Geertz, C. (1986) Anti-anti-relativism. *American Anthropologist*, 86, 263–78

Geertz, H. (1968) Latah in Java: a theoretical paradox. *Indonesia*, 3, 93–104

Gellner, E. (1992) *Post-modernism, Reason and Religion*. London: Routledge

German, A. A. (1972) Aspects of clinical psychiatry in sub-Saharan Africa. *British Journal of Psychiatry*, 121, 461–79

Geyer, F. and Van der Zouwen, J. (1986) *Sociocybernetic Paradoxes: Observation, Control and Evolution of Self-Steering Systems*. London: Sage

Gibbens, T. C. N. and Prince, J. (1962) *Shoplifting*. London: Institute for the Study and Treatment of Delinquency

Giddens, A. (1985) *The Constitution of Society: Outline of the Theory of Structuration*. Cambridge: Polity Press

Giddens, A. (1992) *The Transformation of Intimacy: Sexuality, Love and Eroticism in Modern Societies*. Cambridge: Polity Press

Gilman, C. P. (1892) *The Yellow Wallpaper*. 1988 edn. London: Virago

Gilman, S. L. (1985) *Difference and Pathology: Stereotypes of Sexuality, Race and Madness*. Ithaca: Cornell University Press

Gilman, S. L. (1993) *Freud, Race and Gender*. Princeton: Princeton University Press

Ginsberg, G. P. (1971) Public conceptions and attitudes about suicide. *Journal of Health and Social Behaviour*, 12, 200–1

Girard, R. (1977) *Violence and the Sacred*. Baltimore: Johns Hopkins University Press

Girard, R. (1978) *To Double Business Bound: Essays on Literature, Mimesis and Anthropology*. Baltimore: Johns Hopkins University Press

Gledhill, R. (1988) Alcohol and advertising. *The Times*, 26 October

Gluckman, M. (1954) *Rituals of Rebellion in South East Africa*. Manchester: Manchester University Press

Goffman, E. (1971) *Relations in Public: Microstudies of the Public Order*. New York: Basic Books

Goldstein, A. J. (1970) Some aspects of agoraphobia. *Behaviour Therapy and Experimental Psychiatry*, 1, 305–9

Goldstein, A. J. (1973) Learning theory insufficiency in understanding agoraphobia. *Proceedings of the European Association of Behaviour Therapy.* Munich: Schwarzenberg

Goldstein, A. J. and Chambless, D. L. (1978) A re-analysis of agoraphobic behaviour. *Behaviour Therapy, 9,* 47–59

Gonyo, B. (1987) Genetic sexual attraction. *American Adoption Congress Newsletter, 4,* No.2, 1

Good, B. J. and Good, M.-J. D. (1981) The meaning of symptoms: a cultural hermeneutic model for clinical practitioners. In L. Eisenberg and A. Kleinman (eds), *The Relevance of Social Science for Medicine.* Dordrecht: Reidel

Good, B. J. and Good, M.-J. D. (1988) Ritual, the state and the transformation of emotional discourse in Iranian society. *Culture, Medicine and Psychiatry, 12,* 43–63

Good, B. J. and Good, M.-J. D. (1992) The comparative study of Graeco-Islamic medicine: the integration of medical knowledge into local symbolic contexts. In C. Leslie and A. Young (eds), *Paths to Asian Medical Knowledge.* Berkeley: University of California Press

Goodall, J. (1986) *The Chimpanzees of Gombe.* Cambridge, MA: Harvard University Press

Goody, J. (1982) *Cooking, Cuisine and Class.* Cambridge: Cambridge University Press

Goody, J. (1990) *The Oriental, the Ancient and the Primitive: Systems of Marriage and the Family in the Pre-Industrial Societies of Eurasia.* Cambridge: Cambridge University Press

Goody, J. (1995) *The Expansive Moment: Anthropology in Britain and Africa 1918– 1970.* Cambridge: Cambridge University Press

Gottlieb, A. (1988) American premenstrual tension: a mute voice. *Anthropology Today, 4,* 10–13

Gould, M. S. and Shaffer, D. (1986) The impact of suicide in television movies: evidence of imitation. *New England Journal of Medicine, 315,* 690–4

Gove, W. R. and Tudor, J. F. (1973) Adult sex roles and mental illness. *American Journal of Sociology, 78,* 812–35

Gray, J. J., Ford, K. and Kelly, L. M. (1987) The prevalence of bulimia in a Black College population. *International Journal of Eating Disorders, 6,* 733–40

Gremillion, H. (1992) Psychiatry as social ordering: anorexia nervosa, a paradigm. *Social Science and Medicine, 35,* 57–71

Grimm, V. A. (1997) *From Fasting to Feasting: Attitudes to Food in Late Antiquity.* London: Routledge

Grinberg, L. and Grinberg, R. (1984) A psychoanalytic study of migration: its normal and pathological aspects. *Journal of the American Psychoanalytical Association, 32,* 13–38

Grottanelli, C. (1982) The King's grace and the helpless woman: a comparative study of the stories of Ruth, Charilla, Sita. *History of Religions, 22,* 1–24

Grottanelli, C. (1985) Archaic forms of rebellion and their religious background. In B. Lincoln (ed.), *Religion, Rebellion and Revolution.* London: Macmillan

Gruenberg, E. (1957) Socially shared psychopathology. In A. H. Leighton (ed.), *Explorations in Social Psychiatry.* New York: Basic Books

Guelke, A. (1995) *The Age of Terrorism and the International Political System.* London: Tauris

Guinan, M. E. (1993) War crimes of the twentieth century: rape as a strategy. *Journal of the American Medical Women's Association, 48,* 59

Guzder, J. and Krishna, M. (1991) Sita-Shakti: cultural paradigms for Indian women. *Transcultural Pychiatric Research Review, 28,* 257–301

Hacking, I. (1991a) The making and molding of child abuse. *Critical Inquiry, 17,* 253–8

Hacking, I. (1991b) Two souls in one body. *Critical Inquiry, 17,* 838–67

Hacking, I. (1992a) Multiple personality disorder and its hosts. *History of the Human Sciences, 5,* 3–31

Hacking, I. (1992b) Severals (Review of Braude 1991). *London Review of Books,* 22 June, 21–2

Hacking, I. (1995) *Rewriting the Soul: Multiple Personality and the Sciences of Memory.* Princeton: Princeton University Press

Hage, P. and Harary, F. (1983) *Structural Models in Anthropology.* Cambridge: Cambridge University Press

Hahn, R. A. (1985) Culture-bound syndromes unbound. *Social Science and Medicine, 21,* 165–80

Hahn, R. A. and Gaines, A. D. (eds) (1985) *Physicians of Western Medicine: Anthropological Approaches to Theory and Practice.* Dordrecht: Reidel

Hall, J. A. and Jarvie, I. C. (eds) (1992) *Transition to Modernity: Essays on Power, Wealth and Belief.* Cambridge: Cambridge University Press

Hallam, R. (1984) Agoraphobia: deconstructing a clinical syndrome. *Bulletin of the British Psychological Society, 3,* 337–40

Haller, J. S. (1970) The physician versus the Negro: medical and anthropological concepts of race in the nineteenth century. *Bulletin of the History of Medicine, 44,* 154–67

Hanson, V. D. (1989) *The Western Way of War.* Oxford: Oxford University Press

Haraway, D. (1989) *Primate Visions: Gender, Race and Nature in the World of Modern Science.* New York: Routledge

Haraway, D. (1991) *Simians, Cyborgs and Women: The Reinvention of Nature.* London: Free Association Books

Hardy, J. (1997) *Stalking: Towards a New Understanding.* Unpublished MSc thesis, University College London

Harlan, L. (1992) *Religion and Rajput Women: The Ethic of Protection in Contemporary Narratives.* Berkeley: University of California Press

Harré, R. (1983) *Personal Being: A Theory for Individual Psychology.* Oxford: Blackwell

Harré, R. (ed.) (1986) *The Social Construction of Emotions.* Oxford: Blackwell

Harrington, A. (1987) *Medicine, Mind and the Double Brain: A Study in Nineteenth-Century Thought.* Princeton: Princeton University Press

Harris, C. (1957) Possession 'hysteria' in a Kenyan tribe. *American Anthropologist, 59,* 1046–66

Harris, R. (1985) Murder under hypnosis in the case of Gabrielle Bompard: psychiatry in the courtroom in Belle Epoque Paris. In W. F. Bynum, R. Porter and M. Shepherd (eds), *The Anatomy of Madness*, Vol.2. London: Tavistock

Harvey, P. and Gow, P. (eds) (1994) *Sex and Violence: Issues in Representation and Experience*. London: Routledge

Has, J. (ed.) (1990) *The Anthropology of War*. Cambridge: Cambridge University Press

Hausman, B. L. (1997) *Changing Sex: Transsexualism, Technology and the Idea of Gender*. Durham: Duke University Press

Hawthorn, J. (1983) *Multiple Personality and the Disintegration of Literary Character*. New York: St Martin's Press

Hawton, K., Marsack, P. and Fagg, J. (1981) The attitudes of psychiatrists to deliberate self-poisoning: comparison with physicians and nurses. *British Journal of Medical Psychology*, 54, 341–8

Hawton, K., O'Grady, J., Osborne, M. and Cole, D. (1982) Adolescents who take overdoses: their characteristics, problems and contacts with helping agencies. *British Journal of Psychiatry*, 140, 118–25

Hayashi, S. and Kimura, T. (1978) Effects of exposure to males on sexual preference in female mice. *Animal Behaviour*, 26, 290–5

Heelas, P. (1981) The model applied: anthropology and indigenous psychologies. In P. Heelas and A. Lock (eds), *Indigenous Psychologies: The Anthropology of the Self*. London: Academic Press

Heelas, P. (1997) *The New Age Movement: The Celebration of the Self and the Sacralisation of Modernity*. Oxford: Blackwell

Heelas, P. and Lock, A. (eds) (1981) *Indigenous Psychologies: The Anthropology of the Self*. London: Academic Press

Heim, M. (1994) *The Metaphysics of Virtual Reality*. Oxford: Oxford University Press

Helman, C. (1985) Disease and pseudo-disease: a case history of pseudo-angina. In R. A. Hahn and A. D. Gaines (eds), *Physicians of Western Medicine: Anthropological Approaches to Theory and Practice*. Dordrecht: Reidel

Henderson, V. (1978) The concept of nursing. *Journal of Advanced Nursing*, 3, 113–30

Herdt, G. (1982) *Rituals of Manhood: Male Initiation in Papua New Guinea*. Berkeley: University of California Press

Herdt, G. (1984) *Ritualized Homosexuality in Melanesia*. Berkeley: University of California Press

Herman, J. L. (1992) *Trauma and Recovery*. New York: Basic Books

Hershman, P. (1977) Virgin and Mother. In I. M. Lewis (ed.), *Symbols and Sentiments: Cross-Cultural Studies in Symbolism*. London: Academic Press

Hilgard, E. R. (1977) *Divided Consciousness: Multiple Controls in Human Thought and Action*. New York: Wiley

Hobsbawm, E. (1994) *Age of Extremes: The Short Twentieth Century 1914–1991*. London: Michael Joseph

Hodes, M. (1990) Overdosing as communication: a cultural perspective. *British Journal of Medical Psychology*, 63, 319–33

Hofstadter, R. (1995) The paranoid style in American politics. In R. Hofstadter, *The Paranoid Style in American Politics and Other Essays*. New York: Knopf

Holland, D. C. (1992) How cultural systems become desire: a case study of American romance. In R. D'Andrade and C. Strauss (eds), *Human Motives and Cultural Models*. Cambridge: Cambridge University Press

Hollender, M. (1976) Hysteria: the culture-bound syndromes. *Papua New Guinea Medical Journal*, *19*, 24–9

Holmes, R. (1994) *Firing Line*. London: Pimlico

Holy, L. and Stuchlik, M. (1981) *The Structure of Folk Models*. London: Academic Press

Horn, M. (1993) Memories lost and found. *U.S. News and World Report*, 19 November, 52–63

Horton, R. (1983) Social psychologies: African and Western. In M. Fortes, *Oedipus and Job in West African Religion*. Cambridge: Cambridge University Press

Horwitz, A. V. (1977) The pathways into psychiatric treatment: some differences between men and women. *Journal of Health and Social Behaviour*, *18*, 169–78

Horwitz, A. V. (1982) *The Social Control of Mental Illness*. New York: Academic Press

Howard, M., Andreopoulos, G. J. and Shulman, M. R. (1995) *The Laws of War: Constraints on Warfare in the Western World*. New Haven: Yale University Press

Hubert, H. and Mauss, M. (1964) *Sacrifice: Its Nature and Function*. (1898) Trans. London: Cohen and West

Hudson, B. (1974) The families of agoraphobics treated by behaviour therapy. *British Journal of Sociology*, *4*, 51–9

Huenemann, R. L., Shapiro, L. R., Hampton, M. C. and Mitchell, B. W. (1966) A longitudinal study of gross body composition and the association with food and activity in a teenage population. *American Journal of Clinical Nutrition*, *18*, 325–38

Hughes, C. C. (1985) Culture-bound or construct-bound? The syndromes and DSM-III. In R. C. Simons and C. C. Hughes (eds), *The Culture-bound Syndromes: Folk Illnesses of Psychiatric and Anthropological Interest*. Dordrecht: Reidel

Hughes, R. (1992) *Culture of Complaint: The Fraying of America*. Oxford: Oxford University Press

Human Rights Watch (1994) *Easy Prey: Child Soldiers in Liberia*. New York: Human Rights Watch

Human Rights Watch (1995) *Global Report on Women's Human Rights*. New York: Human Rights Watch

Human Rights Watch/Africa (1990) *Shattered Lives: Sexual Violence during the Rwandan Genocide and Its Aftermath*. New York: Holt

Human Rights Watch/Asia (1995) *Rape for Profit: Trafficking of Nepali Girls and Women to India's Brothels*. New York: Holt

Humphrey, N. and Dennett, D. C. (1989) Speaking for ourselves: an assessment of multiple personality disorder. *Raritan*, *9*, 68–98

Hutnik, N. (1991) *Ethnic Minority Identity: A Social Psychological Perspective*. Oxford: Clarendon Press

Hutt, R. (1985) *Chief Nursing Officer Career Profiles: A Study of Backgrounds*. Brighton: Institute of Management Studies

Ilen, C. and Gardwin-Gill, G. S. (1994) *Child Soldiers: The Role of Children in Armed Conflict*. Oxford: Clarendon Press

Immigration and Refugee Board (1993) *Women in Sri Lanka*. Ottawa: IRF

Independent (1996) Shame of Bosnia's raped PoWs. 28 April, 7.

Ingelby, D. (1982) The social construction of mental illness. In P. Wright and A. Treacher (eds), *The Problem of Medical Knowledge*. Edinburgh: Edinburgh University Press

Ingold, T. (1986) *The Appropriation of Nature: Essays on Human Ecology and Social Relations*. Manchester: Manchester University Press

Ingold, T. (1989) Culture and the perception of the environment, 6th EIDOS Workshop on Culture Understandings of the Environment. London: School of Oriental and African Studies (Rev. ms. 1990)

Jack, R. (1992) *Women and Attempted Suicide*. Hove: Erlbaum

Jack, R. and Williams, J. M. G. (1994) Attribution and intervention in self-poisoning. *British Journal of Medical Psychology*, 64, 359–73

Jackson, J. H. (1884) *Croonian Lectures on the Evolution and Dissolution of the Nervous System*. Cambridge: Cambridge University Press

Jahoda, G. (1982) *Psychology and Anthropology*. London: Academic Press

James, C. W. B. (1963) Psychology and gynaecology. In A. Cloge and A. Bourne (eds), *British Gynaecological Practice*. London: Heinemann

James, D. and Hawton, K. (1985) Overdoses: explanations and attitudes in self-poisoners and significant others. *British Journal of Psychiatry*, 146, 481–5

Jameson, F. (1991) *Postmodernism, or, The Cultural Logic of Late Capitalism*. London: Verso

Janet, P. (1925) *Psychological Healing*. London: Allen and Unwin

Janzen, J. M. (1978) *The Quest for Therapy: Medical Pluralism in Lower Zaire*. Berkeley: University of California Press

Janzen, J. M. (1979) Drums anonymous: towards an understanding of structures of therapeutic maintenance. In M. De Vries *et al.* (eds), *The Use and Abuse of Medicine*. New York: Praeger

Jaroff, L. (1993) Lies of the mind. *Time*, 29 November, 56–61

Jaspers, K. (1923) *General Psychopathology*. 7th edn. 1958, trans. Manchester: Manchester University Press

Jaynes, J. (1990) *The Origin of Consciousness in the Breakdown of the Bicameral Mind*. 2nd edn. Boston: Houghton Mifflin

Jilek, W. G. (1982) *Indian Healing: Shamanic Ceremonialism in the Pacific Northwest Today*. Surrey (Canada): Hancock House

John XXI, Pope (1550) Folk remedies against madness. Trans. In R. Hunter and I. MacAlpine (eds), *Three Hundred Years of Psychiatry 1535–1860*. London: Oxford University Press

Johnson, C. L. and Johnson, F. A. (1983) A micro-analysis of senility: the response of the family and the health professionals. *Culture, Medicine and Psychiatry*, 7, 77–96

Johnson, M. (1987) *The Body in the Mind: The Bodily Basis of Meaning, Imagination and Reason*. Chicago: University of Chicago Press

Johnson, M. (1993) *Moral Imagination: Implications of Cognitive Science for Ethics*. Chicago: University of Chicago Press

Jones, E. (1924) Mother-right and the sexual ignorance of savages. Reprinted in E. Jones, *Psycho-myths Psycho-history: Essays in Applied Psychoanalysis*, 1974. New York: Stonehill

Jones, I. J. (1971) Stereotyped aggression in a group of Australian Western Desert Aborigines. *British Journal of Medical Psychology*, 44, 259–65

Jordanova, L. J. (1980) Natural facts: a historical perspective on science and sexuality. In C. MacCormack and M. Strathern (eds), *Nature, Culture and Gender*. Cambridge: Cambridge University Press

Jordanova, L. (1981) Mental illness, mental health. In Cambridge Women's Studies Collective (eds), *Women in Society*. London: Virago

Jukes, A. (1993) *Why Men Hate Women*. London: Free Association Books

Jung, C. G. (1930) Your Negroid and Indian behaviour. *Forum*, 83, 193–9

Kagan, D. (1996) *On the Origins of War and the Preservation of Peace*. London: Hutchinson

Kakar, S. (1978) *The Inner World: A Psychoanalytic Study of Childhood and Society in India*. Delhi: Oxford University Press

Kakar, S. (1988) Female identity in India. In R. Ghadially (ed.), *Women in India*. Delhi: Sage

Kalisch, B., Kalisch, P. and Scobey, M. (1983) *Images of the Nurse on Television*. Berlin: Springer

Kamphris, J. H. and Emmelkamp, P. M. S. (2000) Stalking: a contemporary challenge for forensic and clinical psychiatry. *British Journal of Psychiatry*, 176, 206–9

Kanitkar, H. (1994) 'Real true boys': moulding the cadets of imperialism. In A. Cornwall and N. Lindisfarne (eds), *Dislocating Masculinity: Comparative Ethnographies*. London: Routledge

Kapferer, B. (1979) Mind, self and other in demonic illness: the negation and reconstruction of self. *American Ethnologist*, 6, 110–33

Keegan, J. (1995) If you won't, we won't. *Times Literary Supplement*, 24 November, 11–12

Keen, D. (1996) War: what is it good for? In T. Allen, K. Hudson and J. Seaton (eds), *War, Ethnicity and the Media*. London: South Bank University

Keillor, G. (1993) *The Book of Guys*. London: Faber

Kelly, K. (1994) *Out of Control: The New Biology of Machines*. London: Fourth Estate

Kendell, R. E. (1975) The concept of disease and its implications for psychiatry. *British Journal of Psychiatry*, 122, 305–15

Kennedy, H. and Dyer, D. E. (1992) Parental hostage-takers. *British Journal of Psychiatry*, 160, 410–12

Kennedy, P. (1993) *Preparing for the Twenty-first Century*. London: HarperCollins.

Kenny, M. G. (1978) Latah: the symbolism of a putative mental disorder. *Culture, Medicine and Psychiatry*, 2, 209–31

Kenny, M. G. (1981) Multiple personality and spirit possession. *Psychiatry*, 44, 327–58

Kenny, M. G. (1983) Paradise lost: the latah problem revisited. *Journal of Nervous and Mental Disorders*, 171, 159–67

Kenny, M. G. (1986) *The Passion of Ansel Bourne: Multiple Personality in American Culture*. Washington: Smithsonian Institution Press

Kerrigan, J. (1996) *Revenge Tragedy: Aeschylus to Armageddon*. Oxford: Oxford University Press

Kiev, A. (1964) The study of folk psychiatry. In A. Kiev, *Magic, Faith and Healing*. New York: Free Press

Kiev, A. (1972) *Transcultural Psychiatry*. Harmondsworth: Penguin

Kilshaw, S. (2000) Gulf War Syndrome: The emergence, construction and moulding of a new disorder (ms.)

King, M. B. and Bhugra, D. (1989) Eating disorders: lessons from a cross-cultural study. *Psychological Medicine, 19*, 955–8

Kirmayer, L. J. (1992a) Social constructions of hypnosis. *International Journal of Clinical and Experimental Hypnosis, 11*, 276–300

Kirmayer, L. J. (ed.) (1992b) Trance and Possession Disorders in DSM-IV. *Transcultural Psychiatric Research Review, 29*, No.4, special issue

Klein, R. (1997) *Eat Fat*. London: Picador

Kleinman, A. (1986) *Social Origins of Distress and Disease: Depression, Neurasthenia and Pain in Modern China*. New Haven: Yale University Press

Kleinman, A. (1987) Anthropology and psychiatry: the role of culture in cross-cultural research on illness. *British Journal of Psychiatry, 151*, 447–54

Kleinman, A. (1988a) *The Illness Narratives: Suffering, Healing and the Human Condition*. New York: Basic Books

Kleinman, A. (1988b) *Rethinking Psychiatry: From Cultural Category to Personal Experience*. New York: Free Press

Kleinman, A. and Good, A. (eds) (1985) *Culture and Depression: Studies in the Anthropology and Cross-Cultural Psychiatry of Affect and Disorder*. Berkeley: University of California Press

Kobetz, R. W. (1975) Hostage incidents: the new police priority. *Police Chief*, May, 32–5

Koch, F. (1968) On 'possession' behaviour in New Guinea. *Journal of Polynesian Society, 77*, 135–46

Koch, K. E. (1972) *Christian Counselling and Occultism: The Counselling of the Psychically Disturbed and Those Oppressed Through Involvement in Occultism*. Grand Rapids: Kregel

Kraepelin, E. (1904) Vergleichende Psychiatrie. Trans. as 'Comparative Psychiatry'. In S. R. Hirsch and M. Shepherd (eds), *Themes and Variations in European Psychiatry*. Bristol: Wright

Kreitman, N. and Schreiber, M. (1979) Parasuicide in young Edinburgh women. *Psychological Medicine, 9*, 469–79

Kreitman, N., Smith, P. and Tan, E. S. (1970) Attempted suicide as language. *British Journal of Psychiatry, 116*, 465–73

Krippner, S. (1987) Cross-cultural approaches to multiple personality disorder: practices in Brazilian spiritism. *Ethos, 15*, 273–95

Krohn, A. (1978) *Hysteria: The Elusive Neurosis*. New York: International University Press

Kroker, A. (1992) *The Possessed Individual: Technology and Postmodernity*. London: Macmillan

Kroker, A. and Kroker, M. (1987) *Body Invaders: Panic Sex in America*. New York: St Martin's Press

Kupperman, D. and Trent, D. (1979) *Terrorism: Threat, Reality and Response*. Stanford: Stanford University Press

La Fontaine, J. (1981) The domestication of the savage male. *Man* (n.s.), *16*, 333–49

La Fontaine, J. (1988) Child sexual abuse and the incest taboo: practical problems and theoretical issues. *Man* (n.s.), *23*, 1–18

La Fontaine, J. (1990) *Child Sexual Abuse*. Cambridge: Polity

La Fontaine, J. (1994) *The Extent and Nature of Organised and Ritual Abuse*. London: HMSO

La Fontaine, J. (1998) *Speak of the Devil: Tales of Satanic Abuse in Contemporary England*. Cambridge: Cambridge University Press

Laber, J. (1993) Bosnia: questions about rape. *New York Review of Books*, 25 March, 3–6

Lacan, J. (1977) The significance of the phallus, In *Ecrits: A Selection*. London: Tavistock

Lakoff, G. (1987) *Women, Fire and Dangerous Things: What Categories Reveal about the Mind*. Chicago: University of Chicago Press

Lambek, M. (1981) *Human Spirits: A Cultural Account of Trance in Mayotte*. Cambridge: Cambridge University Press

Lambo, T. A. (1955) The role of cultural factors in paranoid psychoses among the Yoruba tribe. *Journal of Mental Science*, *101*, 239–66

Lane, H. (1988) *When the Mind Hears: A History of the Deaf*. Harmondsworth: Penguin

Langness, L. L. (1968) Hysterical psychosis in the New Guinea Highlands: a Bena Bena example. *Psychiatry*, *28*, 258–77

Langness, L. L. and Levine, H. G. (eds) (1986) *Culture and Retardation: Life Histories of Mildly Mentally Retarded Persons in American Society*. Dordrecht: Reidel

Larose, S. (1977) The meaning of Africa in Haitian vodu. In I. M. Lewis (ed.), *Symbols and Sentiments: Cross-Cultural Studies in Symbolism*. London: Academic Press

Lasch, C. (1978) *The Culture of Narcissism: American Life in an Age of Diminishing Expectations*. New York: Norton

Laubscher, B. J. F. (1937) *Sex, Custom and Psychopathology: A Study of South African Pagan Natives*. London: Routledge

Laughlin, C. D., McManus, J. and D'Aquili, E. G. (1993) *Brain, Symbol and Experience: Towards a Neurophenomenology of Human Consciousness*. New York: Columbia University Press

Lazarus, A. (1972) Phobias: broad spectrum behavioural views. *Seminars in Psychiatry*, *4*, 85–90

Leach, E. R. (1961) *Rethinking Anthropology*. London: Athlone

Leach, E. R. (1970) The epistemological background to Malinowski's empiricism. In R. Firth (ed.), *Man and Culture: An Evaluation of the Work of Bronislaw Malinowski*. London: Routledge and Kegan Paul

Leach, E. (1991) The social anthropology of marriage and mating. In V. Reynolds and J. Kellett (eds), *Mating and Marriage*. Oxford: Oxford University Press

Lears, T. J. (1983) From salvation to self-realisation: advertising and the therapeutic roots of the consumer culture, 1880–1930. In R. W. Fox and T. J. Lears (eds) *The Culture of Consumption*. New York: Random House

Lebra, W. P. (ed.) (1976) *Culture-bound Syndromes, Ethnopsychiatry and Alternate Therapies*. Honolulu: University of Hawaii Press

Lee, R. L. M. (1981) Structure and anti-structure in the culture-bound syndromes: the Malay case. *Culture, Medicine and Psychiatry*, 5, 233–48

Lee, S. (1996) Reconsidering the status of anorexia nervosa as a Western culture-bound syndrome. *Social Science and Medicine*, 42, 21–34

Lee, S., Hus, L. K. G. and Wing, Y. K. (1992) Bulimia nervosa in Hong Kong Chinese patients. *British Journal of Psychiatry*, 161, 545–51

Lee, S. and Kleinman, A. (2000) Suicide as resistance in Chinese society. In *Chinese Society: Change, Conflict and Resistance*. London: Routledge

Leff, J. (1990a) The 'new cross-cultural psychiatry': a case of the baby and the bathwater (editorial), *British Journal of Psychiatry*, 156, 305–7

Leff, J. (1990b) Correspondence. *British Journal of Psychiatry*, 157, 296

Leff, J., Wigg, N. N., Ghosh, A., Bedi, H., Menon, D. K., Kuipers, L., Korten, A., Ernberg, G., Day, R., Sartorius, N., Jablensky, A. (1987) Influence of relatives' expressed emotion on the course of schizophrenia in Chandigarh. *British Journal of Psychiatry*, 151, 166–73

Leslie, J. (1991) Suttee or sati: victim or victor? In J. Leslie (ed.), *Roles and Rituals for Hindu Women*. London: Pinter

Levine, S. (1980) Crime or affliction? Rape in an African community. *Culture, Medicine and Psychiatry*, 4, 151–65

Lévi-Strauss, C. (1949) *The Elementary Structures of Kinship*. 1969 edn. Boston: Beacon

Levy, S. (1994) *Artificial Life: The Quest for a New Creation*. London: Cape

Lewis, I. M. (1966) Spirit possession and deprivation cults. *Man*, 1, 307–29

Lewis, I. M. (1969) Spirit possession in Northern Somaliland. In J. Beattie and J. Middleton (eds), *Spirit Mediumship and Society in Africa*. London: Routledge and Kegan Paul

Lewis, I. M. (1970) A structural approach to witchcraft and spirit possession. In M. Douglas (ed.), *Witchcraft Confessions and Accusations*. London: Tavistock

Lewis, I. M. (1971) *Ecstatic Religion: An Anthropological Study of Spirit Possession and Shamanism*. Harmondsworth: Penguin

Lewis-Fernández, R., González, C. A., Griffith, E. E. H., Littlewood, R. and Castillo, R. (1993) Dissociative disorders. In J. E. Mezzich *et al.*, *Revised Cultural Proposals for DSM-IV* (Unpublished report by the NIMH-Sponsored Group on Culture and Diagnosis submitted to the DSM-IV Task Force)

Lewontin, R. C. (1983) Gene, organism and environment. In D. S. Bendall (ed.), *Evolution from Molecules to Men*. Cambridge: Cambridge University Press

Lewontin, R. C., Rose, S. and Kamin, L. J. (1984) *Not in Our Genes: Biology, Ideology and Human Nature*. New York: Pantheon

Lienhardt, G. (1961) *Divinity and Experience: The Religion of the Dinka*. Oxford: Clarendon Press

Lifton, R. J. (1986) *The Nazi Doctors: A Study of the Psychology of Evil*. London: Macmillan

Littlewood, R. (1980) Anthropology and psychiatry: an alternative approach. *British Journal of Medical Psychology*, 53, 213–24

Littlewood, R. (1984) The individual articulation of shared symbols. *Journal of Operational Psychiatry*, 15, 17–24

Littlewood, R. (1985) An indigenous conceptualisation of reactive depression in Trinidad. *Psychological Medicine*, 15, 275–81

Littlewood, R. (1986) Russian dolls and Chinese boxes: an anthropological approach to the implicit models of comparative psychiatry. In J. Cox (ed.), *Transcultural Psychiatry*. London: Croom Helm

Littlewood, R. (1988) From vice to madness: the semantics of naturalistic and personalistic understandings in Trinidadian local medicine. *Social Science and Medicine*, 27, 129–48

Littlewood, R. (1991) Artichokes and entities: or, how new is the new cross-cultural psychiatry? *Transcultural Psychiatric Research Review*, 28, 343–56

Littlewood, R. (1992a) Psychiatric diagnosis and racial bias: empirical and interpretive approaches. *Social Science and Medicine*, 34, 141–9

Littlewood, R. (1992b) DSM-IV and culture: is the classification internationally valid? *Psychiatric Bulletin*, 16, 257–61

Littlewood, R. (1992c) Humanism and engagement in a metapsychiatry. *Culture, Medicine and Psychiatry*, 16, 395–405

Littlewood, R. (1992d) Towards an inter-cultural therapy. In J. Kareem and R. Littlewood (eds), *Inter-Cultural Therapy: Themes, Interpretations and Practice*. Oxford: Blackwell

Littlewood, R. (1993a) Ideology, camouflage or contingency? Racism in British psychiatry. *Transcultural Psychiatric Research Review*, 30, 243–90

Littlewood, R. (1993b) *Pathology and Identity: The Work of Mother Earth in Trinidad*. Cambridge: Cambridge University Press

Littlewood, R. (1993c) Culture-bound syndromes: cultural comments. In J. E. Mezzich, A. Kleinman, H. Fabrega and D. Parron (eds), *Working Papers for the DSM-IV Cultural Committee*. New York: American Psychiatric Press

Littlewood, R. (1994) Verticality as the idiom for mood and disorder: a note on an eighteenth-century representation. *British Medical Anthropology Review*, (n.s.), 2:1, 44–8

Littlewood, R. (1996a) Ethnopsychiatry. In A. Barnard and J. Spencer (eds), *Encyclopaedic Dictionary of Social and Cultural Anthropology*. London: Routledge

Littlewood, R. (1996b) 'Moments of Creation': Pregnancy and Parturition as Cosmological Idiom. Fyssen Symposium on Culture and the Uses of the Body, Paris

Littlewood, R. (2001) *Religion, Agency, Restitution*. Oxford: Oxford University Press

Littlewood, R. and Dein, S. (1994) The effectiveness of myths: religion and healing among the Lubavitch of Stamford Hill. *Culture, Medicine and Psychiatry*, 19, 339–83

Littlewood, R. and Lipsedge, M. (1982) *Aliens and Alienists: Ethnic Minorities and Psychiatry*. Harmondsworth: Penguin. 3rd rev. edn, 1993. London: Routledge

Littlewood, R. and Lipsedge, M. (1987) The Butterfly and the Serpent: culture, psychopathology and biomedicine. *Culture, Medicine and Psychiatry*, 11, 289–335

Lloyd, S. E. R. (1990) *Demystifying Mentalities*. Cambridge: Cambridge University Press

Lock, M. (1992) The fragile Japanese family: narratives about individualism and the post-modern state. In C. Leslie and A. Young, *Path to Asian Medical Knowledge*. Berkeley: University of California Press

Lock, M. (1993) *Encounters with Aging: Mythologies of the Menopause in Japan and North America*. Berkeley: University of California Press

Loftus, E. and Ketcham, K. (1994) *The Myth of Repressed Memory: False Memories and Allegations of Sexual Abuse*. New York: St Martin's Press

Long, E. R. (1965) *A History of Pathology*. New York: Dover

Loudon, J. R. (1959) Psychogenic disorders and social conflict among the Zulu. In M. K. Opler (ed.), *Culture and Mental Health*. New York: Macmillan

Lugard, F. D. (1929) *The Dual Mandate in British Tropical Africa*. Edinburgh: Blackwood

Lumsden, C. J. and Wilson, E. O. (1983) *Promethean Fire: Reflections on the Origin of Mind*. Cambridge, MA: Harvard University Press

Lyons, M. (1992) *The Colonial Disease: A Social History of Sleeping Sickness in Northern Zaire 1900–1940*. Cambridge: Cambridge University Press

MacCormack, C. and Strathern, M. (eds) (1980) *Nature, Culture and Gender*. Cambridge: Cambridge University Press

MacCrae, D. G. (1975) The body and social metaphor. In T. Polhemus (ed.), *The Body as a Medium of Expression*. London: Allen Lane

MacFarlane, J., Allen, L. and Honzik, M. (1954) *A Developmental Study of the Behaviour Problems of Normal Children*. Berkeley: University of California Press

Mack, J. (1994) *Abductions: Human Encounters with Aliens*. New York: Simon and Schuster

MacPherson, M. (1988) The hostage-takers: an epidemic of people gone mad. *Washington Post*, 20 February

Madden, R. R. (1857) *Phantasmata or Illusions and Fanaticisms of Protean Forms Productive of Great Evils*. London: Newby

Maddox, G. L., Black, K. W. and Liederman, V. R. (1968) Overweight as social deviance and disability. *Journal of Health and Social Behaviour*, 4, 287–98

Maggs, C. (1983) *The Origins of General Nursing*. London: Croom Helm

Main, M. and Solomon, J. (1990) Procedures for identifying infants as disorganized/disorientated during the Ainsworth Strange Situation. In M. T. Greenberg, D. Cicchetti and E. H. Cummings (eds), *Attachment in the Preschool Years*. Chicago: University of Chicago Press

Mair, G. (1995) *Star Stalkers*. New York: Pinnacle

Malhotra, H. K. and Wig, T. (1975) Dhat syndrome: a culture-bound sex neurosis. *Archives of Sexual Behaviour*, 4, 519–28

Malinowski, B. (1927) *Sex and Repression in Savage Society*. London: Routledge

Malinowski, B. (1941) An anthropological analysis of war. *American Journal of Sociology*, 46, 521–50

Mandelbaum, D. G. (1988) *Women's Seclusion and Men's Honour: Sex Roles in North India, Bangladesh and Pakistan*. Tucson: Arizona University Press

Mannoni, O. (1950) *Psychologie de la colonisation*. Paris: Seuil

Maranhao, T. (1986) *Therapeutic Discourse and Socratic Dialogue*. Madison: Wisconsin University Press

Margulis, L. (1982) *Symbiosis in Cell Evolution*. California: Freeman

Markham-Smith, I. (1987) Career women struck down by yuppie plague. *Sunday Express*, 22 March

Marks, T. M. (1970) Agoraphobic syndrome (phobic anxiety state). *Archives of General Psychiatry*, 23, 538–53

Mars, L. (1946) *La Lutte contre la folie*. Port-au-Prince: Imprimerie de l'Etat

Marsella, A. J. and White, G. M. (eds.) (1982) *Cultural Conceptions of Mental Health and Therapy*. Dordrecht: Reidel

Martin, E. (1992) The end of the body? *American Ethnologist*, 12, 121–40

Martin, J. (1993) *Scram: Relocating under a New Identity*. Washington, DC: Loompanics Unlimited. (Cited in *The Times*, 9 September 1993)

Martindale, C. (1980) Subselves. The internal representation of situational and personal dispositions. In L. Wheeler (ed.), *Review of Personality and Social Psychology*. San Francisco: Sage

Masson, J. (1970) The psychology of the ascetic. *Journal of Asian Studies*, 35, 611–25

Masson, J. (1984) *The Assault on Truth: Freud's Suppression of the Seduction Theory*. New York: Farrar, Strauss and Giroux

Masterton, G. and Platt, S. (1989) Parasuicide and General Elections. *British Medical Journal*, 298, 803–4

Matthews, G. B. (1992) *Thought's Ego in Augustine and Descartes*. Ithaca: Cornell University Press

Mauss, M. (1926) A definition of the collective suggestion of the idea of death. Trans. In M. Mauss, *Sociology and Psychology*, 1979. London: Routledge and Kegan Paul

Mauss, M. (1950) *Sociology and Psychology*, Trans. 1979. London: Routledge and Kegan Paul

Mayr, E. (1982) *The Growth of Biological Thought*. Cambridge, MA: Harvard University Press

Mayr, E. (1988) *Towards a New Philosophy of Biology*. Cambridge, MA: Harvard University Press

McClelland, J. L., Rumelhart, D. E. and the PDP Research Group (1986) *Parallel Distributed Processing: Explorations in the Microstructure of Cognition*, Vol.2: Psychological and Biological Models. Cambridge, MA: MIT Press

McCulloch, J. (1994) *Colonial Psychiatry and the African Mind*. Cambridge: Cambridge University Press

McDougall, W. (1911) *Body and Mind: A History and a Defence of Animism*. London: Methuen

McEvedy, C. P. and Beard, A. W. (1970) The Royal Free epidemic of 1955: a reconsideration. *British Medical Journal*, 3 January, 7–11

McGinn, C. (1990) *The Problem of Consciousness*. Oxford: Blackwell

McKee, V. (1992) Fathers close to the brink. *The Times*, 16 March

McKinlay, S. and Jeffreys, M. (1974) The menopausal syndrome. *British Journal of Preventive and Social Medicine*, 28, 108–15

McManners, H. (1994) *The Scars of War*. London: HarperCollins

Mead, G. H. (1934) *Mind, Self and Society*. Chicago: University of Chicago Press

Meadows, R. (1984) Factitious illness – the hinterland of child abuse. In R. Meadows, *Recent Advances in Paediatrics*. Edinburgh: Churchill Livingston

Melberg, A. (1995) *Theories of Mimesis*. Cambridge: Cambridge University Press

Mercer, K. (1986) Racism and transcultural psychiatry. In P. Miller and N. Rose (eds), *The Power of Psychiatry*. London: Polity Press

Merleau-Ponty, M. (1962) *Phenomenology of Perception*. Trans. London: Routledge and Kegan Paul

Merrill, J. and Owens, J. (1988) Self-poisoning among four immigrant groups. *Acta Psychiatrica Scandinavica*, *77*, 77–80

Merskey, H. M. (1992) The manufacture of personalities: the production of multiple personality disorder. *British Journal of Psychiatry*, *160*, 327–40

Métraux, A. (1959) *Voodoo*. Oxford: Oxford University Press

Metzger, T. A. (1981) Selfhood and authority in Neo-Confucian political culture. In A. Kleinman and T. Y. Lin (eds), *Normal and Abnormal Behaviour in Chinese Culture*. Dordrecht: Reidel

Mezzich, J. E., Kleinman, A., Fabrega, H. and Parron, D. L. (eds) (1996) *Culture and Psychiatric Diagnosis*. Proceedings of the Conference on Cultural Issues and Psychiatric Diagnosis, APA/NIMH, Pittsburgh, American Psychiatric Press. Washington, DC: American Psychiatric Press

Micale, M. S. (1993) Henri F. Ellenberger and the origins of European psychiatric historiography. Introduction in H. F. Ellenberger, *Beyond the Unconscious: Essays*. Princeton: Princeton University Press

Micale, M. S. (1995) *Approaching Hysteria: Disease and Its Interpretations*. Princeton: Princeton University Press

Michaelis, J. D. (1814) *Commentaries on the Law of Moses*. Trans. London: Rivington

Miles, A. (1988) *The Neurotic Woman: The Role of Gender in Psychiatric Illness*. New York: New York University Press

Miller, K. (1985) *Doubles: Studies in Literary History*. Oxford: Oxford University Press

Millman, M. (1980) *Such a Pretty Face: Being Fat in America*. New York: Norton

Minear, L. and Weiss, L. (1995) *Mercy under Fire: War and the Global Humanitarian Community*. Boulder, Co: Westview

Minuchin, S., Baker, L., Rosman, B., Liebman, R., Milman, L. and Todd, T. (1975) A conceptual model of psychosomatic illness in children. *Archives of General Psychiatry*, *32*, 1031–8

Moravec, H. (1989) *Mind Children: The Future of Robot and Human Intelligence*. Cambridge: Harvard University Press

Morel, B. A. (1860) *Traité des maladies mentales*. Paris: Masson

Morgan, G. H., Burns-Cox, C. J., Pocock, H. and Pottle, S. (1975) Deliberate self-harm: clinical and socio-economic characteristics of 368 patients. *British Journal of Psychiatry*, *127*, 574–9

Morris, A. (1985) Sanctified madness: the God-intoxicated saints of Bengal. *Social Science and Medicine*, *21*, 221–330

Morris, J. and Windsor, R. A. (1985) Personal health practices of urban adults in Alabama: the Davis Avenue community study. *Public Health Reports*, *100*, 531–9

Morsy, S. (1978) Sex roles, power and illness in an Egyptian village. *American Ethnologist*, 5, 137–50

Moscovici, S. (1976) *La Psychoanalyse, son image et son public*. Paris: Presses Universitaires de France

Mulhern, S. (1994) Satanism, ritual abuse, and multiple personality disorder: a sociohistorical perspective. *International Journal of Clinical and Experimental Hypnosis*, 42, 265–88

Muller-Hill, B. (1988) *Murderous Science: Elimination by Scientific Selection of Jews, Gypsies and Others. Germany 1933–1945*. Oxford: Oxford University Press

Mulvey, L. (1987) Changes: thoughts on narrative and historical experience. *History Workshop*, 23, 3–19

Mumford, D. and Whitehouse, A. M. (1988) Increased prevalence of bulimia nervosa among Asian schoolchildren. *British Medical Journal*, 297, 718

Mumford, D. M., Whitehouse, A. M. and Choudry, I. Y. (1992) Survey of eating disorders in English-medium schools in Lahore, Pakistan. *International Journal of Eating Disorders*, 11, 173–84

Mumford, D. M., Whitehouse, A. M. and Platts, M. (1991) Socio-cultural correlates of eating disorders among Asian schoolgirls in Bradford. *British Journal of Psychiatry*, 158, 222–8

Munch, R. (1985) Differentiation, consensus and conflict. In J. C. Alexander (ed.), *Neofunctionalism*. London: Sage

Murphy, H. B. M. (1973) History and evolution of syndromes: the striking case of latah and amok. In M. Hammer (ed.), *Psychopathology*. New York: Wiley

Murphy, H. B. M. (1982) *Comparative Psychiatry: The International and Intercultural Distribution of Mental Illness*. Berlin: Springer

Murphy, H. B. M. (1983) Commentary on 'The Resolution of the Latah Paradox'. *Journal of Nervous and Mental Disease*, 171, 176–7

Myers, F. R. (1976) Emotions and the self: a theory of personhood and political order among the Pintupi. *Ethos*, 7, 342–70

Nadel, S. F. (1946) A study of shamanism in the Nuba mountains. *Journal of the Royal Anthropological Institute*, 76, 25–37

Nandy, A. (1995) *The Savage Freud and Other Essays on Possible and Retrievable Selves*. Delhi: Oxford University Press

Nasser, M. (1986) Comparative study of the prevalence of abnormal eating attitudes among Arab female students of both London and Cairo Universities. *Psychological Medicine*, 16, 621–5

Nasser, M. (1993) The psychometric properties of the Eating Attitude Scale in a non-Western population (personal communication).

National Organisation for Women Task Force (1974) *Dick and Jane as Victims: A Survey of 134 Elementary School Readers*. London: Blackstock

National Task Force on Chronic Fatigue Syndrome (CFS), Post-Viral Fatigue Syndrome (PVFS) and Myalgic Encephalomyelitis (ME) (1994) Bristol: Westcare

Needham, R. (1981) Inner states as universals: sceptical reflections on human nature. In P. Heelas and A. Lock (eds), *Indigenous Psychologies: The Anthropology of the Self*. London: Academic Press

Ness, R. (1985) The Old Hag phenomenon. In R. C. Simons and C. C. Hughes (eds), *The Culture-bound Syndromes: Folk Illnesses of Psychiatric and Anthropological Interest.* Dordrecht: Reidel

Netanyahu, B. (1995) *Fighting Terrorism: How Democracies Defeat Domestic and International Terrorists.* New York: Farrar, Strauss and Giroux

Neutra, R., Levy, J. E. and Parker, D. (1977) Cultural expectations versus reality in Navajo seizure patterns and sick roles. *Culture, Medicine and Psychiatry, 1,* 255–75

Newman, P. L. (1964) 'Wild man' behaviour in a New Guinea Highlands community. *American Anthropologist, 66,* 1–19

Ngui, P. G. (1969) The koro epidemic in Singapore. *Australian and New Zealand Journal of Psychiatry, 3,* 263–6

Nin, A. (1993) *Incest: The Diary of Anaïs Nin 1932–1934.* London: Owen

Nordstrom, C. and Robben, A. C. G. (eds.) (1995) *Fieldwork under Fire: Contemporary Studies of Violence and Survival.* Berkeley: University of California Press

Norman, M. (1993) Soldiers of misfortune. *Evening Standard,* 29 October

Nuckolls, C. (ed.) (1992) The cultural construction of diagnostic categories: the case of American Psychiatry. *Social Science and Medicine* (special issue), *35,* 37–49

Nursing Times (1987a) *Man Appeal* (supplement), *83,* No.20, 24–30

Nursing Times (1987b) First among equals? *83,* No.32, 27

Nye, R. A. (1984) *Crime, Madness and Politics in Modern France: The Medical Concept of National Decline.* Princeton: Princeton University Press

Nylander, I. (1971) The feeling of being fat and dieting in the school population. *Acta Sociomedica Scandinavica, 3,* 17–26

O'Brien, H. A. (1883) Latah. *Journal of the Royal Asiatic Society (Straits Branch), 11,* 143–53

O'Brien, S. (1986) *The Negative Scream: A Story of Young People Who Took an Overdose.* London: Kegan Paul

O'Connell, R. (1995) *Ride of the Second Horseman: The Birth and Death of War.* New York: Oxford University Press

October (1995) *War and Rape,* Winter, Special Issue, 72, Cambridge, MA

O'Dwyer, J. M. and Friedman, T. (1993) Multiple personality following childbirth. *British Journal of Psychiatry, 162,* 831–3

Ogrizek, M. (1982) Mami wata: de hystérie à la femininité en Afrique. *Confrontations Psychiatriques, 21,* 213–37

Olujic, M. B. (1995) The Croatian war experience. In C. Nordstrom and A. C. G. Robben (eds), *Fieldwork under Fire: Contemporary Studies of Violence and Survival.* Berkeley: University of California Press

Orbach, S. (1978) *Fat Is a Feminist Issue.* London: Paddington

Orbach, S. (1986) *Hunger Strike.* London: Faber

Ornstein, R. C. (1985) *The Roots of the Self.* San Francisco: Harper

Ortner, S. B. (1974) Is female to male as nature is to culture? In: M. A. Rosaldo and L. Lamphere (eds), *Women, Culture and Society.* Stanford: Stanford University Press

Osborne, M. A. (1994) *Nature, the Exotic and the Science of French Colonialism.*

Bloomington: Indiana University Press

Otterbein, K. F. (1994) *Feuding and Warfare*. New York: Gordon and Breach

Owen, A. (1989) *The Darkened Room: Women, Power and Spiritualism in Late Victorian England*. London: Virago

Oxley, T. (1849) Malay amoks. *Journal of the Indian Archipelago and Eastern Asia*, 3, 532–3

Padilla, A. M. (ed.) (1980) *Acculturation: Theory, Models and Some New Findings*. Boulder: Westview

Palmer, C. E. and Noble, D. N. (1984) Child-snatching: motivations, mechanisms and melodrama. *Journal of Family Issues*, 5, 27–45

Parfit, D. (1984) *Reasons and Persons*. Oxford: Clarendon Press

Parker, S. (1960) The windigo psychosis. *American Anthropologist*, 62, 602–55

Parker, S. and Parker, H. (1986) Father–daughter sexual abuse: an emerging perspective. *American Journal of Orthopsychiatry*, 56, 531–49

Parkin, D. (1992) Introduction. In D. De Coppet (ed.), *Understanding Rituals*. London: Routledge

Parkin, D. (1993) Nemi in the modern world: return of the exotic. *Man* (n.s.), 28, 79–99

Parnell, T. F. and Day, D. O. (eds) (1997) *Munchausen by Proxy Syndrome*. New York: Sage

Parry, H. J., Balter, M. B., Mellinger, G. D., Cisin, I. H. and Manheimer, D. I. (1973) National patterns of psychotherapeutic drug use. *Archives of General Psychiatry*, 28, 769–83

Parsons, T. (1951) Illness and the role of the physician: a sociological perspective. *American Journal of Orthopsychiatry*, 21, 452–60

Parsons, T. (1952) *The Social System*. London: Routledge and Kegan Paul

Parsons, T. (1954) The incest taboo in relation to social structure and the socialisation of the child. *British Journal of Sociology*, 5, 101–5

Parsons, T. and Fox, R. (1952) Illness, therapy and the modern urban American family. *Journal of Social Issues*, 8, 31–44

Pattison, E. M., Wintrob, R. M. (1981) Possession and exorcism in contemporary America. *Journal of Operational Psychiatry*, 12, 12–30

Patton, G. C., Johnson-Sabine, E., Wood, K., Mann, A. H. and Wakeling, A. (1990) Abnormal eating attitudes in London schoolgirls – a prospective epidemiological study: outcome at twelve months follow-up. *Psychological Medicine*, 20, 383–94

Peacock, J. L. (1975) *Consciousness and Change: Symbolic Anthropology in Evolutionary Perspective*. Oxford: Blackwell

Peters, L. G. and Price-Williams, D. (1983) A phenomenological overview of trance. *Transcultural Psychiatric Research Review*, 20, 5–39

Philen, R. M. *et al.* (1989) Mass sociogenic illness by proxy: parentally reported epidemic in an elementary school. *Lancet*, *ii*, 1372–6

Phillips, D. L. and Segal, B. (1969) Sexual status and psychiatric symptoms. *American Sociological Review*, 29, 678–87

Pinquet, M. (1993) *Voluntary Death in Japan*. Cambridge: Polity Press

Piper, A. (1994) Multiple personality disorder. *British Journal of Psychiatry, 164*, 600–12

Platt, S. (1987) The aftermath of Angie's overdose: is soap (opera) damaging to your health? *British Medical Journal, 294*, 954–7

Podrabinek, A. (1980) *Punitive Medicine*. Ann Arbor: Karoma

Polhemus, T. (1978) *Social Aspects of the Human Body*. Harmondsworth: Penguin

Prather, J. and Fidell, L. (1975) Sex differences in the content and style of medical advertisements. *Social Science and Medicine, 9*, 23–6

Price, A. W. (1995) *Mental Conflict*. London: Routledge

Price, G. B. (1913) Discussion on the causes of invaliding from the tropics. *British Medical Journal, ii*, 1290–7

Prince, M. (1905) *The Dissociation of a Personality: The Hunt for the Real Miss Beauchamp*. Oxford: Oxford University Press (Republished 1978 with an introduction by C. Rycroft).

Prince, R. (1960) The 'brain-fag' syndrome in Nigerian students. *Journal of Mental Science, 106*, 559–70

Prince, R. (1983) Is anorexia nervosa a culture-bound syndrome? *Transcultural Psychiatric Research Review, 20*, 299–300

Prince, R. (1985) The concept of culture-bound syndromes: anorexia nervosa and brain-fag. *Social Science and Medicine, 22*, 197–203

Prince, R. (1991) Review. *Transcultural Psychiatric Research Review, 28*, 44–55

Proust, M. (1958) *A la recherche du temps perdu*. Paris: Gallimard

Pumariega, A. J. (1986) Acculturation and eating attitudes in adolescent girls: a comparative and correlational study. *Journal of the American Academy of Child Psychiatry, 25*, 276–9

Putnam, F. W. (1989) *Diagnosis and Treatment of Multiple Personality Disorder*. New York: Guilford

Radcliffe-Brown, A. R. (1951) *Structure and Function in Primitive Society*. London: Routledge and Kegan Paul

Raleigh, V. S. and Balarajan, R. (1992) Suicide and self-burning among Indians and West Indians in England and Wales. *British Journal of Psychiatry, 161*, 365–8

Ramon, S., Bancroft, J. H. J. and Skrimshire, A. M. (1975) Attitudes to self-poisoning among physicians and nurses in a general hospital. *British Journal of Psychiatry, 127*, 257–64

Rampling, D. (1985) Ascetic ideals and anorexia nervosa. *Journal of Psychiatric Research, 19*, 89–94

Ramsay, A. M. (1986) *Postviral Fatigue Syndrome: The Saga of the Royal Free Disease*. London: Glover

Rawnsley, K. and Loudon, J. B. (1964) Epidemiology of mental disorder in a closed community. *British Journal of Psychiatry, 110*, 830–9

Raymond, J. G. (1982) Medicine as a patriarchal religion. *Journal of Medicine and Philosophy, 7*, 197–216

Reay, M. (1977) Ritual madness observed: a discarded pattern of faith in Papua New Guinea. *Journal of Pacific History, 12*, 55–79

Reich, W. (1975) *The Mass Psychology of Fascism*. Harmondsworth: Penguin

Reyna, S. P. and Downs, R. E. (eds) (1994) *Studying War: Anthropological*

Perspectives. New York: Gordon and Breach

Reynolds, E. H. (1990) Structure and function in neurology and psychiatry. *British Journal of Psychiatry*, *157*, 481–90

Reynolds, V. (1980) *The Biology of Human Action*. Oxford: Freeman

Reynolds, V. (1991) The biological basis of human patterns of mating and marriage. In V. Reynolds and J. Kellett (eds), *Mating and Marriage*. Oxford: Oxford University Press

Richards, A. (1982) *Chisungu: A Girls' Initiation Ceremony among the Bemba of Zambia*. London: Tavistock

Richards, P. (1996) *Fighting for the Rain Forest: War, Youth and Resources in Sierra Leone*. London: International African Institute

Rieff, P. (1966) *The Triumph of the Therapeutic*. London: Chatto and Windus

Rip, C. M. (1973) *Contemporary Social Pathology*, 3rd edn. Pretoria: Academica

Ritenbaugh, C. (1982a) Obesity as a culture-bound syndrome. *Culture, Medicine and Psychiatry*, *6*, 347–64

Ritenbaugh, C. (1982b) New approaches to old problems: interactions of culture and nutrition. In N. J. Chrisman and T. W. Maretzki (eds), *Clinically Applied Anthropology*. Dordrecht: Reidel

Ritenbaugh, C. and Shisslak, C. (1994) Eating disorders: a cross-cultural review in regard to DSM-IV. In J. E. Mezzich, A. Kleinman, H. Fabrega and D. L. Parron (eds), *Culture and Psychiatric Diagnosis*. Washington, DC: American Psychiatric Press.

Ritenbaugh, W. and Simons, R. C. (1985) Gentle interrogation: inquiry and interaction in brief initial psychiatric evaluations. In R. A. Hahn and A. D. Gaines (eds), *Physicians of Western Medicine: Anthropological Approaches to Theory and Practice*. Dordrecht: Reidel

Rivers, W. H. R. (1924) *Medicine, Magic and Religion*. London: Kegan Paul, Trench and Trubner

Robben, A. C. G. M. (1995) The politics of truth and emotion among victims and perpetrators of violence. In C. Nordstrom and A. C. G. Robben (eds), *Fieldwork under Fire: Contemporary Studies of Violence and Survival*. Berkeley: University of California Press

Robins, J. (1986) *Fools and Mad: A History of the Insane in Ireland*. Dublin: Institute of Public Administration

Robins, L. N., Meizer, G. E. and Weissman, M. M. (1984) Lifetime prevalence of specific psychiatric disorders. *Archives of General Psychiatry*, *41*, 949–58

Roheim, G. (1950) *Psychoanalysis and Anthropology: Culture, Personality and the Unconscious*. New York: International Universities Press

Roland, A. (1988) *In Search of the Self in India and Japan*. Princeton: Princeton University Press

Ronell, A. (1989) *The Telephone Book: Technology, Schizophrenia, Electric Speech*. Lincoln: University of Nebraska Press

Rooth, F. G. (1971) Indecent exposure and exhibitionism. *British Journal of Hospital Medicine*, April, 521–33

Rooth, F. G. (1974) Exhibitionism outside Europe and America. *Archives of Sexual Behaviour*, *2*, 351–62

Rorty, A. O. (1985) Self-deception, akrasia and irrationality. In J. Elster (ed.), *The Multiple Self*. Cambridge: Cambridge University Press

Roscoe, P. B. (1994) Amity and aggression: a symbolic theory of incest. *Man* (n.s.), *29*, 49–76

Rosen, G. (1968) *Madness in Society: Chapters in the Historical Sociology of Mental Illness*. London: Routledge and Kegan Paul

Ross, C. A. (1994) *The Osiris Complex: Case Studies in Multiple Personality Disorder*. Toronto: University of Toronto Press

Ross, C. A. (1995) *Satanic Ritual Abuse: Principles of Treatment*. Toronto: University of Toronto Press

Rowan, J. (1990) *Subpersonalities: The People inside Us*. London: Routledge

Rubenstein, J. (1996) *Tangled Loyalties: The Life and Times of Ilya Ehrenburg*. London: Tauris

Rush, B. (1799) Observations intended to favour a supposition that the black colour (as it is called) of the Negroes is derived from the Leprosy. *Transactions of the American Philosophical Society*, *4*, 289–97

Russell, D. E. H. (1984) *Sexual Exploitation: Rape, Child Sexual Abuse and Workplace Harassment*. San Francisco: Sage

Russell, G. F. M. (1990) Metamorphose de l'anorexie nerveuse et implications pour la prevention des troubles du comportement alimentaire. In J.-L. Venisse (ed.), *Les Nouvelles Addictions*. Paris: Masson

Ryan, J. (1994) *The Vanishing Subject: Early Psychology and Literary Modernism*. Chicago: University of Chicago Press

Sachdev, P. S. (1990) *Studies in Maori Ethnopsychiatry*. Unpublished PhD thesis, University of New South Wales

Sachs, O. (1989) *Seeing Voices: A Journey into the World of the Deaf*. Berkeley: University of California Press

Sachs, W. (1937) *Black Hamlet*. London: Bles

Sahlins, M. (1976) *Culture and Practical Reason*. Chicago: University of Chicago Press

Sahlins, M. (1983) Raw women, cooked men and other 'great things' of the Fiji Islands. In P. Brown and D. Tuzin (eds), *The Ethnography of Cannibalism*. Washington, DC: SPA

Sakinofsky, I., Roberts, R. S., Brown, Y., Cumming, C. and James, P. (1990) Problem resolution and repetition of parasuicide. *British Journal of Psychiatry*, *156*, 395–9

Salisbury, R. (1966) Possession in the New Guinea Highlands: review of literature. *Transcultural Psychiatric Research Review*, *3*, 103–8

Salisbury, R. (1967) Reply to Langness. *Transcultural Psychiatric Research Review*, *4*, 130–4

Salmons, P. H., Lewis, V. J., Rogers, P., Gatherer, A. J. H. and Booth, D. A. (1988) Body shape dissatisfaction in schoolchildren. *British Journal of Psychiatry*, *153*, Supplement 2, 27–31

Samuel, G. (1990) *Body, Mind and Culture: Anthropology and the Biological Interface*. Cambridge: Cambridge University Press

Sargant, W. (1973) *The Mind Possessed: From Ecstasy to Exorcism*. London: Heinemann

Sartorius, N., Jablensky, A., Korten, A., Ernberg, G., Anker, M., Cooper, J. E. and

Day, R. (1986) Early manifestations and first-contact incidence of schizophrenia in different cultures. *Psychological Medicine*, *16*, 909–28

Sawbridge, P. (1988) The post-adoption centre: what are the users teaching us? *Adoption and Fostering*, *12*, 5–12

Scambler, G. and Hopkins, A. (1986) Being epileptic: coming to terms with stigma. *Sociology of Health and Illness*, *8*, 26–43

Scheff, T. J. (1979) *Catharsis in Healing, Ritual and Drama*. Berkeley: University of California Press

Scheper-Hughes, N. (1979) *Saints, Scholars and Schizophrenics: Mental Illness in Rural Ireland*. Berkeley: University of California Press

Scheper-Hughes, N. (1990) Three propositions for a critically-applied medical anthropology. *Social Science and Medicine*, *30*, 189–97

Scheper-Hughes, N. and Lock, M. M. (1987) The mindful body: A prolegomenon to future work in medical anthropology. *Medical Anthropology Quarterly* (n.s.), *1*, 6–39

Schmidt, U., Hodes, M. and Treasure, J. (1993) Early onset bulimia nervosa: who is at risk? *Psychological Medicine*, *22*, 623–8

Schmidtke, A. and Hafner, H. (1988) The Werther effect after television films: new evidence for an old hypothesis. *Psychological Medicine*, *18*, 665–76

Schnabel, J. (1994) *Dark White: Aliens, Abductions and the UFO Obsession*. London: Hamish Hamilton

Schneider, K. (1959) *Clinical Psychopathology*. 5th edn. Trans. M. W. Hamilton. New York: Grune and Stratton

Schreiber, F. R. (1973) *Sybil*. Chicago: Regnery

Schrödinger, E. (1944) *What Is Life?* Cambridge: Cambridge University Press

Schutz, A. (1976) *The Phenomenology of the Social World*. Rev. edn. London: Heinemann

Schwartz, H. (1996) *The Culture of the Copy: Striking Likenesses, Unreasonable Facsimiles*. New York: Zone

Scott, J. C. (1990) *Domination and the Arts of Resistance: Hidden Transcripts*. New Haven: Yale University Press

Scott, P. D. (1978) The psychiatry of kidnapping and hostage-taking. In R. N. Gaind and B. L. Hudson (eds), *Current Themes in Psychiatry*. London: Macmillan

Seaford, R. (1995) *Reciprocity and Ritual: Homer and Tragedy in the Developing City State*. Oxford: Clarendon Press

Searle, J. (1984) *Minds, Brain, Science*. Harmondsworth: Penguin

Searle, J. (1992) *The Rediscovery of the Mind*. Cambridge: MIT Press

Sedgwick, P. (1982) *Psycho Politics*. London: Pluto

Seidenberg, R. (1974) Images of health, illness and women in drug advertising. *Journal of Drug Issues*, *4*, 264–7

Seligman, C. G. (1928) Anthropological perspectives and psychological theory. *Journal of the Royal Anthropological Institute*, *62*, 193–228

Seligman, C. S. (1929) Sex, temperament, conflict and psychosis in a Stone Age population. *British Journal of Medical Psychology*, *9*, 187–202

Shah, J. H. (1960) Causes and prevention of suicide. *Indian Journal of Social Work*, *21*, 167–75

Sharp, L. A. (1993) *The Possessed and the Dispossessed: Spirits, Identity and Power in a Madagascar Migrant Town*. Berkeley: University of California Press

Shauer, K. G. (1975) *An Introduction to Attribution Processes*. Cambridge: Winthrop

Shaw, B. D. (1992) Explaining incest: brother-sister marriage in Graeco-Roman Egypt. *Man* (n.s.), *27*, 267–99

Shaw, R. P. and Wong, Y. (1989) *Genetic Seeds of Warfare: Evolution, Nationalism and Patriotism*. Boston: Unwin Hyman

Shepher, J. (1983) *Incest: A Biosocial View*. New York: Academic Press

Shook, E. V. (1985) *Ho'oponopono: Contemporary Uses of a Hawaiian Problem-solving Process*. Hawaii: East-West Center

Shore, B. (1993) Feeling our way: towards a bio-cultural model of emotion. Paper presented at the Emory/Mellon Symposium on Emotions, Emory University, Georgia

Shorter, E. (1983) *A History of Women's Bodies*. London: Allen Lane

Showalter, E. (1987a) *The Female Malady: Women, Madness and English Culture 1830–1980*. London: Virago

Showalter, E. (1987b) Review of Kenny 1986. *Times Literary Supplement*, 22 May, 537

Showalter, E. (1990) *Sexual Anarchy: Gender and Culture at the Fin de Siècle*. New York: Viking

Showalter, E. (1993) Hysteria, feminism and gender. In S. L. Gilman, H. King, R. Porter, G. S. Rousseau and E. Showalter, *Hysteria beyond Freud*. Berkeley: University of California Press

Showalter, E. (1998) *Hysterias: Hysterical Epidemics and Modern Culture*. London: Picador

Shweder, R. A. (1985) Menstrual pollution, soul loss and the comparative study of emotions. In A. Kleinman and A. Good, *Culture and Depression: Studies in the Anthropology and Cross-Cultural Psychiatry of Affect and Disorder*. Berkeley: University of California Press

Shweder, R. A. and Bourne, E. J. (1982) Does the concept of the person vary cross-culturally? In A. J. Marsella and G. M. White (eds), *Cultural Conceptions of Mental Health and Therapy*. Dordrecht: Reidel

Sidel, R. (1973) The role of revolutionary optimism in the treatment of mental illness in the People's Republic of China. *American Journal of Orthopsychiatry, 43*, 732–6

Simnet, A. (1986) The pursuit of respectability: women and the nursing profession 1860–1900, In R. White, *Political Issues in Nursing*. Chichester: Wiley (Quoting *The Englishwoman*, 1913, No.53)

Simons, R. C. (1980) The resolution of the Latah paradox. *Journal of Nervous and Mental Disease, 168*, 195–206

Simons, R. C. (1983a) *Latah: A Culture-specific Elaboration of the Startle Reflex*. 16mm film, Michigan State University

Simons, R. C. (1983b) Latah II – problems with a purely symbolic interpretation. *Journal of Nervous and Mental Disease, 171*, 168–75

Simons, R. C. (1983c) Latah III – how compelling is the evidence of a psychoanalytic interpretation? *Journal of Nervous and Mental Disease, 171*, 178–81

Simons, R. C. (1985) Culture-bound syndromes unbound. In R. C. Simons and C. C. Hughes (eds), *The Culture-bound Syndromes: Folk Illnesses of Psychiatric and Anthropological Interest*. Dordrecht: Reidel

Simons, R. C. and Hughes, C. C. (eds.) (1985) *The Culture-bound Syndromes: Folk Illnesses of Psychiatric and Anthropological Interest*. Dordrecht: Reidel

Sinason, V. (ed.) (1994) *Treating Survivors of Satanist Abuse*. London: Routledge

Skultans, V. (1987) The management of mental illness among Maharastrian families: a case study of a Mahanubhav healing temple. *Man, 22*, 661–79

Smith-Rosenberg, C. (1972) The hysterical woman: sex roles and role conflict in nineteenth-century America. *Social Research, 39*, 652–78

Smith-Rosenberg, C. (1973) Puberty to menopause: the cycle of femininity in nineteenth-century America. *Feminist Studies, 1*, 58–72

Smuts, B. (1992) Male aggression against women: an evolutionary perspective. *Human Nature, 3*, 1–44

Sneddon, I. B. (1983) Simulated disease. *Journal of the Royal College of Physicians, 17*, 199–205

Sontag, S. (1979) *Illness as Metaphor*. London: Allen Lane

Sorosky, A. D., Baran, A. and Pannor, R. (1975) Identity conflicts in adoptees. *American Journal of Orthopsychiatry, 45*, 18–27

Spanos, N. P. (1989) Hypnosis, demonic possession and multiple personality: strategic enactments and disavowals of responsibility for actions. In C. A. Ward (ed.), *Altered States of Consciousness and Mental Health: A Cross-Cultural Perspective*. Newbury Park: Sage

Spanos, N. P. and Gottlieb, J. (1979) Demonic possession, mesmerism and hysteria: a social psychological perspective on their historical interrelationship. *Journal of Abnormal Psychology, 88*, 527–46

Sperber, D. (1985) Anthropology and psychology: towards an epidemiology of representations. *Man (n.s.), 20*, 73–89

Spiegel, D. (ed.) (1994) *Dissociation: Culture, Mind and Body*. Washington: American Psychiatric Press

Spiegel, M. (1996) *The Dreaded Comparison: Human and Animal Slavery*. New York: Mirror Books

Spring, A. (1978) Epidemiology of spirit possession among the Luvale of Zambia. In J. Hoch-Smith and A. Spring (eds), *Women in Ritual Symbolic Roles*. New York: Plenum

Stearns, P. N. (1994) *American Cool: Constructing a 20th-Century Emotional Style*. New York: State University of New York Press

Stein, H. F. (1986) 'Sick people' and 'trolls': a contribution to the understanding of the dynamics of physician explanatory models. *Culture, Medicine and Psychiatry, 10*, 221–9

Stephen, P. (1987) Career patterns of women medical graduates 1974–1934. *Medical Education, 21*, 255–9

Sternberg, R. J. and Barnes, M. L. (eds) (1988) *The Psychology of Love*. New Haven: Yale University Press

Stevenson, J. (1979) *Popular Disturbances in England 1700–1870*. London: Longman

Stimson, G. (1975) Women in a doctored world. *New Society, L2*, 265–6

Stocking, G. (1987) *Victorian Anthropology*. New York: Free Press

Stoller, P (1989) *Fusion of the Worlds: An Ethnography of Possession among the Songhay of Niger*. Chicago: University of Chicago Press

Strachan, H. (1996) Who deters, wins sometimes. *TLS*, 12 April, 25

Strachey, L. (1918) *Eminent Victorians*. London: Folio Society, 1967

Strathern, M. (1992) *After Nature: English Kinship in the Late Twentieth Century*. Cambridge: Cambridge University Press

Strickland, S. (1993) A love that does not know its true name. *Independent on Sunday*, 3 January, 20

Strozier, C. B. (1994) *Apocalypse: On the Psychology of Fundamentalism in America*. Boston: Beacon Press

Stuart, R. B. and Jacobson, B. (1979) Sex differences in obesity. In E. S. Gomberg and V. Franks (eds), *Gender and Disordered Behaviour: Sex Differences in Psychopathology*. New York: Brunner/Mazel

Swartz, L. (1985) Anorexia nervosa as a culture-bound syndrome. *Social Science and Medicine 20*, 725–30

Swartz, L. (1987) Illness negotiation: the case of eating disorders. *Social Science and Medicine, 24*, 613–18

Swartz, L. (1989) *Aspects of Culture in South African Psychiatry*. Unpublished Ph D thesis, Cape Town University

Symonds, A. (1971) Phobias after marriage: women's declaration of independence. *American Journal of Psychoanalysis, 31*, 144–52

Szasz, T. (1961) *The Myth of Mental Illness*. New York: Hoeber/Harper

Szasz, T. (1977) *Karl Kraus and the Soul-Doctors: A Pioneer Critic and His Criticism of Psychiatry and Psychoanalysis*. London: Routledge and Kegan Paul

Taguieff, P. A. (1988) *La Force du préjugé: Essai sur le racisme et ses doubles*. Paris: La Découverte

Tan, E. K. and Carr, J. E. (1977) Psychiatric sequelae of amok. *Culture, Medicine and Psychiatry, 1*, 59–67

Tanner, T. (1993) In two voices. *Times Literary Supplement*, July, 12

Tart, C. (1980) A systems approach to altered states of consciousness. In J. M. Davidson and R. J. Davidson (eds), *The Psychobiology of Consciousness*. New York: Plenum

Tate, T. (1991) *Children for the Devil: Ritual Abuse and Satanic Crime*. London: Methuen

Taussig, M. (1980) Reification and the consciousness of the patient. *Social Science and Medicine, 14*, 3–13

Taussig, M. (1987) *Shamanism, Colonialism and the Wild Man: A Study in Terror and Healing*. Chicago: University of Chicago Press

Taussig, M. (1993) *Mimesis and Alterity*. New York: Routledge

Taylor, C. (1990) *Sources of the Self: The Making of the Modern Identity*. Cambridge: Harvard University Press

Taylor, C. (1992) *The Ethics of Authenticity*. Cambridge: Harvard University Press

Teish, L. (1985) *Jambalaya*. San Francisco: Harper and Row

Teoh, L. (1972) The changing psychopathology of amok. *Psychiatry, 35*, 345–53

Terr, L. (1994) *Unchained Memories: True Stories of Traumatic Memories Lost and Found*. New York: Basic Books

Thigpen, C. H. and Cleckley, H. M. (1957) *The Three Faces of Eve.* New York: McGraw-Hill

Thomas, A. (dir.) (1993) *In Satan's Name.* ITV documentary, 30 June

Thomas, K. (1984) *Man and the Natural World: Changing Attitudes in England 1500–1800.* Harmondsworth: Penguin

Tilt, E. J. (1862) *Ovarian Inflammation and the Physiology and Diseases of Menstruation.* London: Churchill

The Times (1984) The kind and gentle bank robber – aged 70. 6 October

The Times (1987) (untitled) 14 July

The Times (1990) (untitled, on collective overdoses) 12 June

The Times (1994) The lessons of war. Magazine, 5 February, p. 21

The Times (1995) Iranians 'raped on death row'. 31 January, p. 13

The Times (1996a) Bosnian women tell of wartime rape. 27 January, p. 9

The Times (1996b) Serb war crimes suspect goes on hunger strike. 7 May, p. 10

The Times (1996c) Enemies' blunders. 14 September, P. 12

The Times (1996d) Prosecutor of war crimes to pursue rapists. 15 October, p. 12

Timerman, J. In E. Stover and E. O. Nightingale (eds) (1985) *The Breaking of Minds and Bodies.* New York: Freeman

Tomas, D. (1989) The technophilic body: on technicity in William Gibson's cyborg culture. *New Formations, 8,* 111–29

Tooth, G. (1950) *Studies in Mental Illness in the Gold Coast.* Colonial Research Publication No.6. London: HMSO

Toren, C. (1993) Making history: the significance of childhood cognition for a comparative anthropology of mind. *Man* (n.s.), *28,* 461–78

Townsend, J. M. and Carbone, C. L. (1980) Menopausal syndrome: illness or social role: a transcultural analysis. *Culture, Medicine and Psychiatry, 4,* 229–48

Triseolitis, J. (1973) *In Search of Origins: The Experience of Adopted People.* London: Routledge and Kegan Paul

Turner, B. (1984) *The Body and Society: Explorations in Social Theory.* Oxford: Blackwell

Turner, V. (1969) *The Ritual Process: Structure and Anti-Structure.* London: Routledge and Kegan Paul

Turner, V. (1974) *Dramas, Fields and Metaphors.* Ithaca: Cornell University Press

Twitchell, J. B. (1987) *Forbidden Partners: The Incest Taboo in Modern Culture.* New York: Columbia University Press

US Department of State (1993) *Country Reports on Human Rights Practices.* Washington, DC: Department of State

Usher, J. (1991) *Women's Madness: Misogyny or Mental Illness?* New York: Harvester Wheatsheaf

Van der Waals, F., Mohrs, J. and Foets, M. (1993) Sex differences among recipients of benzodiazepines in Dutch general practice. *British Medical Journal, 307,* 7 August, 363–6

Van Gennep, A. (1960) *The Rites of Passage.* London: Routledge and Kegan Paul

Van Sant, A. J. (1993) *Eighteenth-Century Sensibility and the Novel: The Senses in Social Context.* Cambridge: Cambridge University Press

Victor, J. S. (1993) *Satanic Panic: The Creation of a Contemporary Legend*. London: Open Court

Vidal, J.-M. (1985) Explications biologiques et anthropologiques de l'interdit de l'inceste. *Nouvelle Revue d'Ethnopsychiatrie*, No.3, 75–107

Vint, F. W. (1932) A preliminary note on the cell content of the prefrontal cortex of the East African native. *East African Medical Journal*, 9, 30–55

Vitebsky, P. (1992) *Dialogues with the Dead: The Discussion of Mortality, Loss and Continuity among the Sora of Central India*. Cambridge: Cambridge University Press

Vonnegut, M. (1976) *The Eden Express*. London: Cape

Walker, M. (1993) *Surviving Secrets*. Buckingham: Open University Press

Walter, N. (1950) *The Sexual Cycles of Human Warfare*. London: Mitre

Ward, C. A. (ed.) (1989) *Altered States of Consciousness and Mental Health: A Cross-Cultural Perspective*. Newbury Park: Sage

Wardle, J. and Marshland, L. (1990) Adolescent concerns about weight and eating: a social developmental perspective. *Journal of Psychosomatic Research*, 34, 377–91

Warner, M. (1983) *Joan of Arc: The Image of Female Heroism*. Harmondsworth: Penguin

Warner, M. (1985) *Monuments and Maidens: The Allegory of the Female Form*. London: Weidenfeld and Nicolson

Warner, R. (1985) *Recovery from Schizophrenia: Psychiatry and Political Economy*. New York: Routledge and Kegan Paul

Watkins, J. G. and Johnson, R. J. (1982) *We, the Divided Self*. New York: Irvington

Weinstein, E. (1962) *Cultural Aspects of Delusion*. New York: Free Press

Weissman, C. S. and Teitelbaum, M. A. (1985) Physician gender and the physician–patient relationship. *Social Science and Medicine*, 20, 119–27

Werbner, R. (1991) *Tears of the Dead*. Edinburgh: Edinburgh University Press

Wessely, S. (1987) Mass hysteria: two syndromes? *Psychological Medicine*, 17, 109–20

Westermarck, E. (1894) *The History of Human Marriage*. 1926 rev. edn. New York: Macmillan

Westermeyer, J. (1973) On the epidemiology of amok violence. *Archives of General Psychiatry*, 28, 873–6

White, G. M. (1982) The role of cultural explanations in 'somatisation' and 'psychologisation'. *Social Science and Medicine*, 16, 1519–30

Wilkes, K. V. (1988) *Real Persons: Personal Identity without Thought Experiments*. Oxford: Clarendon Press

Williams, E. A. (1994) *The Physical and the Moral: Anthropology, Physiology and Philosophical Medicine in France 1750–1850*. Cambridge: Cambridge University Press

Williams, R. (1958) *Culture and Society 1790–1950*. London: Chatto and Windus

Wilson, E. (1988) *Hallucinations: Life in the Post-Modern City*. London: Radius

Wilson, P. J. (1967) Status ambiguity and spirit possession. *Man* (n.s.), 2, 366–78

Wilson, S. and Barber, T. (1981) Vivid fantasy and hallucinatory abilities in the life histories of excellent hypnotic subjects. In E. Klinger (ed.), *Imagery: Concepts, Results and Applications*. New York: Plenum

Winefield, R. (1987) *Never the Twain Shall Meet: Bell, Gallaudet and the Communications Debate*. Washington: Gallaudet University Press

Wing, J. K. (1978) *Reasoning about Madness*. Oxford: Oxford University Press

Winkler, C. (1991) Rape as social murder. *Anthropology Today*, 7, No.3, 12–14

Winokur, G. (1973) The types of affective disorder. *Journal of Nervous and Mental Disease*, 156, 82–96

Winzeler, R. (1990) Amok: historical, psychological and cultural perspectives. In W. J. Karim (ed.), *Emotions of Culture: A Malay Perspective*. Singapore: Oxford University Press

Winzeler, R. L. (1995) *Latah in Southeast Asia*. Cambridge: Cambridge University Press

Wittgenstein, L. (1958) *Philosophical Investigations*. Oxford: Blackwell

Wolf, A. P. (1970) Childhood association and sexual attraction: a further test of the Westermarck hypothesis. *American Anthropologist*, 72, 503–15

Wolf, A. P. (1994) *Sexual Attraction and Childhood Association: A Chinese Brief for Edward Westermarck*. Stanford: Stanford University Press

Wolpe, J. (1970) Identifying the antecedents of an agoraphobic reaction. *Behaviour Therapy and Experimental Psychology*, 1, 299–309

Woolley, B. (1993) *Virtual Worlds*. Harmondsworth: Penguin

Wootton, B. (1959) *Social Science and Social Pathology*. London: Allen and Unwin

World Health Organisation (1983) *Depressive Disorders in Different Cultures: Report of the WHO Collaborative Study on Standardised Assessment of Depressive Disorders*. Geneva: WHO

World Vision (1996) *The Effects of Armed Conflicts on Girls: A Discussion Paper for the UN Study of the Impact of Armed Conflict on Children*. Geneva: World Vision

Wrangham, R. and Peterson, D. (1998) *Demonic Males and the Origins of Human Violence*. London: Bloomsbury

Wright, L. (1993) *Remembering Satan*. New York: Knopf

Wu, D. Y. H. (1982) Psychotherapy and emotion in traditional Chinese medicine. In A. J. Marsella and G. M. White (eds), *Cultural Conceptions of Mental Health and Therapy*. Dordrecht: Reidel

Wyllie, R. W. (1973) Introspective witchcraft among the Effutu of Southern Ghana. *Man* (n.s.), 8, 74–9

Yamazaki, G., Beauchamp, G. K., Kupniowski, D., Bard, J., Thomas, L. and Boyse, E. A. (1988) Familial imprinting determines H-Z selective mating preferences. *Science*, 240, 1331–2

Yap, P. M. (1960) The possession syndrome. *Journal of Mental Science*, 160, 114–37

Yap, P. M. (1967) Classification of the culture-bound reactive syndromes. *Australian and New Zealand Journal of Psychiatry*, 1, 172–9

Yap, P. M. (1974) *Comparative Psychiatry: A Theoretical Framework*. Toronto: University of Toronto Press

Young, A. (1976) Some implications of medical beliefs and practices for social anthropology. *American Anthropologist*, 78, 5–24

Young, A. (1980a) The discourse on stress and the reproduction of conventional knowledge. *Social Science and Medicine*, 14, 133–46

Young, A. (1980b) The creation of medical knowledge: some problems in interpretation. *Social Science and Medicine*, 15, 319–38

Young, A. (1991) Emil Kraepelin and the original American psychiatric diagnosis. In P. Heiderer and G. Bibeau (eds), *Anthropologies of Medicine*. Braunschweig, Germany: Vieweg

Young, A. (1993a) Making facts and marking time in psychiatric research: an essay on anthropology of scientific knowledge (unpublished ms.)

Young, A. (1993b) A description of how ideology shapes knowledge of a mental disorder: post-traumatic stress disorder. In S. Lindenbaum and M. Lock (eds), *Knowledge, Power and Practice: The Anthropology of Medicine and Everyday Life*. Berkeley: University of California Press

Young, A. (1995) *The Harmony of Illusions: Inventing Post-Traumatic Stress Disorder*. Princeton: Princeton University Press

Young, D. (1993) *Origins of the Sacred: The Ecstasies of Love and War*. London: Abacus

Young, I. (1984) Pregnant embodiment: subjectivity and alienation. *Journal of Medicine and Philosophy*, 9, 45–62

Index